The Massachusetts Eye and Ear Infirmary

REVIEW MANUAL FOR OPHTHALMOLOGY

Fourth Edition

The Massachusetts Eye and Ear Infirmary

REVIEW MANUAL FOR OPHTHALMOLOGY

■ Fourth Edition

Veeral S. Sheth, MD
Clinical Assistant Professor
Department of Surgery
University of Chicago
Chicago, Illinois

Vitreoretinal Surgeon
Eye and Vision Center
NorthShore University HealthSystem
Glenview, Illinois

Marcus M. Marcet, MD
Clinical Assistant Professor
Eye Institute
University of Hong Kong
Hong Kong, China

Paulpoj Chiranand, MD
Retina Fellow
Department of Ophthalmology
University of Chicago
Chicago, Illinois

Harit K. Bhatt, MD
Attending Physician
University of Retina and Macula Associates
Advocate Christ Medical Center
Oak Lawn, Illinois

Jeffrey C. Lamkin, MD
Assistant Professor
Department of Ophthalmology
Northeast Ohio University College of Medicine
Kent, Ohio

Rama D. Jager, MD, MBA, FACS
University Retina & Macula Associates, P.C.
Oak Forest, Illinois

Clinical Assistant Professor
Department of Surgery, Section of Ophthalmology
    and Visual Science
University of Chicago
Chicago, Illinois

All author royalties are donated directly to the Joslin Diabetes Center and the Massachusetts Eye and Ear Infirmary to support research and the advancement of ophthalmology.

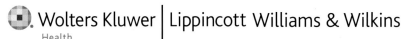

Wolters Kluwer | Lippincott Williams & Wilkins
Health

Philadelphia · Baltimore · New York · London
Buenos Aires · Hong Kong · Sydney · Tokyo

Senior Executive Editor: Jonathan W. Pine, Jr.
Product Managers: Emilie Moyer and Ashley Fischer
Vendor Manager: Bridgett Dougherty
Senior Manufacturing Manager: Benjamin Rivera
Marketing Manager: Lisa Lawrence
Design Coordinator: Teresa Mallon
Production Service: SPi Global

Library of Congress Cataloging-in-Publication Data
The Massachusetts Eye and Ear Infirmary review manual for ophthalmology /
Veeral S. Sheth ... [et al.]. — 4th ed.
      p. ; cm.
   Review manual for ophthalmology
   Red. ed. of: The Massachusetts Eye and Ear Infirmary review manual for ophthalmology / Rama D. Jager, Jeffrey C. Lamkin.
3rd ed. c2006.
   Includes bibliographical references and index.
   ISBN 978-1-4511-1136-1 (alk. paper)
   1. Ophthalmology—Examinations, questions, etc. 2. Eye—Diseases—Examinations,
questions, etc. I. Sheth, Veeral S. II. Jager, Rama D. Massachusetts Eye and Ear Infirmary
review manual for ophthalmology. III. Massachusetts Eye and Ear Infirmary. IV. Title:
Review manual for ophthalmology.
   [DNLM: 1. Eye Diseases—Examination Questions. 2. Eye—Examination Questions. WW 18.2]

   RE49.L35 2011
   617.7'15—dc23

                                                                                          2011014078

Dedicated to

To our mentors—past, present, and future—who guide us.

To our daughters, born during the production of this edition:

Simryn, Sophia, and Margaux.

Contents

Foreword to the Fourth Edition

It is very gratifying once again to write a foreword for the latest *Massachusetts Eye and Ear Infirmary Review Manual for Ophthalmology*. Dr. Rama D. Jager, joined by Dr. Veeral Sheth, along with their colleagues, have expended great effort creating and revising this new edition. The text is superbly designed to help physicians maintain and update their fund of knowledge in the ever-changing landscape of ophthalmology. The greatly enhanced photographic content in this edition acknowledges the importance of pattern recognition in our field.

Ophthalmology continues to change rapidly, and there have been significant advances in the 6 years since the previous edition. Maintaining familiarity with new findings in diagnosis and treatment is a requisite for any well-rounded practitioner or trainee. Self-assessment, a major feature of this review, offers an effective pathway for new learning. Coupled with continuing medical education, this exercise forms the cornerstone for continuous updating of our fund of knowledge.

As in earlier editions, the self-assessment questions in this book have been carefully prepared to help the reader identify the clinically significant areas within ophthalmology and the basic science concepts which underpin the latest advances. No effort has been made to reconstruct questions from current or previous board examinations; rather, the editors aim to capture the essentials of the latest developments in all areas of ophthalmology for the practitioner or trainee who wishes to be informed of recent scientific progress and the refashioned foundations of clinical science.

I congratulate Drs. Sheth and Jager for their contribution to ophthalmology through this fourth edition of the *Review*.

Joan W. Miller, MD
Henry Willard Williams Professor of Ophthalmology
Chief and Chair, Department of Ophthalmology
Harvard Medical School
Massachusetts Eye and Ear Infirmary

Foreword to the First Edition

It is a great pleasure to write a brief foreword to *The Massachusetts Eye and Ear Infirmary Review Manual for Ophthalmology*. Dr. Jeffrey Lamkin, the primary organizer and executor of this project with the secondary help of the residents of the Massachusetts Eye and Ear Infirmary, initially conceived it as part of his teaching obligation to the residents while serving as Chief Resident. A highly professional and scholarly set of questions was prepared. It became apparent that many other residents and ophthalmologists seeking to identify the strengths and weaknesses in their ophthalmic knowledge could profit from the dissemination of the material.

The past decade witnessed an explosion in ophthalmic knowledge that was truly daunting and unprecedented. We can expect this expansion to accelerate in the future at an exponential rate. How does one keep abreast of new developments, and how does one form judgments as to what is clinically relevant knowledge and what is of more theoretical or marginal interest at the moment? Most of us are highly specialized in either the knowledge industry or in our clinical practice patterns. If we wish to stay in touch with other specialties of ophthalmology, we tend to need help. Self-assessment and continuing medical education should by now be cornerstones of our professional lives, but these tasks will also be progressively shared with others! We will be increasingly held to higher quality assurance standards, and recertification examinations are to be put in place. Furthermore, the ability to practice medicine in the future may become aligned with profiles of the clinical outcomes of the patients we treat, as could be mandated by federal agencies and insurance payers. Sound and constantly remodeled knowledge will thus be the best basis for protecting and advancing our clinical practices.

The questions in this publication have been prepared with great care, in order to achieve balance among the various subspecialties of our field and to highlight clinically significant subjects and basic scienceconcepts and findings that under-gird them. No effort has been made to reconstruct questions from Board or OKAP examinations; rather, the questions have been created in a way that proceeds from what one group of people has determined to be an essential database for the practicing ophthalmologist who wishes to be informed of recent scientific discoveries and the refashioned foundations of clinical science.

As they say in the movies, any resemblance to questions that appear on formal examinations is completely coincidental and reflects the fact that people who are serious students of the subject have independently identified topics that should be within the purview and common fund of knowledge of a contemporary clinician. The questions themselves are less important than the subjects they represent. A well-positioned cadre that can serve as an arbiter for this fund of knowledge is residents-in-training who are eager to equip themselves for their impending clinical professional lives, and who daily critically assess and internalize the rivulets of information that are flowing toward them from their teachers and clinical preceptors.

This textbook is the distinctive product of a unique mind and constellation of talents possessed by Jeffrey Lamkin. I can think of nobody bette r suited to shepherd this project than Jeffrey because he is guided by an insightful and retentive mind, a capacity for detail and global integration, and an ardent love of knowledge and its transmission to those around him. Due to the depth of his commitment to resident education and that of other colleagues, he has made a tremendous gift of his energies and time to our entire field.

Frederick A. Jakobiec, MD

Preface

More than 6 years have passed since the release of the third edition of the *Massachusetts Review Manual for Ophthalmology*. During this period, the field of ophthalmology has continued to evolve at a breakneck pace. This evolution has led not only to a better understanding of the pathophysiologic processes responsible for several blinding diseases, but also to better outcomes for our patients. Therefore, maintaining a *current* and deep fund of knowledge in ophthalmology, however challenging, remains a crucial requisite for excellent patient care.

The fourth edition of the *Massachusetts Eye and Ear Infirmary Review Manual for Ophthalmology* differs from the third in several ways. The new edition has been updated with an extensive number of new questions and images to reflect the latest teachings in the field. Although this edition is markedly different from its predecessor, the intent of this book remains constant: to humbly attempt to help our fellow colleagues—whether they are attending physicians, fellows-in-training, residents, or medical students—assimilate useful information in the vast and ever-expanding field of ophthalmology. We posit that "learning"—remembering what is important—is often better accomplished through self-assessment with questions and answers, rather than with elaborative rote memorization. This hypothesis has not only been tested with our own empirical experience but has also been partially validated by recent scientific research.[1]

However, we do want to emphasize that this book should *not* serve as the *sole* method of preparation for any specific examination and is no way intended to duplicate the American Board of Ophthalmology (ABO) certification exam or any other ophthalmology examination, for that matter. Instead, we hope to help you retain knowledge *already* gleaned from reading, as well as provide a tool for accurate self-assessment.

I (RDJ), would like to recognize my fellow coauthors who have collaborated with me on this book. First and foremost, my friend and former fellow Dr. Veeral Sheth graciously agreed to take the lead in organizing this edition, and he has done an outstanding job. Drs. Harit K. Bhatt, Paul Chiranand, Marcus Marcet, and Jeffrey Lamkin have been great friends to work with, and they have done an incredible job going through each question, ensuring its appropriateness, and creating new and relevant questions with many more clinical images for this new edition. Finally, we would like to sincerely thank Jonathan Pine, the Senior Executive Editor at Lippincott who supported this project from the start, and Emilie Moyer and Ashley Fischer who have been extraordinarily patient and have been instrumental in creating this revised edition.

Working with friends to revise a book, which will help in the practice of ophthalmology, has been a truly wonderful experience. We hope that you, the reader, will benefit from our efforts.

Rama D. Jager, M.D., M.B.A., F.A.C.S.
Veeral S. Sheth, M.D.
Harit K. Bhatt, M.D.
Paul Chiranand, M.D.
Marcus M. Marcet, M.D.
Jeffrey C. Lamkin, M.D.
Chicago, Illinois

---

[1] Science. 2011 Feb 11;331 (6018):772–5

General Medicine

▮ Questions

1. Which of the following statements about the normal microbial flora is false?
   a. The microorganisms on the epithelial surfaces of the body remain in place chiefly through adherence.
   b. When mechanical defenses of the epithelial layers are breached so as to expose normally sterile areas, severe infections can result from the normal microbial flora.
   c. There is little benefit of these microorganisms to humans.
   d. If antimicrobial agents eliminate normal flora, the host's susceptibility to normally excluded pathogenic microorganisms is increased.

2. Which of the following statements about *Staphylococcus aureus* is false?
   a. 25% of tertiary care isolates are resistant to beta-lactam antibiotics.
   b. Transmission of organisms is by direct contact.
   c. Resistance of organisms to antimicrobials is usually plasmid determined and varies by institution.
   d. First-generation cephalosporins are the treatment of choice for life-threatening infections.

3. Which of the following is true of *Staphylococcus epidermidis*?
   a. *Staphylococcus epidermidis* is present in up to 90% of skin cultures and cannot produce local infections.

   b. Its characteristic adherence to prosthetic devices makes it the most common cause of prosthetic heart infections and is a common infectious organism of intravenous catheters and cerebrospinal fluid shunts.
   c. Most isolates are not resistant to methicillin or cephalosporins; therefore, the drugs of choice are first-generation cephalosporins.
   d. Management of an infected prosthetic device or vascular catheter only requires appropriate antibiotic administration.

4. Which of the following associations regarding *Streptococcus* is incorrectly paired?
   a. *Streptococcus pneumoniae*: Lancet-shaped diplococci that cause alpha-hemolysis on blood agar.
   b. Group A beta-hemolytic streptococci: Acute suppurative infections transmitted through droplets mediated by an opsonizing antibody.
   c. *Streptococcus pyogenes*: Highly sensitive to Penicillin G.
   d. *Streptococcus pneumoniae*: Can lead to pneumococcal pneumonia that is highly sensitive to penicillin and has a low mortality rate in the elderly.

5. Which of the following patients would not require endocarditis prophylaxis during invasive surgery?
   a. a patient with a history of severe coronary artery disease.
   b. a patient with a prosthetic heart valve.
   c. a patient with a previous history of bacterial endocarditis.
   d. a patient with acquired valvular dysfunction such as rheumatic heart disease.

6. What type of ocular surgery would require endocarditis prophylaxis?
   a. cataract surgery.
   b. vitrectomy.
   c. tear duct reconstruction.
   d. corneal transplant.

7. Which of the following is a false statement regarding pseudomembranous enterocolitis?
   a. It is most commonly caused by *Clostridium difficile*.
   b. *Clostridium difficile* is an anaerobic gram-negative bacterium.
   c. Typically occurs within 1 to 14 days of starting antibiotic therapy in which patients develop fever and diarrhea.
   d. Treatment includes discontinuing the causative antibiotic and administering metronidazole for 10 days.

8. Which of the following is true regarding *Haemophilus influenzae*?
   a. Long-term immunity follows with the development of bactericidal antibodies to the type B capsule in the presence of complement.
   b. *Haemophilus influenzae* is uncommonly found in the respiratory tracts of children.
   c. Macrolides, such as erythromycin, are the treatment of choice.
   d. Immunized patients are no longer susceptible to all strains of *Haemophilus influenza*.

9. Which of the following statements regarding *Neisseria gonorrhoeae* is false?
   a. Gonococci are not part of the normal microbial flora.
   b. 50% of women and 95% of men infected with gonococci are symptomatic.

c. *Chlamydia trachomatis* is found in as many as half of all women and one-third of all men infected with gonococci.
   d. Macrolides and quinolones are generally not good agents to treat gonococcal infections.

10. Which of the following is true regarding *Neisseria meningitidis*?
    a. Infection with *Neisseria meningitidis* is limited to meningitis.
    b. Meningitis with a petechial or puerperal exanthema is the classic presentation.
    c. The routine administration of meningococcal vaccine is recommended.
    d. The treatment of choice for meningococcal meningitis is vancomycin.

11. Which of the following statements about syphilis is false?
    a. The treatment of choice for patients with neurosyphilis is Penicillin G 2.4 million units intramuscularly weekly for 3 weeks.
    b. Transplacental transmission from an untreated pregnant female to her fetus before 16 weeks' gestation can result in congenital syphilis.
    c. Serum FTA-ABS titers do not decrease with successful treatment.
    d. Serum VDRL becomes negative after successful therapy.

12. Which of the following spirochetes causes Lyme disease?
    a. *Treponema pallidum*.
    b. *Ixodes scapularis*.
    c. *Borrelia burgdorferi*.
    d. *Leptospira interrogans*.

13. Which statement is true regarding *Chlamydia trachomatis*?
    a. *Chlamydia trachomatis* is the most common sexually transmitted infection.
    b. Chlamydial infections are treated with third-generation cephalosporins.
    c. Chlamydia is a small extracellular parasite.
    d. *Chlamydia trachomatis* can survive long periods outside the body and it is essential to avoid contact with patients that are infected.

14. Which of the following regarding tuberculosis is false?
    a. Infection usually occurs through inhalation of infective droplets and rarely by way of the skin or gastrointestinal tract.
    b. Treatment of active infection often involves use of two or three drugs because of the emergence of resistance.
    c. Laboratory diagnosis involves culture of infective material on Lowenstein-Jensen medium for 6 to 8 weeks and use of the acid-fast type of Ziehl-Neelsen stain.
    d. A positive PPD reaction is defined as an area of induration of 5 mm or greater read 48 to 72 hours after administration.

15. Which of the following is part of the normal flora that is present in the oral cavity, lower gastrointestinal tract, and female genital tract?
    a. *Histoplasma capsulatum.*
    b. *Candida albicans.*
    c. *Aspergillus fumigatus.*
    d. *Blastomyces dermatitidis.*

16. Toxoplasmosis is most commonly caused by
    a. exposure to cat feces.
    b. exposure to dog feces.
    c. eating raw eggs.
    d. exposure to human feces.

17. Which of the following statements about herpesviruses is false?
    a. EBV is associated with nasopharyngeal carcinoma.
    b. EBV is associated with Burkitt's lymphoma.
    c. Resolution of lesions caused by herpes simplex may be followed by postherpetic neuralgia.
    d. Untreated neonatal herpes infection carries an 80% mortality rate.

18. Which of the following methods of transmission of hepatitis viruses is incorrect?
    a. hepatitis A: fecal–oral route.
    b. hepatitis B: fecal–oral route.
    c. hepatitis C: blood transfusions.
    d. hepatitis D: sexual transmission.

19. Which of the following is false of these viruses or viral conditions?
    a. Severe acute respiratory syndrome (SARS) originated in China and rapidly spread by air travel to other countries.
    b. The hantavirus is a highly virulent respiratory pathogen transmitted by ticks.
    c. The Ebola virus can cause severe hemorrhage, generally occurring from the gastrointestinal tract.
    d. The West Nile virus is transmitted by a mosquito vector, and illness may vary from a flu-like syndrome to meningitis and encephalitis.

20. Which of the following statements regarding AIDS is true?
    a. Approximately 200 million people in the world have AIDS.
    b. The majority of individuals infected with HIV live in the United States.
    c. The ELISA test for HIV is 99% sensitive, but only 75% specific for HIV.
    d. Breast milk can also be a method of transmission of HIV.

21. *Pneumocystis carinii* pneumonia is generally treated with
    a. trimethoprim–sulfamethoxazole.
    b. ceftriaxone.
    c. doxycycline.
    d. penicillin.

22. Ganciclovir is used in the treatment of CMV retinitis and colitis in immunocompromised patients. Ganciclovir's major toxicity is
    a. hepatotoxicity.
    b. bone marrow suppression.
    c. nephrotoxicity.
    d. encephalopathy.

23. Hypertension is defined as
    a. systolic blood pressure of 140 mm Hg or higher.
    b. a single blood pressure reading of 140/80.
    c. diastolic pressure of 80 mm Hg or higher.
    d. systolic blood pressure of 130 mm Hg or higher.

24. Causes of secondary hypertension include all of the following, except
    a. pheochromocytoma.
    b. hypothyroidism.
    c. hyperaldosteronism.
    d. Cushing's syndrome.

25. Which of the following statements about lifestyle factors affecting blood pressure is false?
    a. Processed foods account for 75% of sodium intake in the United States.
    b. Patients with mild hypertension who smoke a pack of cigarettes a day have a fivefold higher risk of coronary artery disease.
    c. Alcohol consumption of more than 1 oz of ethanol (10 oz of wine or 24 oz of beer) is associated with resistance to antihypertensive therapy.
    d. Regular aerobic exercise contributes to reduced mortality and morbidity from hypertension.

26. Which medication is incorrectly paired with a common side effect?
    a. doxazosin: postural hypotension.
    b. atenolol: bronchospasm.
    c. spironolactone: gynecomastia.
    d. amlodipine: drug-induced lupus.

27. What types of antihypertensive agent should be used to start initial therapy for hypertension in a newly diagnosed patient without other comorbidity?
    a. thiazide diuretics.
    b. calcium channel blockers.
    c. angiotensin II receptor blockers (ARBs).
    d. alpha-adrenergic antagonists.

28. What is the definition of a transient ischemic attack (TIA)?
    a. a loss of neurologic function caused by ischemia that lasts for <24 hours and clears without residual signs.
    b. a progressively enlarging cerebral infarct that produces neurological deficits, which worsen over 24 to 48 hours.
    c. an ischemic event that produces a stable permanent neurological disability.
    d. an ischemic, but not infarcted area of the brain, which has been shown to have some plasticity with regard to recovery.

29. Which of the following statements with regard to stroke is false?
    a. Clopidogrel has a better side effect profile than ticlopidine with regard to bone marrow suppression.
    b. The use of tissue plasminogen activator (TPA) within 24 hours of the onset of symptoms improves outcome in patients with stroke.
    c. Aspirin offers a moderate benefit in the prevention of recurrent stroke.
    d. Hypertension should be controlled, although blood pressure reduction during acute ischemic stroke may cause harmful decreases in local perfusion.

30. Which of the following statements regarding intracranial hemorrhage or causes of intracranial hemorrhage is false?
    a. The most common site of berry aneurysms is at the origin of the posterior communicating artery from the internal carotid artery.
    b. Immediate CT examination demonstrates blood in the subarachnoid space in approximately 95% of the cases of ruptured aneurysm or AVM.
    c. The most common symptom of subarachnoid hemorrhage is a generalized seizure.
    d. Initial restoration of normal blood pressure and its maintenance at normal levels are mandatory in the treatment of ruptured aneurysms.

31. Ocular and cerebral conditions associated with carotid stenosis include all of the following, except
    a. amaurosis fugax.
    b. ocular ischemic syndromes.
    c. transient ischemic attack (TIA).
    d. intracranial hemorrhage.

32. Which of the following statements about carotid endarterectomy (CEA) is false?
    a. CEA should only be considered if the surgeon performing the operation has a perioperative morbidity rate of <3%.
    b. In the Asymptomatic Carotid Atherosclerosis Study, patients with asymptomatic carotid stenosis of >60% who underwent CEA did not show a significantly lower risk of having another major ischemic stroke, compared to patients who solely had medical management.
    c. CEA provided a significant benefit in reducing the risk of ipsilateral stroke in patients with symptomatic stenosis of 50% or more.
    d. In the North American Symptomatic Carotid Endarterectomy Trial, CEA was shown to have increasing benefit with higher degrees of carotid stenosis.

33. Folic acid can reduce the risk of stroke in patients by reducing the plasma levels of
    a. high-density cholesterol (HDL).
    b. homocysteine.
    c. triglycerides.
    d. low-density cholesterol (LDL).

34. What is the best procedure for determining a cardiac source in patients presenting with isolated amaurosis fugax or transient vision loss?
    a. transesophageal echocardiography.
    b. transthoracic echocardiography.
    c. MRI of the chest.
    d. CT scan of the chest.

35. What is the number one killer in the United States and around the world?
    a. lung cancer.
    b. breast cancer.
    c. coronary artery disease.
    d. HIV.

36. What is the number one preventable risk factor for cardiovascular disease worldwide?
    a. physical inactivity.
    b. smoking.
    c. obesity.
    d. diet high in saturated fat and cholesterol.

37. All of the following can impede the supply of oxygen to the myocardium except
    a. anemia.
    b. carotid artery stenosis.
    c. reduced mean arterial pressure.
    d. hypoxemia.

38. It has become clear that markers of inflammation are strong risk factors for CAD. What is the best marker that correlates most with future cardiovascular events?
    a. interleukin-6.
    b. TNF-alpha.
    c. high-sensitivity C-reactive protein (hs-CRP).
    d. serum amyloid A (SAA).

39. The metabolic syndrome is characterized by a group of metabolic risk factors in one person that increase the risk of cardiovascular disease. What is not one of these risk factors?
    a. elevated liver function tests (LFTs).
    b. abdominal obesity.
    c. low HDL level.
    d. hypertension.

40. Which of the following is a *clear* risk factor for ischemic heart disease?
    a. female gender.
    b. stress.
    c. personality type.
    d. diabetes.

41. The difference between a non–Q-wave myocardial infarction and unstable angina is
    a. non–Q-wave infarcts will have angina at rest, whereas unstable angina will not.
    b. non–Q-wave infarcts will have elevated cardiac enzymes, whereas unstable angina will not.
    c. non–Q-wave infarcts can have T wave inversions, whereas unstable angina will not.
    d. non–Q-wave infarcts can have ST segment depression on ECG, whereas unstable angina will not.

42. What portion of all myocardial infarctions are painless?
    a. 5%.
    b. 10%.
    c. 25%.
    d. 50%.

43. Dressler's syndrome is characterized by all of the following, except
    a. pleuropericardial pain.
    b. fever.
    c. arthralgias.
    d. vomiting.

44. All of the following can cause sudden cardiac death except
    a. pneumonia.
    b. Wolfe-Parkinson-White syndrome.
    c. long QT syndrome.
    d. ventricular fibrillation.

45. Noninvasive diagnostic testing in patients with ischemic heart disease (IHD) includes all of the following, except
    a. chest CT.
    b. electrocardiography (ECG).
    c. cardiac enzymes.
    d. echocardiography.

46. All of the following are used to treat acute coronary syndrome (ACS), except
    a. metoprolol.
    b. low–molecular-weight heparin.
    c. nitroglycerin.
    d. HCTZ.

47. Percutaneous transluminal coronary angioplasty (PTCA) is usually superior to thrombolytic therapy in acute coronary syndromes in all of the following situations except
    a. initiation of therapy more than 90 minutes after acute coronary syndrome.
    b. patients with an increased risk of intracranial hemorrhage.
    c. patients with a prior history of CABG.
    d. patients with a history of recent extensive abdominal surgery.

48. Clinical signs of acute left ventricular heart failure can include all of the following, except
    a. dyspnea.
    b. hemoptysis.
    c. diaphoresis.
    d. hepatomegaly.

49. The lower limit of normal for ejection fraction is
    a. 30%.
    b. 40%.
    c. 50%.
    d. 60%.

50. What is the most common cause of congestive heart failure (CHF) in the United States?
    a. aortic stenosis.
    b. mitral regurgitation.
    c. myocarditis.
    d. ischemic heart disease (IHD).

51. The most common cause of right-sided heart failure is
    a. left-sided heart failure.
    b. primary pulmonary hypertension.
    c. pulmonary embolism.
    d. coarctation of the aorta.

52. Usually, the most effective way of treating *systolic* dysfunction is to
    a. reduce preload.
    b. increase preload.
    c. reduce afterload.
    d. increase afterload.

53. The calcium channel blocker of choice in CHF patients with IHD is
    a. captopril.
    b. amlodipine.
    c. diltiazem.
    d. doxazosin.

54. Usually, the most effective way of treating *diastolic* dysfunction is to
    a. reduce preload.
    b. increase preload.
    c. reduce afterload.
    d. increase afterload.

55. The primary pacemaker of the heart is the
    a. sinoatrial (SA) node.
    b. atrioventricular (AV) junction.
    c. bundle of His.
    d. chordae tendineae.

56. Which one of the following bradyarrhythmias or conduction disturbances is the most innocuous?
    a. sinus bradycardia.
    b. second-degree AV block.
    c. third-degree AV block.
    d. left bundle branch block.

57. Which of the following supraventricular tachycardias are incorrectly matched with their ECG findings?
    a. Wolff-Parkinson-White syndrome: Delta wave (initial upsloping of QRS complex).
    b. atrial flutter: P waves have saw tooth appearance.
    c. paroxysmal atrial tachycardia: Prolonged PR interval.
    d. atrial fibrillation: No identifiable P wave.

58. The preferred first-line therapy to treat arrhythmias in patients who have had prior cardiac arrest or hemodynamically unstable ventricular tachycardia is
    a. automated implantable cardioverter-defibrillator (ICD).
    b. pacemaker.
    c. amiodarone.
    d. adenosine.

59. Major risk factors in which it is necessary to have lower LDL goals in patients include all of the following except
    a. an age of 45 or greater in males and 55 or greater in females.
    b. cigarette smoking.
    c. high HDL cholesterol (>60 mg/dL).
    d. hypertension.

60. Common adverse reactions from HMG-CoA reductase inhibitors, also known as "statins," include
    a. incontinence and constipation.
    b. muscle soreness.

    c. renal stones and diabetes.
    d. palpitations and anxiety.

61. Which of the following is not an irreversible obstructive disease?
    a. asthma.
    b. emphysema.
    c. chronic bronchitis.
    d. peripheral airway disease.

62. Which of the following is a restrictive lung disease?
    a. chronic bronchitis.
    b. emphysema
    c. fibrosis of the lung parenchyma.
    d. pneumothrorax.

63. What is the single most effective and cost-effective intervention to reduce the risk of COPD and to slow COPD progression?
    a. supplemental oxygen.
    b. smoking cessation.
    c. continuous positive airway pressure (CPAP).
    d. beta adrenergic agonists.

64. Which of the following could be used to manage an acute asthma attack?
    a. subcutaneous epinephrine.
    b. salmeterol.
    c. inhaled beclomethasone.
    d. cromolyn sodium.

65. Which of the following has been proven to increase survival in patients with severe COPD?
    a. oral corticosteroids.
    b. nitroglycerin.
    c. captopril.
    d. supplemental oxygen.

66. The average lifespan of an erythrocyte is
    a. 2 weeks.
    b. 6 weeks.
    c. 120 days.
    d. 1 year.

67. Erythropoiesis is stimulated by erythropoietin which is produced mainly in the
    a. lungs.
    b. liver.
    c. kidney.
    d. bone marrow.

68. What is by far the most common type of anemia worldwide?
    a. iron deficiency anemia.
    b. anemia of chronic disease.
    c. thalassemia.
    d. vitamin B12 deficiency anemia.

69. Which of the following is not a cause of microcytic anemia?
    a. iron deficiency.
    b. thalassemia.
    c. sideroblastic anemia.
    d. pernicious anemia.

70. Manifestations of sickle cell disease include all of the following except
    a. acute painful episodes.
    b. necrosis of the bone.
    c. hematuria.
    d. aphthous ulcers.

71. What blood test is typically used to measure the effect of heparin therapy?
    a. prothrombin time (PT).
    b. partial thromboplastin time (PTT).
    c. bleeding time.
    d. international normalized ratio (INR).

72. What blood test is typically used to measure the effect of warfarin therapy?
    a. prothrombin time (PT).
    b. partial thromboplastin time (PTT).
    c. bleeding time.
    d. international normalized ratio (INR).

73. The most common cause of abnormal bleeding in individuals is
    a. platelet disorders.
    b. hemophilia A.

    c. von Willebrand's disease.
    d. Vitamin K deficiency.

74. All of the following can cause thrombocytopenia except
    a. von Willebrand's disease.
    b. idiopathic thrombocytopenic purpura (ITP).
    c. sulfonamides.
    d. posttransfusion reactions.

75. Which of the following medications irreversibly inhibits platelet aggregation?
    a. antihistamines.
    b. tricyclic antidepressants.
    c. aspirin.
    d. NSAIDs.

76. What is the most common and severe hereditary coagulation disorder?
    a. factor II deficiency.
    b. factor V deficiency.
    c. factor VIII deficiency.
    d. protein C deficiency.

77. Which of the following statements about Vitamin K is false?
    a. Vitamin K is necessary for the production of factors II, VII, IX, and X in the liver.
    b. Vitamin K should not be given intramuscularly because of the risk of sudden death from an anaphylactoid reaction.
    c. Celiac sprue, cystic fibrosis, and biliary obstruction can be causes of Vitamin K deficiency.
    d. Vitamin K is routinely administered to newborns to prevent hemorrhagic disease in newborns.

78. Which of the following is not a primary hypercoagulable state?
    a. antithrombin III deficiency.
    b. protein C deficiency.
    c. hyperhomocysteinemia.
    d. factor IX deficiency.

79. The phospholipid antibody syndrome is characterized by all of the following except
    a. cerebral aneurysms.
    b. recurrent spontaneous abortions.
    c. DVT.
    d. venous and arterial thrombosis.

80. The most common rheumatic disorder is
    a. Behçet's disease.
    b. relapsing polychondritis.
    c. Wegener's granulomatosis.
    d. rheumatoid arthritis.

81. Which of the following is not a seronegative spondylopathy?
    a. relapsing polychondritis.
    b. ankylosing spondylitis.
    c. inflammatory bowel disease.
    d. psoriatic arthritis.

82. The classic triad for Reiter's syndrome includes all of the following except
    a. conjunctivitis.
    b. arthritis.
    c. uveitis.
    d. urethritis.

83. Which of the following findings would lead a clinician to suspicion of ankylosing spondylitis?
    a. atrophy of the distal phalanges ("pencil-in-cup" appearance on radiographic films).
    b. fusion of the spine ("bamboo spine").
    c. knee and ankle pain.
    d. interphalangeal arthritis ("sausage digits").

84. Which of the following is not part of the criteria needed to diagnose systemic lupus erythematosus (SLE)?
    a. oral ulcers.
    b. arthritis.
    c. positive for HLA-DR2.
    d. antinuclear antibody positivity.

85. More than 95% of patients with scleroderma have
    a. calcinosis.
    b. Raynaud's phenomenon.
    c. sclerodactyly.
    d. telangiectasias.

86. A patient who has a Schirmer-1 test of <5 mm in 5 minutes has had recurrent or persistent swollen salivary glands and who is positive for rheumatoid factor probably has
    a. scleroderma.
    b. Sjögren's syndrome.
    c. juvenile rheumatoid arthritis.
    d. relapsing polychondritis.

87. The findings below would make one suspicious for
    a. dermatomyositis.
    b. scleroderma.
    c. polymyositis.
    d. relapsing polychondritis.

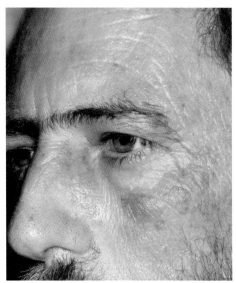

A

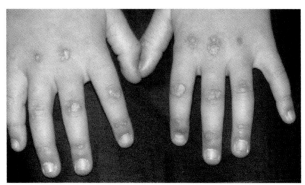

B

88. The most common clinical findings in relapsing polychondritis are
    a. laryngeal collapse.
    b. conjunctivitis and iritis.
    c. aortic insufficiency and vasculitis.
    d. arthropathy, auricular, and nasal chondritis.

89. What is the gold standard for diagnosing giant cell arteritis (GCA)?
    a. ESR.
    b. C-reactive protein (CRP).
    c. temporal artery biopsy.
    d. ESR and CRP.

90. Cogan's syndrome can be associated with which of the following in up to 50% of cases?
    a. Churg-Strauss angiitis.
    b. Wegener's granulomatosis.
    c. polyarteritis nodosa (PAN).
    d. Takayasu's arteritis.

91. What is the most common clinical manifestation of Behçet's syndrome?
    a. oral ulcers.
    b. genital ulcers.
    c. polyarthritis.
    d. erythema nodosum.

92. All of the following are potential side effects from administration of exogenous corticosteroids, except
    a. hypokalemia.
    b. osteoporosis.
    c. peptic ulcer.
    d. orthostatic hypotension

93. What is the most common side effect of oral NSAIDs?
    a. myelosuppression.
    b. gastrointestinal upset.
    c. hepatic toxicity.
    d. corneal melt.

94. The American Diabetes Association recommends a diagnosis of diabetes when 1 of 3 criteria is met. These criteria include all of the following except
    a. fasting glucose level ≥ 126 mg/dL.
    b. fasting glucose level < 126 mg/dL, but ≥ 200 mg/dL 2 hours after ingestion of 75 g of oral glucose.
    c. hemoglobin A1c (HbA1c) ≥ 7.
    d. a glucose level of ≥ 200 mg/dL at any time with classic symptoms of diabetes.

95. Which of the following is true of type 1 diabetes?
    a. Most often due to an immune-mediated destruction of insulin-producing beta cells in the pancreas.
    b. Occurs most commonly after the age of 40.
    c. Monozygotic twins show a concordance rate of having diabetes of >90%.
    d. Obesity is present in 80% to 90% of these patients.

96. Risk factors for developing type 2 diabetes include all of the following except
    a. low socioeconomic status.
    b. hypertension.
    c. obesity.
    d. stress.

97. What is the earliest sign of malignant hyperthermia?
    a. elevated body temperature.
    b. tachycardia.
    c. metabolic acidosis.
    d. muscular rigidity.

98. Which of the following describes the Somogyi phenomenon?
    a. high sugars following episodes of hypoglycemia.
    b. hypoglycemia following episodes of very high sugar levels.
    c. hyperglycemia following insulin administration.
    d. hypoglycemia following insulin administration.

99. The most sensitive and specific screening test for thyroid disease is
    a. free T3.
    b. free T4 and TSH.
    c. transthyretin.
    d. thyroid microsomal antibody detection.

100. 85% to 90% of patients with the disease characterized by findings in the image below have antibodies to
    a. TSH.
    b. TSH receptor.
    c. T3.
    d. T4.

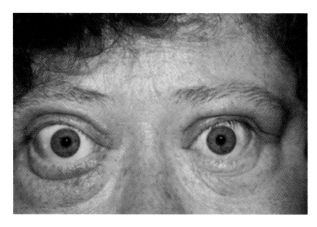

Answers

1. **c.** There is extensive benefit of normal microbial flora to humans through priming of the immune system as well as excluding other pathogenic microorganisms from causing harm.

2. **d.** *Staphylococcus aureus* colonizes the anterior nares and other skin sites in 15% of community isolates. Acute serious staphylococcal infections require immediate intravenous antibiotic therapy. A penicillinase-resistant penicillin or first-generation cephalosporin is normally used. With the emergence of methicillin-resistant staphylococci, vancomycin has become the drug of choice in the treatment of life-threatening infections, pending susceptibility studies.

3. **b.** *Staphylococcus epidermidis* can cause local infection when local defenses are compromised. Most isolates are resistant to methicillin and cephalosporin; therefore, the drug of choice is vancomycin, occasionally in combination with rifampin or gentamicin. Management of an infected prosthetic device or vascular catheter not only involves appropriate antibiotic coverage but often requires removal of the infected prosthetic device or vascular catheter as well.

4. **d.** Pneumococcal virulence is determined by its complex polysaccharide capsule, of which there are 80 distinct serotypes. Pneumococcal pneumonia can cause a very severe pneumonia in the elderly, whose mortality rate approaches 25%. Part of this may be because of the increasing resistance of *Streptococcus pneumoniae* to penicillin. In recent studies, multidrug resistance (MDR) was approaching 20%, and penicillin resistance was over 25%. Prophylaxis is available through use of the 23-valent vaccine.

5. **a.** Patients with a history of coronary artery disease do not routinely require endocarditis prophylaxis for invasive surgeries. In all of the other situations, endocarditis prophylaxis should be considered. Most congenital cardiac malformations also require endocarditis prophylaxis.

6. **c.** Endocarditis prophylaxis for ocular surgeries is usually not necessary except for cases involving the nasolacrimal drainage system or sinuses or for repair of orbital trauma.

7. **b.** Pseudomembranous colitis most commonly occurs from *Clostridium difficile* after the administration of oral antibiotics. *Clostridium difficile* is an endemic anaerobic gram-positive bacillus that is part of the normal gastrointestinal flora. Vancomycin can be used in patients who are in their first trimester of pregnancy or those who cannot tolerate metronidazole.

8. **a.** *Haemophilus influenzae* is a common inhabitant of the upper respiratory tract in 20% to 50% of healthy adults and 80% of children. Infections that could be caused by *Haemophilus influenzae* include meningitis, epiglottitis, orbital cellulitis, arthritis, otitis media, bronchitis, pericarditis, sinusitis, and pneumonia. Most, if not nearly all, strains of *Haemophilus influenzae* are resistant to macrolides. Since *Haemiphilus influenzae* type B vaccines were introduced, *Haemophilus influenza* infection has been nearly eradicated. Immunized patients, however, are still susceptible to infections caused by strains of *Haemophilus influenza* other than type B.

9. **d.** Macrolides and quinolones are generally good agents to treat gonococcal infections. They have an added benefit in that they also can concomitantly treat *Chlamydia trachomatis* infection, which is often found in patients with concurrent gonococcal infections.

10. **b.** Meningococcal infections include meningitis, respiratory tract infections, endocarditis, arthritis, pericarditis, pneumonia, endophthalmitis, and purpura fulminans. The treatment of choice for meningococcal meningitis has been high-dose penicillin or in the case of allergy or resistance, chloramphenicol or third-generation cephalosporin. Routine administration of meningococcal vaccines

is not recommended except in patients who have undergone splenectomy, complement-deficient persons, military personnel, travelers to endemic regions, and close contacts of infected patients.

11. **a.** The treatment of choice for neurosyphilis is 2.4 million units of Penicillin G *intravenously* every 4 hours for 10 days. Early-stage syphilis (e.g., within 1 year of infection) is treated with 1 dose of 2.4 million units of Penicillin G intramuscularly. In patients who have neurosyphilis, the serum VDRL may be negative, but the CSF VDRL will be positive. False-positive VDRLs can occur in patients with systemic lupus erythematosus, liver disease, pregnancy, or other treponemal infections.

12. **c.** *Ixodes scapularis* is the deer tick that transmits the spirochete *Borrelia burgdorferi* to deer and humans. Lyme disease is the most common vector-borne disease in the United States.

13. **a.** *Chlamydia* is a small, obligate, intracellular parasite that contains DNA and RNA. *C trachomatis* can survive only briefly outside the body. *Chlamydia trachomatis* is the most common sexually transmitted infection, with 4 million new cases per year. Third-generation cephalosporins are used to treat gonococcal infections, which often coexist with chlamydial infections. Treatment of choice for chlamydial infection is the tetracycline family of antibiotics.

14. **d.** A positive PPD is defined as an area of induration 10 mm or greater read 48 to 72 hours after intradermal injection. All of the agents currently used to treat tuberculosis have toxic side effects, especially hepatic and neurologic. Isoniazid and ethambutol can cause optic neuritis, and rifampin may cause pink-tinged tears and blepharoconjunctivitis.

15. **b.** *Candida albicans* is a yeast normally present in the oral cavity, lower gastrointestinal tract, and female genital tract. Under conditions of disrupted local defenses or depressed immunity,

overgrowth or parenchymal invasion can occur. Treatment of serious systemic infections has traditionally involved the use of intravenous amphotericin B.

16. **a.** Toxoplasmosis can be caused by eating undercooked or raw meat. Toxoplasma can also be transmitted to humans by ingestion of oocysts through exposure to cat feces, water, or soil containing the parasite. Pregnant women should avoid changing cat litter as toxoplasma can be transmitted to the fetus and cause severe complications including mental retardation, blindness, and epilepsy. The most commonly used therapeutic regimen includes a combination of pyrimethamine, sulfadiazine, and folinic acid.

17. **c.** Resolution of lesions caused by *Varicella-zoster* may be followed by postherpetic neuralgia. In some patients, tricyclic antidepressants, carbamazepine, and gabapentin have reduced the pain of postherpetic neuralgia.

18. **b.** Hepatitis B is parenterally or sexually transmitted. Hepatitis C can also be transmitted through parenteral drug use, hemodialysis, and occupational exposure to blood. Hepatitis E is transmitted through the fecal–oral route.

19. **b.** Severe acute respiratory syndrome (SARS) emerged in late 2002 and early 2003 and originated in the Guangdong Province of China. Early, the infection was transmitted primarily through household contacts and in health care facilities and was rapidly spread by air travel to other countries. The hantavirus is a virulent respiratory pathogen transmitted from rodent carriers, particularly deer mice.

20. **d.** By 2003, more than 35 million people in the world were living with HIV/AIDS. The majority of these individuals (more than 95%) live in developing countries. The ELISA test is 99% sensitive and 99% specific for HIV, but false-negatives can occur in the first few weeks after initial infection.

21. **a.** *Pneumocystis carinii* is generally treated with trimethoprim–sulfamethoxazole (trade names Bactrim, Septra).

22. **b.** Ganciclovir's major toxicity is reversible bone marrow suppression. One-third of patients using systemic ganciclovir develop significant granulocytopenia. Foscarnet is also used to treat CMV and its main side effect is nephrotoxicity.

23. **a.** The Seventh Report of the Joint National Committee on Prevention, Detection, Evaluation, and Treatment of High Blood Pressure has defined hypertension as a systolic blood pressure 140 mm Hg or higher or a diastolic blood pressure of 90 mm Hg or higher. The classification is based on the average of two or more properly measured seated blood pressure readings on each of two or more office visits.

24. **b.** Hypothyroidism is often associated with *hypo*tension. All of the other conditions listed are causes of secondary hypertension. Approximately 90% of cases of hypertension are primary, in which the etiology is unknown, and 10% are secondary to identifiable causes. Other causes of secondary hypertension include polycystic kidney disease, renovascular disease, and coarctation of the aorta.

25. **b.** Cigarette smoking is associated with a 25-fold higher risk of coronary artery disease in patients with mild hypertension. In patients without hypertension, cigarette smoking increases the risk fivefold.

26. **d.** Hydralazine is commonly reported to have drug-induced lupus as a side effect. Doxazosin and other alpha-blockers can result in postural hypotension. Beta-blockers often can cause bronchoconstriction and should be avoided in patients with asthma. ACE inhibitors also commonly have the common side effect of a dry cough.

27. **a.** Thiazide-type diuretics are the treatment of choice for initial hypertension. Special considerations should be taken into account in patients with certain conditions. ACE inhibitors and beta-blockers are recommended as first-line drugs in patients with acute coronary syndromes and patients with ventricular dysfunction. ACE inhibitors and ARBs are beneficial for those with diabetic nephropathy. ACE inhibitors and ARBs are contraindicated in pregnancy because of teratogenic effects.

28. **a.** A TIA lasts <24 hours but must be taken as a harbinger for repeat strokes. Answer B is the definition of an *evolving stroke*. Answer C defines a *completed stroke*. Answer D is the definition of the penumbra, a term used to describe the ischemic area of brain tissue surrounding the main infarct. The penumbra has been shown to recover in some cases.

29. **b.** TPA is best used within 3 hours of onset of symptoms and is associated with improved outcomes in select patients. Unfortunately, TPA is often underutilized because of the lack of availability and awareness and because patients can present to the hospital or emergency department several hours after the onset of symptoms.

30. **c.** The most common symptom of subarachnoid hemorrhage is the sudden development of a violent, usually localized headache.

31. **d.** Ischemic stroke is also associated with carotid stenosis. The annual stroke rate among patients with isolated amaurosis fugax, retinal infarcts, or TIAs is approximately 2%, 3%, and 8%, respectively. Untreated patients with amaurosis fugax, retinal infarcts, or TIAs have a 30% risk of myocardial infarction and an 18% risk of death over a 5-year period.

32. **c.** 4% of individuals over the age of 40 have asymptomatic carotid bruits. Patients with TIA or previous stroke in the territory of the carotid circulation are judged to be "symptomatic."

CEA was shown to be effective in symptomatic patients with high-grade stenosis, 70% to 99%.

There is still uncertainty regarding the benefit of CEA for symptomatic stenosis in the range of 30% to 69%.

33. **b.** High homocysteine levels have been associated with an increased risk of stroke and vascular disease. Folic acid helps reduce homocysteine levels and can be recommended to all patients with cardiovascular or atherosclerotic disease.

34. **a.** Transesophageal echocardiography is the best procedure for determining the cardiac source of an embolus.

35. **c.** Atherosclerotic coronary artery disease (CAD) remains by far the number one killer in the United States and around the world. CAD accounts for approximately a third of all deaths in the United States. The number of people that die from CAD is far greater than the number of people that die from all types of cancers combined.

36. **b.** Smoking remains the number one preventable risk factor for cardiovascular disease worldwide. The risk of CAD can be decreased by 50% in just 1 year after an individual stops smoking.

37. **b.** Coronary artery stenosis, not carotid artery stenosis, can lead to myocardial ischemia. The balance between arterial supply and myocardial demand for oxygen determines whether ischemia occurs. Coronary stenosis, thrombosis, reduced arterial pressure, hypoxemia, or severe anemia can impede the supply of oxygen to the myocardium. On the demand side, an increase in heart rate, ventricular contractility, or wall tension may each increase utilization of oxygen.

38. **c.** All of the answer choices are inflammatory markers. Hs-CRP is the best marker of inflammation for cardiovascular disease. C-reactive protein levels <1, between 1 and 3, and >3 μg/mL identify patients at low, medium, and high risk, respectively, for future cardiovascular events.

39. **a.** The metabolic syndrome is defined as a constellation of three or more of the following: abdominal obesity, hypertriglyceridemia, low HDL level, fasting glucose level of 110 mg/dL or more, and hypertension.

40. **d.** A family history of ischemic heart disease, hypertension, elevated serum cholesterol, smoking, and diabetes are risk factors for ischemic heart disease.

41. **b.** Both unstable angina and non–Q-wave MI can have very similar presentations. The presence of elevated cardiac enzymes can serve to differentiate non–Q-wave MI from unstable angina.

42. **c.** Painless myocardial infarcts are more common in patients with diabetes and elderly patients, and painless MI can present as syncope or congestive heart failure. Women can also present with atypical symptoms of an MI (e.g., stomach upset, malaise) instead of the classic "chest pain radiating down the arm" presentation.

43. **d.** Dressler's syndrome occurs after myocardial infarction, typically 2 to 3 days later, and is caused by a postinfarct pericarditis. Dressler's syndrome, or *post-MI*, is characterized by a pericardial friction rub. This rub can be accompanied by fever, arthralgias, and pleuropericardial pain. Dressler's syndrome is typically treated with NSAIDs, aspirin, or corticosteroids.

44. **a.** Sudden cardiac death is defined as unexpected nontraumatic death occurring within 1 hour after onset of symptoms in clinically stable patients. Arrhythmias, such as ventricular tachycardia or fibrillation, are usually the cause of sudden cardiac death. Other causes include torsade de pointes, hypertrophic cardiomyopathy, Wolfe-Parkinson-White syndrome, long QT syndrome, and pulmonary embolism.

45. **a.** Noninvasive diagnostic testing in ischemic heart disease includes ECG, serum enzyme measurement, echocardiography, and various types of stress testing. During angina or myocardial infarction (MI), ST segments become elevated

or depressed, and T waves may be inverted or become peaked. Cardiac enzymes are released into the bloodstream when myocardial necrosis occurs. CK-MB and troponins T and I are important cardiac enzymes in detecting myocardial infarction. Troponins T and I have been shown to be more cardiac specific and sensitive than CK-MB. Troponin levels remain elevated from 3 hours to 14 days after MI, whereas CK-MB levels rise approximately 4 hours after MI, peaking between 12 and 24 hours after the event.

Echocardiography is used to image the ventricles and atria, the heart valves, left ventricular contraction and wall-motion abnormalities, left ventricular ejection fraction, and the pericardium. Patients with IHD, particularly following infarction, commonly have regional wall-motion abnormalities that correspond to the areas of myocardial injury.

46. d. HCTZ is used in the treatment of hypertension, not ACS. Beta-blocker therapy reduces myocardial oxygen demands and should be considered for all patients with evolving MI. ACE inhibitors given orally during the acute phase of MI can decrease the risk of mortality when initiated within the first 24 hours of acute MI. Nitrates and an antithrombin agent are also commonly given in patients with ACS.

47. a. Optimal myocardial salvation requires that nearly complete reperfusion be achieved as soon as possible. If significant delay occurs (>90 minutes) before PTCA can be performed, thrombolysis is preferable. Contraindications to thrombolysis using intravenous thrombolytic agents include known sites of potential bleeding, a history of prior cerebrovascular accident, recent surgery, or prolonged cardiopulmonary resuscitation efforts.

48. d. Hepatomegaly, pedal edema, and cyanosis are signs of right ventricular failure. The most frequent symptoms of left ventricular failure are dyspnea with exertion or at rest, orthopnea, paroxysmal nocturnal dyspnea, diaphoresis, generalized weakness, fatigue, anxiety, and lightheadedness.

49. c. In patients without CHF, the ejection fraction (EF) is more than 0.50. EF of <0.50 indicates impairment. Echocardiography is the most useful and least invasive method of determining ejection fraction.

50. d. All of the other answers listed can also be causes of CHF as well, but IHD is the most common cause.

51. a. The most common cause of right-sided heart failure is left-sided heart failure.

52. c. Preload refers to the amount of stretch to which muscle fibers are subjected at the end of diastole or refilling. Afterload is the amount of tension or force in the ventricular muscle mass just after onset of contraction. Reducing afterload is usually the most effective way of treating systolic dysfunction. Reducing vascular resistance and lowering arterial blood pressure decrease the burden on the left ventricle and enhance contraction and ejection. ACE inhibitors are the medication of choice to accomplish this, although angiotensin receptor blockers, hydralazine, and other medications can be considered if the patient is unable to tolerate ACE inhibitors.

53. b. Amlodipine has been shown to be safe in patients with CHF. Other calcium channel blockers such as diltiazem have shown to actually increase mortality in patients with CHF. Doxazosin and prazosin are alpha-adrenergic blockers. Captopril is an ACE inhibitor.

54. a. Diastolic function can be improved by reducing preload, which in turn lowers filling pressures in the ventricle. Preload can be reduced by reducing circulating blood volume, by increasing the capacitance of the venous bed, and by improving systolic function to more effectively empty the ventricle. Diuretics are the most effective agents

for reducing blood volume. Oral thiazide or loop diuretics are effective for long-term diuresis, but intravenous loop diuretics such as furosemide or bumetanide are more potent for severe CHF or pulmonary edema.

55. **a.** The SA node is the primary pacemaker of the heart and is located in the right atrium just inferior to the entrance to the superior vena cava. The electrical impulse that originates in the SA node is conducted down through the atria and ventricles. If the SA node function is absent, secondary pacemakers in the AV junction, the bundle of His, or the ventricle can generate stimuli and maintain the heartbeat. Normally, stimulus formation in these other secondary pacemaker sites is slower than that of the SA node.

56. **a.** A bradyarrhythmia is any rhythm resulting in a ventricular rate of <60 beats per minute (bpm). Sinus bradycardia is a sinus rhythm (initiated by the SA node) that is slower than 60 bpm. Sinus bradycardia is usually harmless and can be found in normal individuals and athletes. Treatment is usually not indicated.

AV block is caused by a delay or block in conduction through the AV junction. First-degree AV block is asymptomatic and is diagnosed by prolongation of the PR interval. There are two types of second-degree AV block. In the Wenckebach type, the ECG reveals progressive PR prolongation prior to a nonconducted P wave. In Mobitz type II AV block, the QRS complex is dropped at regular intervals. In complete, or third-degree, AV block, all of the atrial stimuli are blocked at the AV node, so the P waves from the atria and the QRS complexes are completely asynchronous. Complete AV block is usually more ominous. The right ventricle and left ventricle receives its electrical impulse from the bundle of His from the right bundle branch and left bundle branch respectively. Conduction deficits in either of these can lead to either a right bundle branch block or left bundle branch block and should be evaluated for cardiac disease.

57. **c.** In paroxysmal atrial tachycardia (PAT), the P waves have an abnormal configuration and axis. The treatment of choice for PAT is intravenous adenosine, which has a very short half-life and success rate of converting to sinus rhythm of over 90%. In atrial fibrillation, atrial thrombi may accumulate from stagnation of blood. Anticoagulation is indicated for patients with chronic atrial fibrillation associated with valvular disease, cardiomyopathy, or cardiomegaly and before conversion to sinus rhythm is attempted.

58. **a.** Automated ICDs are now the first-line therapy to treat arrhythmias in patients with prior cardiac arrest or prior episodes of hemodynamically unstable ventricular tachycardia.

59. **c.** High HDL cholesterol is actually a "negative" risk factor and allows one to remove one risk factor from the total count. The other answer choices are major risk factors that lower LDL goals. Low HDL level (<40 mg/dL) and family history of premature CHD also make it necessary to have lower LDL goals. Anyone with coronary heart disease or diabetes should have an LDL of <100. Anyone with two or more risk factors listed in the answers should have an LDL goal of <130. Anyone with zero to one risk factor should have an LDL of <160.

60. **b.** HMG-CoA reductase inhibitors, or "statins," can cause muscle soreness, tenderness, and pain. It is important to evaluate baseline muscle symptoms and CK prior to initiating therapy, every 6 to 12 weeks, and when the patient is having muscle soreness or pain. These medications can also cause diarrhea and increase liver transaminases. Baseline liver function tests as well as subsequent measurements should be taken in anyone who is starting a statin.

61. **a.** In obstructive lung disease, changes in the bronchi, bronchioles, and lung parenchyma can cause airway obstruction. Asthma is a reversible obstructive disease secondary to bronchospasm. In asthma, the airways are hyperresponsive and

develop an inflammatory response to various stimuli. Irreversible obstructive disease, also referred to as chronic obstructive pulmonary disease (COPD), is the fourth leading cause of death in the United States.

62. c. Restrictive lung diseases are a diffuse group of conditions that cause diffuse parenchymal damage. The consequences of this damage include a reduction in total lung volume, diffusing capacity, and vital capacity.

63. b. Although all of the answer choices can reduce the symptoms in patients with COPD, smoking cessation is still the most effective means of reducing the risks and slowing progression of COPD.

64. a. Subcutaneous epinephrine can be used to manage an acute asthma attack. More commonly used medications for an acute asthma attack are the short-acting beta-2 adrenergic agonists such as albuterol and terbutaline. Salmeterol is a long-acting beta-2 adrenergic agonist and is helpful for maintenance treatment of asthma, not for acute exacerbations. Cromolyn is a mast cell stabilizer and is not used acutely. Inhaled steroids such as beclomethasone can be used for long-term therapy for reducing bronchial hyperreactivity.

65. d. The Nocturnal Oxygen Therapy Trial (NOTT), a multicenter randomized trial, demonstrated that continuous low-flow oxygen therapy for patients with severe COPD resulted in improved survival. Patients receiving supplemental oxygen, however, must be carefully monitored because such treatment may decrease the respiratory drive to eliminate carbon dioxide.

66. c. Circulating RBCs have a lifespan of about 120 days.

67. c. Erythropoietin is produced mainly in the kidneys. Any reduction in oxygen tension in the kidneys, for example, hypoxemia, low hemoglobin level, or arterial insufficiency, stimulates production of erythropoietin.

68. a. Anemia is diagnosed in adults if the hematocrit is <13.5 g/dL in males and <12 g/dL in females. Iron deficiency anemia is by far the most common type of anemia worldwide. A source of blood loss must be ruled out in any patient with iron deficiency anemia. Menstrual blood loss plays a major role in females. Gastrointestinal blood loss plays a major role in both men and women.

69. d. The usual classification of anemias is based on their pathophysiologic mechanism, for example, iron deficiency or folic acid deficiency anemia. However, the anemias can also be classified according to the size of the RBC. Possible causes of microcytic anemia include iron deficiency, thalassemia, and anemia of chronic disease. Possible causes of macrocytic anemia include vitamin B12 or folate deficiency.

70. d. In sickle cell anemia, an abnormal hemoglobin leads to a chronic hemolytic anemia. One out of every 400 African Americans born in the United States has sickle cell anemia. Chronic hemolytic anemias can produce jaundice, gallstones, splenomegaly, and poorly healing ulcers over the lower tibia. A manifestation of sickle cell disease is acute painful episodes that are caused by the sickling of the RBCs. These painful episodes are precipitated by infection, dehydration, or hypoxia.

71. b. The PTT is most commonly used to measure the effect of heparin therapy. However, blood tests are not typically used to measure the effects of low–molecular-weight heparin.

72. d. While the PT does change with warfarin, the INR is a more useful test to measure the therapeutic effect of warfarin. For deep vein thromboses and tissue replacement heart valves, the INR typically is maintained between 2.0 and 3.0; for mechanical prosthetic replacement heart valves, the INR is maintained between 2.5 and 3.5.

73. a. Platelet disorders are by far the most common cause of abnormal bleeding. Platelet disorders

may result from an insufficient number of platelets, inadequate function, or both. Mild platelet dysfunction may be asymptomatic or may cause minor bruising, menorrhagia, or bleeding after surgery. More severe dysfunction leads to petechiae, purpura, and gastrointestinal bleeding.

74. **a.** Von Willebrand's disease is caused by deficiency or abnormality of a portion of the factor VIII molecule, called von Willebrand factor, which causes platelet adhesion abnormalities, not thrombocytopenia. ITP is the result of platelet injury by antiplatelet antibodies. Many drugs can also cause immunologic platelet destruction. These include quinine, quinidine, digitalis, procainamide, sulfonamides, and gold to name a few.

75. **c.** Aspirin irreversibly inhibits platelet aggregation for the lifespan of the circulating platelets present. This causes a prolongation in the bleeding time for at least 48 to 72 hours following ingestion. NSAIDs cause reversible inhibition of platelet function. The other answer choices can have an effect on platelet function as well.

76. **c.** The most common and most severe is factor VIII deficiency, called hemophilia A. Typical manifestations of this X-linked disease include severe and protracted bleeding after minor trauma and spontaneous bleeding into joints (hemarthroses), the central nervous system, and the abdominal cavity. Treatment involves infusion of coagulation factor VIII.

77. **b.** Vitamin K should not be given intravenously because of the risk of an anaphylactoid reaction. Vitamin K deficiency leads to prolongation of both the PT and PTT.

78. **d.** Factor IX deficiency, also called hemophilia B, leads to a bleeding disorder. This is much less common than hemophilia A, which is caused by a factor VIII deficiency. Protein S deficiency, prothrombin gene mutation, and factor V Leiden (which is a point mutation in the factor V gene) are all also primary hypercoagulable states.

Factor V Leiden mutation is found in 3% to 7% of the white population and is far less prevalent or even absent in the black and Asian populations.

79. **a.** The phospholipid antibody syndrome can also lead to cerebrovascular arterial thrombotic events, not cerebral aneurysms. Ophthalmic complications include retinal vein and artery occlusion, retinal vasculitis, choroidal infarction, and anterior ischemic optic neuropathy. Tests for patients with this syndrome include anticardiolipin antibodies and lupus anticoagulants.

80. **d.** Rheumatoid arthritis (RA) is the most common rheumatic disorder, affecting approximately 1% of adults. RA is a symmetrical, deforming, peripheral polyarthritis characterized by synovial membrane inflammation. Approximately 80% of patients with RA are positive for rheumatoid factor. Human leukocyte antigen DR4 (HLA-DR4) is found in 70% of Caucasian seropositive patients.

81. **a.** The term spondyloarthropathy refers to a spectrum of diseases that share certain clinical features, including axial inflammation, asymmetric arthritis, genital lesions, skin lesions, eye inflammation, and bowel inflammation. The seronegative spondyloarthropathies are ankylosing spondylitis, reactive arthritis (also known as Reiter's syndrome), inflammatory bowel disease (Crohn disease and ulcerative colitis), psoriatic arthritis, and juvenile idiopathic arthritis (JIA). These diseases all share an association with HLA-B27. The most common ophthalmic finding in patients with seronegative spondyloarthropathies is a nongranulomatous anterior uveitis. They are termed "seronegative" because of the lack of IgG antibodies to rheumatoid factor in serum.

82. **c.** While uveitis does occur in 15% to 25% of patients with reactive arthritis, it is not part of the classic triad. There is a clear genetic predisposition in that 63% to 95% of these patients are positive for HLA-B27. The male-to-female ratio is at least 5:1. Precipitating agents include

Chlamydia trachomatis in the genitourinary tract and *Salmonella*, *Shigella*, *Yersinia*, and *Campylobacter* organisms in the gastrointestinal tract.

83. **b.** The classic features of ankylosing spondylitis are inflammatory low back pain, fusion of the axial skeleton, and sacroiliitis. The last stage of this process is a completely fused and immobilized spine, also known as "bamboo" or "poker spine." Men are affected three times more often than women in this disease. There is a strong association with HLA–B27 (90% of patients). In Reiter's syndrome, the arthritis typically appears within 1 to 3 weeks after the inciting urethritis or diarrhea. It is an episodic oligoarthritis primarily affecting the lower extremities, particularly the knees and ankles. Interphalangeal arthritis of the toes and fingers can lead to "sausage digits" in Reiter's syndrome. Whittling of the distal phalanges is seen in psoriatic arthritis.

84. **c.** Even though HLA types DR2 and DR3 are associated with SLE suggesting a genetic predisposition, they are not used as part of the criteria for diagnosing SLE. Other criteria include malar rash, discoid rash, photosensitivity, serositis, renal disorder, neurologic disorder, hematologic disorder, and immunologic disorder. Four of these criteria are required to make the diagnosis of SLE. Also, the ANA test is virtually positive in all SLE patients but not very specific. Two antibodies that are highly specific for SLE are anti–double-stranded DNA (dsDNA) antibodies and anti-Smith (anti-SM) antibodies.

85. **b.** Scleroderma, also known as progressive systemic sclerosis, is characterized by fibrous and degenerative changes in the viscera, skin, or both. CREST (calcinosis, Raynaud's phenomenon, esophageal involvement, sclerodactyly, and telangiectasias) is a limited form of systemic scleroderma. Renal involvement is often associated with malignant hypertension and can be a major cause of mortality in patients with scleroderma.

86. **b.** Sjögren's syndrome is characterized by rheumatoid arthritis, dry mouth, and dry eyes. The dry mouth and dry eyes is because of an inflammatory infiltrate into the lacrimal and salivary glands. Patients with Sjögren's syndrome often have autoantibodies known as anti-SS-A and anti-SS-B.

87. **a.** A heliotrope rash around the eyelids (image A, violaceous erythema) and Gottron's sign (image B, plaques on finger knuckles) are seen in dermatomyositis. The heliotrope rash is the most specific rash in dermatomyositis, but it is present in only a minority of patients. Dermatomyositis is distinguished from polymyositis by the presence of cutaneous lesions. Laboratory findings include elevated serum levels of skeletal muscle enzymes and abnormal electromyography results.

88. **d.** Laryngotracheobronchial disease may lead to a fatal complication from laryngeal collapse. Cardiovascular lesions include aortic insufficiency and vasculitis. Ocular manifestations occur in approximately 50% of patients with this disease with the most common ocular conditions being conjunctivitis, scleritis, uveitis, and retinal vasculitis.

89. **c.** Caucasians are most commonly affected with GCA. It is particularly common in northern European countries such as Scandinavia. Clinical features include headache, polymyalgia rheumatica, jaw claudication, constitution symptoms, and ophthalmic symptoms. Signs include tenderness over the temporal artery, a pulseless temporal artery, scalp tenderness, fever, and loss of vision. The most common laboratory result in GCA is an elevated ESR. Temporal artery biopsy is suggested for all cases of suspected GCA. Treatment with corticosteroids should not be delayed pending laboratory results.

90. **c.** Cogan's syndrome is a constellation of hearing loss, tinnitus, vertigo, and interstitial keratitis. Polyarteritis nodosa (PAN) is characterized by necrotizing vasculitis of the medium-sized and

small-muscular arteries. Takayasu arteritis affects large arteries, particularly branches of the aorta. Other names for Takayasu arteritis are aortic arch arteritis, aortitis syndrome, and pulseless disease. It occurs primarily in children and young women and is common in the Far East, particularly Japan. Wegener's granulomatosis is a necrotizing granulomatous vasculitis of both the upper and lower respiratory tract and can lead to a focal segmental glomerulonephritis; 80% of patients with Wegener's granulomatosis are serum positive for a cytoplasmic pattern of antineutrophil cytoplasmic antibodies (c-ANCA). In Churg-Strauss syndrome, eosinophilia is generally present and asthma is the principal feature.

91. **a.** Behçet's syndrome was initially described as a triad of oral ulcers, genital ulcers, and uveitis with hypopyon. Oral ulcers are the most common clinical feature, affecting over 98% of patients. Genital ulcers occur in 80% to 87% of these patients and skin disease occurs in 69% to 90% of these patients. Pathergy, which is a pustular response to skin injury, and dermatographism can also be seen. Behçet's syndrome is most common in the Middle East and Far East. HLA-B51 is associated with this disease.

92. **d.** Orthostatic hypotension can be an effect of rapid exogenous steroid withdrawal, which can lead to adrenal insufficiency. One important mechanism in which corticosteroids have anti-inflammatory effects is through the inhibition of prostaglandin synthesis. This results from preventing the release of the prostaglandin precursor arachidonic acid from membrane phospholipids. Systemic complications include peptic ulceration, osteoporosis, aseptic necrosis of the femoral head, muscle and skin atrophy, hyperglycemia, hypertension, edema, weight gain, mental status changes, and hypokalemia.

93. **b.** Corneal melts and punctate keratopathy have been reported to be associated with topical NSAID administration. The most significant adverse effects from use of oral NSAIDs are

gastrointestinal bleeding, renal failure, worsening hypertension, and heart failure. They can also interfere with platelet function and cause bone marrow suppression, hepatic toxicity, and CNS symptoms.

94. **c.** Diabetes mellitus is now defined as a group of metabolic diseases characterized by hyperglycemia resulting from defects in insulin secretion, insulin action, or both. All of the conditions are diagnostic of having diabetes except answer choice c. Note that HbA1c measurement is not currently recommended for diagnosing diabetes.

95. **a.** Type 1 diabetes was previously called insulin-dependent diabetes mellitus or juvenile-onset diabetes. The peak incidence of diabetes is around the time of puberty. This form of diabetes is due to a deficiency in endogenous insulin secretion secondary to destruction of insulin-producing beta cells in the pancreas. Most type 1 diabetes is due to immune-mediated destruction characterized by the presence of various autoantibodies. One or more autoantibodies are present in 90% of patients at initial presentation, and these patients are prone to other autoimmune disorders. It appears that environmental factors play a role in this disease as well, as studies of monozygotic twins have shown that both twins develop diabetes only 30% to 50% of the time. Obesity is present in 80% to 90% of type 2 diabetics.

96. **d.** Type 2 diabetes accounts for 90% of Americans with diabetes. Type 2 diabetics are usually older than 40 at presentation, and obesity is a frequent finding. Other risk factors include hypertension, gestational diabetes, physical inactivity, and low socioeconomic status. There is also a strong genetic tendency for developing type 2 diabetes, though no specific genetic locus has been associated with the disease. Autoimmune destruction of beta cells does not usually occur in type 2 diabetes. Instead, there is insulin resistance in target tissues and a gradual loss of compensatory insulin production by the beta cells.

97. b. Volatile anesthetics such as halothane, enflurane, isofulrane, and most notably intravenous succinylcholine are all known to trigger malignant hyperthermia. Tachycardia and elevated carbon dioxide levels at end-tidal volumes are the earliest signs of malignant hyperthermia. Labile blood pressure, tachypnea, sweating, muscle rigidity, blotchy discoloration of the skin, cyanosis, and dark urine all signal progression of the disorder. This disorder can be fatal if diagnosis is delayed.

98. a. The Somogyi phenomenon is the occurrence of posthypoglycemic rebound hyperglycemia. Growth hormone and catecholamines are thought to cause the Somogyi phenomenon. Recognition of this process is important because patients may incorrectly decide to increase their longer-acting insulin dose to treat the hyperglycemia and thereby increase the hypoglycemia that precipitated the problem.

99. b. In screening for thyroid disease, the combination of free T4 and sensitive TSH assays has a sensitivity of 99.5% and a specificity of 98%.

100. b. Patients with Graves hyperthyroidism exhibit various combinations of hypermetabolism, diffuse enlargement of the thyroid gland, ophthalmopathy (exophthalmos and lid retraction seen in the figure), and infiltrative dermopathy. Although the exact cause is not known, Graves hyperthyroidism is thought to be an autoimmune disorder, with 85% to 90% of patients having circulating TSH receptor antibodies. This disease is common with a 10:1 female preponderance. The incidence peaks in the third and fourth decades of life. Current smoking is associated with an increased incidence of ophthalmopathy.

CHAPTER 2

Fundamentals of Ophthalmology

▪ Questions

1. What are the average dimensions in height and width of the orbital opening?
   a. 30 mm h × 35 mm w.
   b. 35 mm h × 40 mm w.
   c. 35 mm h × 45 mm w.
   d. 45 mm h × 35 mm w.

2. What is the average volume of the human orbit?
   a. 30 mL.
   b. 35 mL.
   c. 40 mL.
   d. 45 mL.

3. Which bones comprise the orbital roof?
   a. greater wing of the sphenoid and frontal bone.
   b. frontal bone and sphenoid bone (lesser wing).
   c. greater wing of sphenoid bone and palatine bone.
   d. ethmoid bone and frontal bone.

4. Which one of the following bones is not part of the medial orbital wall?
   a. maxilla.
   b. ethmoid.
   c. sphenoid.
   d. palatine.

5. Which orbital wall is the strongest?
   a. medial.
   b. inferior.
   c. lateral.
   d. superior.

6. How many axons compose a healthy adult optic nerve?
   a. 3 million.
   b. 3.6 million.
   c. 600,000.
   d. 1.2 million.

7. Which of the following is an eccrine gland?
   a. Krause.
   b. Moll.
   c. Wolfring.
   d. lacrimal.

8. Which of the following about Müller's muscle is not true?
   a. It consists of smooth muscle fibers.
   b. It receives parasympathetic innervation.
   c. It originates from the levator muscle.
   d. It attaches to the tarsus.

9. The conjunctiva
   a. contains two geographical zones—palpebral and bulbar.
   b. contains lymphoid tissue.
   c. fuses with the optic nerve sheath.
   d. is composed of keratinized squamous epithelium.

2

10. Which of the following is not true?
    a. Vortex veins drain the uveal system.
    b. Vortex veins are located radially posterior to the rectus muscles.
    c. Most eyes have at least four vortex veins.
    d. The location of the vortex veins correspond to the equator of the eye.

11. What is the correct order of tear components from anterior to posterior?
    a. mucin, aqueous, lipid.
    b. lipid, aqueous, mucin.
    c. aqueous, mucin, lipid.
    d. aqueous, lipid, mucin.

12. Which of the following is not true about the cornea?
    a. The tear-corneal epithelium surface forms a positive lens of approximately 40 D.
    b. The central cornea is steeper than the peripheral cornea.
    c. The average central corneal thickness is 500 to 550 μm.
    d. The anterior surface of the cornea is less curved than the posterior surface of the cornea.

13. What are average adult corneal diameters?
    a. 11 mm horizontally and vertically.
    b. 12 mm horizontally and vertically.
    c. 12 mm horizontally and 11 mm vertically.
    d. 11 mm horizontally and 12 mm vertically.

14. The corneal stroma does not contain
    a. type II collagen.
    b. type I collagen.
    c. type V collagen.
    d. type III collagen.

15. The correct order of angle structures, from anterior to posterior, is
    a. scleral spur (SS), pigmented trabecular meshwork (TM), nonpigmented TM, Schwalbe's line (SL), and ciliary body band (CBB).
    b. SL, pigmented TM, nonpigmented TM, CBB, and SS.
    c. SL, pigmented TM, nonpigmented TM, SS, and CBB.
    d. SL, nonpigmented TM, pigmented TM, SS, and CBB.

16. The trabecular meshwork
    a. contains cells with contractile properties.
    b. is divided into four separate layers.
    c. is not affected by HSV.
    d. is the only area of egress for ocular fluid.

17. The site of greatest resistance to aqueous outflow is the
    a. corneoscleral meshwork.
    b. uveal meshwork.
    c. posterior, pigmented trabecular meshwork.
    d. juxtacanalicular trabecular meshwork.

18. The locations of attachment of the uveal tract to the sclera do NOT include
    a. optic nerve.
    b. scleral spur.
    c. entry of the vortex veins.
    d. exit of the vortex veins.

19. The iris does not
    a. contain dilator muscle derived from mesoderm.
    b. have a posterior pigmented layer, which is continuous with the ciliary body and subsequently the retina.
    c. contain a sphincter muscle, which is derived from neuroectoderm.
    d. have both parasympathetic and sympathetic innervations.

20. The ciliary body
    a. does not affect intraocular pressure.
    b. is lined by a double layer of nonpigmented and pigmented epithelium.
    c. contains large nonfenestrated capillaries, fibroblasts, and collagen.
    d. is an avascular tissue.

21. The ciliary muscle
    a. contains striated muscle fibers.
    b. is mainly innervated by the parasympathetic system.
    c. is responsible for the development of presbyopia.
    d. has two major divisions.

22. Which of the following in regard to the iris is correct?
    a. The iris is composed of six layers, three of which are epithelial.
    b. Clump cells are part of the anterior border layer of the iris.
    c. The iris dilator and iris sphincter are posterior to the iris pigment epithelium.
    d. The cell bodies of the anterior iris pigment epithelium give rise to the iris dilator muscle.

23. The lens contributes ___ D of focusing power to the ocular system.
    a. 10.
    b. 20.
    c. 40.
    d. 60.

24. Select the correct description of autonomic innervation to the eye.
    a. The iris sphincter muscle receives sympathetic innervation via the short ciliary nerves; the iris dilator muscle receives parasympathetic innervation via the short ciliary nerves.
    b. The iris sphincter muscle receives parasympathetic innervation via the short ciliary nerves; the iris dilator muscle receives sympathetic innervation by the short ciliary nerves.
    c. The iris sphincter muscle receives parasympathetic innervation via the short ciliary nerves; the iris dilator muscle receives sympathetic innervation via the long ciliary nerves.
    d. The iris sphincter muscle receives parasympathetic innervation via the long ciliary nerves; the iris dilator muscle receives sympathetic innervation via long ciliary nerves.

25. The choriocapillaris
    a. contains a large nonfenestrated vascular network.
    b. allows passage of fluorescein dye.
    c. is devoid of pericytes.
    d. is located posterior to the retina and anterior to Bruch's membrane.

26. The newborn equatorial lens diameter in a normal eye is
    a. 4.5 mm.
    b. 5.5 mm.
    c. 6.5 mm.
    d. 7.5 mm.

27. Choose the correct statement.
    a. The inner plexiform layer is anterior to the inner nuclear layer.
    b. The external limiting membrane is posterior to the rod/cone segments.
    c. The ganglion cell layer carries the axons of the ganglion cells.
    d. The outer plexiform layer contains the nuclei of the photoreceptors.

28. Which one of the following concerning retinal photoreceptors is correct?
    a. Rods contain photopigment discs that are not attached to the cell membrane and synapse with bipolar cells at a rod pedicle.
    b. Cones contain photopigment discs that are not connected to the cell membrane and synapse with bipolar cells at a cone pedicle.
    c. Rods contain photopigment discs that are attached to the cell membrane and synapse with bipolar cells at the rod spherule.
    d. Cones contain photopigment discs that are attached to the cell membrane and synapse with bipolar cells at a cone pedicle.

29. Select the correct neuronal sequence for intraretinal processing.
    a. photoreceptor to Müller cell to ganglion cell.
    b. photoreceptor to bipolar cell to ganglion cell.
    c. photoreceptor to horizontal cell to amacrine cell.
    d. photoreceptor to horizontal cell to ganglion cell.

30. In the entire retina, rods outnumber cones by a ratio of approximately
    a. 2:1.
    b. 5:1.
    c. 20:1.
    d. 50:1.

2

31. Which one of the following regarding Müller cells is correct?
   a. The footplates of the Müller cells form the internal limiting membrane.
   b. Müller cells are the only nonneural (glial) cellular element found within the neural retina.
   c. Müller cells do not generate any detectable light-induced transretinal voltages.
   d. Müller cells intimately envelop virtually all retinal neurons.

32. A cilioretinal artery contributes to some portion of the macular circulation in approximately
   a. 5% of individuals.
   b. 15% of individuals.
   c. 50% of individuals.
   d. 90% of individuals.

33. The inner retinal circulation's deepest level of penetration is the
   a. ganglion cell layer.
   b. inner plexiform layer.
   c. inner nuclear layer.
   d. outer plexiform layer.

34. Which of the following statements regarding the retinal pigment epithelium is incorrect?
   a. The RPE absorbs light.
   b. The RPE cells are involved in active transport and have no polarity.
   c. Photoreceptor outer segments are phagocytized by RPE cells.
   d. Vitamin A metabolism is a key function of RPE cells.

35. Which of the following is not true about the macula?
   a. It is clinically located between the superior and inferior arcade.
   b. It can be affected by diabetes and cause vision loss.
   c. Histologically, it contains only one layer of ganglion cells.
   d. Zeaxanthin and lutein pigments are present in the macula.

36. Upon entering the cranial cavity, the optic nerve runs
   a. lateral to the internal carotid artery and inferior to the anterior cerebral artery.
   b. medial to the internal carotid artery and inferior to the anterior cerebral artery.
   c. medial to the internal carotid artery and superior to the anterior cerebral artery.
   d. lateral to the internal carotid artery and superior to the anterior cerebral artery.

37. Which of the following concerning ganglion axon decussation is true?
   a. Greater than fifty percent of fibers cross in the chiasm.
   b. Fewer numbers of ganglion cells cross than do not cross in the chiasm.
   c. A much greater proportion of macular fibers cross than peripheral fibers.
   d. A much greater proportion of peripheral fibers cross than macular fibers.

38. Which one of the extraocular muscles is served by a single nucleus that is shared by both oculomotor nerve nuclei?
   a. superior rectus.
   b. medial rectus.
   c. inferior oblique.
   d. levator palpebrae superioris.

39. Which is the only muscle supplied by the oculomotor nerve that receives crossed innervation?
   a. superior rectus.
   b. medial rectus.
   c. inferior oblique.
   d. levator palpebrae superioris.

40. Which one of the following concerning the pupillomotor fibers of the third cranial nerve is true?
   a. They run central in the nerve, in the superior division.
   b. They run central in the nerve, in the inferior division.
   c. They run peripheral in the nerve, in the superior division.
   d. They run peripheral in the nerve, in the inferior division.

41. Which one of the following is true regarding cranial nerve V?
    a. The supratrochlear nerve is a terminal division of V1.
    b. V2 exits the skull base at the foramen ovale.
    c. V3 exits the skull base through the foramen rotundum.
    d. V2 supplies sensation to the external ear.

42. Which of the following is true about ocular development?
    a. The secondary vitreous has vascularity.
    b. In the fetal nucleus, the inverted Y suture is located anterior to upright Y suture.
    c. During gestation, the number of axons present in the optic nerve increases and then decreases several weeks prior to birth.
    d. Alcohol intake during gestation has no affect on optic nerve development.

43. Which segment of the optic nerve is the longest?
    a. intraocular.
    b. intracanalicular.
    c. intracranial.
    d. intraorbital.

44. Mesenchymal structures of the head, including the eye, are all derived from
    a. mesoderm.
    b. neural crest cells.
    c. a combination of neural crest cells and mesoderm.
    d. a combination of neural crest cells and ectoderm.

45. Neural crest cells give rise to the following structures:
    a. optic nerve sheath, uveal melanocytes, choroidal stroma, ciliary muscle, and iris stroma.
    b. the entire sclera, optic nerve sheath, uveal melanocytes, entire choroid.
    c. orbital bones, fat, trochlear cartilage, extraocular muscles, and orbital connective tissues.
    d. ciliary body, ciliary epithelium, iris stroma, orbital bones, and orbital connective tissues.

46. The mesoderm gives rise to
    a. the pupillomotor muscles, ciliary muscle, and extraocular muscles.
    b. all vascular endothelia, extraocular muscles, and the trochlea.
    c. all vascular endothelia, pupillomotor muscles, and all blood vessels.
    d. all vascular endothelia, all extraocular muscles, and temporal sclera.

47. All of the following structures originate from the surface ectoderm except
    a. the lacrimal gland.
    b. the lens.
    c. the substantia propria of the conjunctiva.
    d. the corneal epithelium.

48. What factor distinguishes anophthalmia from microphthalmia?
    a. stage of globe development.
    b. the presence or absence of a globe.
    c. globe size.
    d. the presence or absence of organic abnormalities of a globe.

49. What factor distinguishes microphthalmia from nanophthalmia?
    a. the size of the globe.
    b. the presence or absence of a globe.
    c. the presence or absence of lid fusion.
    d. the presence or absence of organic abnormalities of a globe.

50. Cystic protrusion in the palpebral fissure may be all of the following except
    a. cystic coloboma.
    b. orbital encephalocele.
    c. microphthalmos.
    d. nanophthalmos.

51. In reference to dermoids, which of the following is not true?
    a. Dermoids are epidermal hamartomas.
    b. Locations include the orbit and conjunctiva.
    c. The solid variety is most frequently found at the limbus.
    d. There is an association with Goldenhar's syndrome.

52. Which one of the following statements regarding anterior segment dysgenesis is incorrect?
    a. All varieties may be inherited as autosomal dominant traits and may be either unilateral or bilateral.
    b. Posterior embryotoxon is the mildest form of the peripheral varieties.
    c. In Peters' anomaly, the central cornea is always opacified, and the lens is always densely adherent to the posterior corneal surface.
    d. Rieger's syndrome is Rieger's anomaly plus facial and musculoskeletal anomalies.

53. Which one of the following concerning aniridia is false?
    a. Rudimentary iris can be seen.
    b. Aniridia is always familial.
    c. Retinal abnormalities can be present in this condition.
    d. There is an association of aniridia with Wilms' tumor, genitourinary anomalies, and mental retardation.

54. The following statements refer to childhood lens disorders. Choose the correct answer.
    a. Microspherophakia is commonly associated with Marfan syndrome.
    b. Cataracts, glaucoma, aminoaciduria, and female gender are characteristic findings in Lowe's syndrome.
    c. Cataracts in the congenital rubella syndrome are generally dense nuclear cataracts.
    d. Defects in the rubella syndrome are typically limited to the eye.

55. All of the following regarding persistent fetal vasculature (PFV) are true except
    a. It is most often unilateral in presentation.
    b. It portends good long-term visual prognosis.
    c. It is differentiated from retinoblastoma by the presence of microphthalmos or cataract.
    d. It may calcify.

56. Choose the incorrect statement regarding tear secretion apparatus and function.
    a. ACTH and androgens can stimulate tear secretion from the main lacrimal gland.
    b. The glands of Wolfring are located along the orbital margin of each tarsus, with the glands of Krause in the conjunctival fornix.
    c. The accessory glands of Krause and Wolfring account for approximately 50% of total lacrimal secretory mass.
    d. Both sympathetic and parasympathetic nerve stimuli are important for reflex tear secretion.

57. In reference to Descemet's membrane/corneal endothelium complex, which of the following is not true?
    a. The endothelial cell count in a young adult with no previous ocular surgery is about 5,000 cells/mm squared.
    b. Posterior keratoconus can be differentiated from Peters' anomaly by the presence of fetal Descemet's membrane.
    c. Fetal Descemet's membrane can be differentiated from adult Descemet's membrane by its banding pattern.
    d. The corneal endothelium actively maintains corneal deturgescence via a pump system dependent on Na^+/K^+-ATPase function and carbonic anhydrase.

58. What is not true regarding prostaglandins?
    a. The cyclooxygenase reaction culminates in the production of prostaglandins, prostacyclin, and thromboxane.
    b. In general, prostaglandins cause mydriasis.
    c. Corticosteroids inhibit both the cyclooxygenase and lipoxygenase pathways of arachidonic acid metabolism.
    d. The effect of prostaglandins on intraocular pressure is complex, with low doses decreasing intraocular pressure and high doses increasing intraocular pressure.

59. Which enzyme is not present normally in the aqueous humor?
    a. carbonic anhydrase.
    b. lysozyme.
    c. hyaluronidase.
    d. lactate dehydrogenase.

60. The partial pressure of oxygen in aqueous humor is
    a. 40 mm Hg.
    b. 55 mm Hg.
    c. 75 mm Hg.
    d. 85 mm Hg.

61. Lens epithelial cells are mitotically most active at which of the following sites?
    a. anterior pole.
    b. posterior pole.
    c. lens equator.
    d. ring around the anterior lens.

62. Which of the following statements is incorrect in regard to lens protein?
    a. Gamma crystallins are the smallest.
    b. Crystallins are only expressed in the lens.
    c. Alpha crystallin is the largest of the lens crystallins.
    d. Beta crystallin is the most abundant of the lens crystallins.

63. Which glands are primarily responsible for secreting the lipid layer of the tear film?
    a. glands of Krause.
    b. glands of Wolfring.
    c. tarsal meibomian glands.
    d. lacrimal gland–palpebral lobe.

64. Choose the incorrect statement.
    a. The glands of Wolfring are located along the proximal tarsal margin.
    b. The tear film contains only IgA.
    c. The lacrimal gland is innervated by sympathetic and parasympathetic nerves.
    d. The levator aponeurosis divides the lacrimal gland.

65. What is amount of aqueous humor produced by humans every minute?
    a. 0.5 µL/min.
    b. 1.0 µL/min.
    c. 2.0 µL/min.
    d. 4.0 µL/min.

66. The normal aging process of vitreous liquefaction is associated with
    a. diffuse decreases in hyaluronic acid concentration.
    b. diffuse decreases in collagen concentration.
    c. focal decreases in collagen concentration.
    d. motion-induced collagen damage.

67. Which of the following statements is true in regard to myopia?
    a. Myopia is associated with alterations in vitreous concentration of collagen and hyaluronic acid.
    b. Myopia cannot be surgically corrected.
    c. Myopia is associated with a decreased incidence of retinal detachment.
    d. Myopia is not associated with choroidal neovascularization.

68. Choose the correct statement regarding posterior vitreous detachment (PVD).
    a. A complete PVD includes detachment of the vitreous from the anterior border of the vitreous base.
    b. PVD frequently presents as a chronic insidious event.
    c. PVD is thought to be protective against retinal detachment secondary to proliferative diabetic retinopathy.
    d. Occurs only under the natural aging process of the eye.

69. Eyes that have undergone removal of the vitreous
    a. have decreased water content.
    b. have increased vitreous viscosity.
    c. may experience accelerated cataract formation.
    d. may have decreased oxygen tension at the retinal surface.

70. Which of the following is true?
    a. Vitamin A is transported in the serum as all-cis retinol.
    b. Trans-to-cis isomerization occurs in the RPE.
    c. Aldehyde and alcohol conversion occurs in the RPE.
    d. The normal retina contains two types of cones.

2

71. Which one of the following concerning the effects of light on rod outer segment metabolism is false?
    a. In the dark, high cyclic guanosine monophosphate (cGMP) levels keep sodium channels open and rod outer segments depolarized.
    b. Light absorption leads to configurational changes in rhodopsin and activation of transducin.
    c. Transducin, through an amplification cascade, activates phosphodiesterase (PDE).
    d. Falling intracellular cGMP leads to closure of sodium channels, with subsequent further depolarization of the rod outer segment.

72. Which of the below is false regarding the retina?
    a. The retina is primarily dependent on anaerobic metabolism (glycolysis).
    b. The retina contains glial elements as well as neural elements.
    c. Phototransduction occurs in outer segment of the photoreceptor cells.
    d. Amacrine cells function as interneurons.

73. All of the following are effective methods of increasing ocular absorption of topically applied materials (without increasing systemic absorption) except
    a. adding a second eyedrop immediately after the first.
    b. waiting 5 to 10 minutes between different medications.
    c. nasolacrimal sac compression.
    d. closing the eyes quietly for 3 to 5 minutes after administration.

74. All of the following factors increase the amount of medication penetrating the cornea except
    a. higher concentration of the drug.
    b. higher viscosity of the vehicle.
    c. higher pH of the drug.
    d. higher lipid solubility of the drug.

75. Unwanted side effects of direct cholinergic agonists include all of the following except
    a. induced hyperopia.
    b. decreased vision in older patients.

c. headache in younger patients.
    d. possible aggravation or induction of angle-closure glaucoma.

76. Which of the following medications must be used with caution in patients taking a monoamine oxidase inhibitor?
    a. cyclopentolate.
    b. brimonidine.
    c. prednisolone.
    d. prostaglandin analog.

77. Following a unilateral dose of apraclonidine, it is easy to identify the eye that received the medication by looking for
    a. lid retraction.
    b. increased conjunctival injection.
    c. miosis.
    d. cell and flare.

78. Beta-adrenergic agonists generally
    a. increase aqueous humor production, decrease outflow facility, and increase intraocular pressure.
    b. increase aqueous humor production, increase outflow facility, and increase intraocular pressure.
    c. increase aqueous humor production, increase outflow facility, and decrease intraocular pressure.
    d. decrease aqueous humor production, decrease outflow facility, and decrease intraocular pressure.

79. In what anatomic location is dipivefrin converted to epinephrine?
    a. angle.
    b. conjunctiva.
    c. cornea.
    d. aqueous humor.

80. Carbonic anhydrase inhibitors (CAIs) should be used with great caution in all of the following types of patients except
    a. patients with a distant history nephrolithiasis that is currently inactive.
    b. patients with chronic liver failure.
    c. patients on thiazide diuretics.
    d. patients on digoxin.

81. Which one of the following concerning glucocorticoid effects is false?
    a. They inhibit capillary formation.
    b. They do not affect IgE titers.
    c. They act through impairing the efferent limb of the immune response.
    d. They impair epithelial healing.

82. Which of the following corticosteroids has the highest relative potency?
    a. dexamethasone 0.1%.
    b. fluorometholone 0.1%.
    c. prednisolone 1%.
    d. hydrocortisone 0.5%.

83. Which of the following corticosteroids has the smallest effect on intraocular pressure elevation?
    a. dexamethasone 0.1%.
    b. hydrocortisone 0.5%.
    c. medrysone 1%.
    d. prednisolone 1%.

84. Given a history of a hypersensitivity reaction to penicillins, the probability of a similar reaction to a cephalosporin is approximately
    a. 1%.
    b. 5%.
    c. 10%.
    d. 15%.

85. Which one of the following concerning antibiotic mechanisms is false?
    a. Sulfonamides act by inhibiting bacterial DNA synthesis.
    b. Tetracycline is poorly water soluble but may be dissolved in eye drops containing mineral oil.
    c. Chloramphenicol use is most strongly associated with aplastic anemia when used orally.
    d. Aminoglycoside efficacy is mostly dependent on anaerobically supported antibiotic uptake.

86. Which class of medication is known to cause auditory/vestibular dysfunction and nephrotoxicity?
    a. aminoglycoside.
    b. sulfonamide.
    c. tetracycline.
    d. penicillin.

87. Which antibiotic has been associated with macular infarction?
    a. penicillin.
    b. gentamicin.
    c. doxycycline.
    d. ceftazidime.

88. Which one of the following concerning vancomycin is false?
    a. It inhibits bacterial replication by blocking cell wall synthesis.
    b. Empirical use in neutropenic patients is recommended for infection prophylaxis.
    c. It is one of the drugs of choice in filtering bleb-related endophthalmitis.
    d. Because of its poor gastrointestinal uptake, it is an excellent drug for pseudomembranous colitis.

89. Which one of the following concerning ocular antiviral agents is false?
    a. Vidarabine is an analog of adenine, whereas idoxuridine and trifluridine are analogs of thymidine.
    b. Trifluridine is more soluble than vidarabine or idoxuridine.
    c. Trifluridine is more effective than vidarabine and idoxuridine.
    d. Cross-resistance to different agents is commonly seen.

90. What is the diameter of the anatomic human fovea?
    a. 0.5 mm (500 μm).
    b. 1.0 mm (1,000 μm).
    c. 1.5 mm (1,500 μm).
    d. 2.0 mm (2,000 μm).

91. Which one of the following agents presents the lowest risk of corneal or conjunctival toxicity as a preoperative antiseptic?
    a. chlorhexidine gluconate 4% (Hibiclens).
    b. povidone-iodine solution.
    c. hydrogen peroxide.
    d. benzalkonium chloride.

92. Which of the following preoperative regimens most effectively reduces conjunctival bacterial colony counts?
   a. topical antibiotic for 3 days preoperatively.
   b. topical povidone-iodine for 3 days preoperatively.
   c. topical antibiotic for 3 days preoperatively, followed by topical povidone-iodine at the time or surgery.
   d. topical povidone-iodine at the time of surgery, followed immediately by vigorous saline flush.

93. Potential side effects of topical prostaglandins or their analogs include each of the following except
   a. bradycardia.
   b. red eye.
   c. iris hyperpigmentation.
   d. uveitis.

94. What does the anterior lamellae of the upper eyelid consist of?
   a. skin, orbicularis, and associated fascial and vascular components.
   b. capsulopalpebral fascia, tarsus, and orbital septum.
   c. Müller's muscle, conjunctiva, and levator aponeurosis.
   d. orbital septum, orbital fat, and levator aponeurosis.

95. All of the following are potential ocular side effects of sildenafil except
   a. photophobia.
   b. decreased color vision or changes in color perception.
   c. conjunctival hyperemia.
   d. miosis.

96. Which is false regarding chronic progressive external ophthalmoplegia (CPEO)?
   a. The eyelids are often involved in CPEO.
   b. CPEO can include muscle paralysis.
   c. CPEO is inherited in an autosomal recessive pattern.
   d. CPEO can be associated with heart block and retinitis pigmentosa.

97. Mitochondrial DNA is implicated in all of the following except
   a. neuropathy, ataxia, and retinitis pigmentosa (NARP) phenotype.
   b. Leber's hereditary optic neuropathy.
   c. Leigh's syndrome.
   d. Duchenne muscular dystrophy.

98. Which of the listed disorders, in their carrier states, do not display ocular findings?
   a. ocular albinism.
   b. choroideremia.
   c. retinitis pigmentosa.
   d. Best disease.

99. Amacrine cells are located in which layer?
   a. outer plexiform layer.
   b. outer nuclear layer.
   c. inner nuclear layer.
   d. inner plexiform layer.

100. Müller cells
   a. extend from the ILM to the photoreceptors.
   b. are neuronal in nature.
   c. do not constitute the external limiting membrane.
   d. play a role in beta-carotene metabolism.

101. The RPE
   a. is a double layer of cuboidal epithelial cells.
   b. contains a cumulative 8 to 12 million cells in a given individual.
   c. has a 100:1 ratio in regard to photorecptors:RPE cells.
   d. has neural function.

102. Major roles of the RPE include all of the following except
   a. regeneration of visual pigment.
   b. consumption of photoreceptor outer segments.
   c. absorption of light.
   d. transmission of neural impulses between photoreceptors and the choroid.

103. Topical drug penetration is increased by
   a. surfactants.
   b. low viscosity.
   c. water solubility.
   d. nonphysiologic pH.

2

104. Side effects of pilocarpine include all of the following except
    a. salivation.
    b. vomiting/diarrhea.
    c. bronchial dilation.
    d. diaphoresis.

105. Pilocarpine is used in the treatment of which of the following?
    a. accommodative esotropia.
    b. chronic control of pupillary-block angle closure glaucoma.
    c. uveitis.
    d. band keratopathy.

106. Which of the following is an indirect-acting muscarinic agonist?
    a. pilocarpine.
    b. carbachol.
    c. phospholine iodide.
    d. isopto carbachol.

107. Which of the following mydriatics is the longest acting?
    a. cyclopentolate.
    b. tropicamide.
    c. scopolamine.
    d. homatropine.

108. Which of the following mydriatics has a duration of action of approximately 2 days?
    a. homatropine.
    b. atropine.
    c. scopolamine.
    d. cyclopentolate.

109. Muscarinic antagonists help in all of the following except
    a. refraction in children.
    b. malignant glaucoma.
    c. angle closure.
    d. iridocyclitis.

110. Adverse effects of cholinergic antagonists include all of the following except
    a. confusion.
    b. mydriasis.
    c. diarrhea.
    d. urinary retention.

111. Which of the following medications can induce uveitis and hypotony?
    a. cidofovir.
    b. valacyclovir.
    c. acyclovir.
    d. zidovudine.

112. Which of the following systemic antibiotics has good intraocular penetration?
    a. penicillin.
    b. moxifloxacin.
    c. gentamicin.
    d. erythromycin.

113. What class of medication has been reported to cause reactivation of herpetic keratitis?
    a. prostaglandins.
    b. carbonic anhydrase inhibitors.
    c. beta adrenergic antagonists.
    d. adrenergic agonists.

114. Which regional anesthetic has the shortest duration of action?
    a. lidocaine.
    b. bupivacaine.
    c. mepivacaine.
    d. procaine.

115. Which drug below is a polyene?
    a. ketoconazole.
    b. natamycin.
    c. fluconazole.
    d. itraconazole.

116. What is a serious side effect of the sulfonamide drug class?
    a. heart block.
    b. ototoxicity.
    c. Stevens-Johnson syndrome.
    d. hypotony.

117. In reference to Down's syndrome, which of the following is true?
    a. It is the second most common chromosomal syndrome in humans.
    b. Maternal age is not a risk factor.
    c. Patients display various forms of congenital heart disease.
    d. Patients do not have an increased risk for development of Alzheimer's disease.

118. Which of the following is true regarding autosomal recessive inheritance?
    a. Males and females are affected in equal proportions.
    b. The mutant gene will cause the clinical disease.
    c. Consanguinity plays no role.
    d. The ratio of normal to affected siblings is usually 4:1.

119. Which of the following medications increases uveoscleral outflow?
    a. apraclonidine.
    b. pilocarpine.
    c. epinephrine.
    d. timolol.

120. What is true about local anesthesia in ocular surgery?
    a. After administration, large nerve fibers are blocked first.
    b. After administration, sensory nerve fibers are blocked before parasympathetic/sympathetic fibers.
    c. Amide local anesthetics are preferred over ester agents for retrobulbar blockade due to longer duration and less toxicity.
    d. Chronic use is not associated with morbidity.

Answers

1. **c.** The average dimensions of the orbital entrance are 35 mm in height and 45 mm in width.

2. **a.** Thirty cubic centimeters (cc or mL for liquid measures) is approximately 2 tablespoons.

3. **b.** The orbital roof is formed by the frontal bone and the lesser wing of the sphenoid bone. A good mnemonic to use is "rooFLESS".

4. **d.** The palatine bone is NOT part of the medial wall.

5. **c.** The lateral wall of the orbit is the thickest and strongest aspect of the bony orbit. It is formed by the zygoma and the greater wing of the sphenoid.

6. **d.** Approximately 1.2 million axons form a normal optic nerve. Each axon originates from the ganglion cell layer of the retina and extends to the lateral geniculate body. Fetal optic nerves contain a greater number of axons (~3.7 million by 16 weeks), some of which regress by birth. Fewer axons may be a feature of certain optic nerve diseases (e.g., glaucoma).

7. **b.** The glands of Moll secrete sweat and are located on the eyelid.

8. **b.** Müller's muscle is a sympathetically innervated muscle. All other answers are true.

9. **b.** The lymphoid tissue is called conjuctiva-associated lymphoid tissue, which is akin to MALT in other mucosa. There are three zones of conjunctiva, palpebral, bulbar, and forniceal. The conjunctiva does NOT fuse with the optic nerve sheath. The epithelium is NON-keratinized squamous epithelium that is two to five cells in thickness.

10. **b.** Vortex veins are usually located in between the rectus muscles in each quadrant 15 to 25 mm

posterior to the limbus. Most eyes have at least four vortex veins. They approximate the equator of the globe. They are responsible for drainage of the uveal system.

11. **b.** From anterior to posterior, the tear film consists of oil, aqueous, and mucin.

12. **a.** The *air–tear* interface at the corneal surface creates a 40 to 43 D positive lens. The other choices are all true. The cornea is 0.5 mm on average in the central cornea and 1.0 mm in the peripheral cornea.

13. **c.** The average adult corneal diameter is reached at approximately 2 years of age.

14. **a.** Type II collagen is not found in the corneal stroma. Types I, III, V, and VI are found in the corneal stroma.

15. **d.** Another way of remembering this is the mnemonic (from peripheral to central): "I Can't See This Stuff!" This corresponds to Iris, Ciliary body, Scleral spur, Trabecular meshwork, and Schwalbe's line.

16. **a.** Trabecular meshwork cells contain contractile properties. The meshwork can be inflamed by the herpes virus causing trabeculitis and increased IOP. The uveoscleral pathway also allows for egress of ocular fluid.

17. **d.** Animal outflow studies have shown that the TM immediately proximal to Schlemm's canal (juxtacanalicular TM) is the primary limiting factor for outflow facility.

18. **c.** The entry of the vortex veins is incorrect.

19. **a.** The dilator and sphincter muscle are both derived from the neuroectoderm. The other answers are true.

45. **a.** Neural crest gives rise to ciliary musculature, corneal stroma and endothelium (but not corneal epithelium), most of the sclera (except for a temporal portion, which is of mesodermal origin), choroidal stroma, some of the orbital bones, orbital cartilage, orbital connective tissue, nerve sheaths, and uveal melanocytes. Extraocular muscles form from paraxial mesoderm.

46. **d.** Blood vessel endothelia, extraocular muscles, and temporal sclera are all mesodermal in origin. The mesoderm also contributes to the formation of the vitreous. The pupillomotor muscles are neuroectodermal in origin. The trochlea is from neural crest.

47. **c.** Conjunctival epithelium is derived from surface ectoderm, but the substantia propria is derived from neural crest.

48. **b.** Anophthalmia is the absence of an identifiable eye. Microphthalmia describes the presence of a small, disorganized eye.

49. **d.** In nanophthalmia, the eye is smaller than normal with a disproportionately large lens, but otherwise unremarkable.

50. **d.** Nanophthalmos is, by definition, a small, but otherwise normal eye. Cysts are not seen in association with it. The other answers are associated with cyst formation.

51. **a.** Dermoids are choristomas: normal cells and/or tissue present in abnormal locations.

52. **c.** In Peters' anomaly, the central cornea is always opacified because of the central defect in Descemet's membrane and the absence of endothelium. The lens may be adherent to the cornea, but this is not always seen. Axenfeld anomaly, Axenfeld's syndrome, Rieger's anomaly, and Rieger's syndrome are now considered a single entity known as Axenfeld-Rieger syndrome, which has been associated with mutations in the RIEG1/PIXT2 gene and the forkhead gene FKHL7. Axenfeld-Rieger syndrome is most commonly inherited in an autosomal dominant fashion, and can lead to glaucoma in 50% of cases.

53. **b.** There is nearly always some rudimentary iris tissue present in aniridia, although it may be difficult to see clinically. Aniridia is caused by a defect of the PAX6 gene on chromosome 11p13, and may be SPORADIC or FAMILIAL. Sporadic aniridia is associated with Wilms' tumor (usually because of deletion of the PAX6 gene and the adjacent Wt1 Wilms' tumor gene). Aniridia is not typically found in patients with autosomal-dominant Wilms' rumor. When aniridia is associated with mental retardation, Wilms' tumor, ambiguous genitalia, or other genitourinary anomalies, there is usually a small deletion in the short arm of chromosome 11. Foveal and optic nerve hypoplasia can be associated with aniridia.

54. **c.** Microspherophakia is observed most often with Weill-Marchesani syndrome, not Marfan's syndrome. Patients with Marfan's syndrome are usually tall and lean, in contrast to patients with Weill-Marchesani syndrome, who are short and stocky. Marfan's syndrome is often associated with ectopia lentis. Lowe's syndrome is inherited in an X-linked recessive fashion and is thus found almost exclusively in men. Any organ in the body may be damaged by rubella, and the rubella syndrome is characterized by the triad of cataracts, deafness, and cardiac defects. Juvenile glaucoma and cataract rarely coincide with congenital rubella infection.

55. **b.** The visual prognosis in PHPV (also known as PFV, or persistent fetal vasculature) is currently poor. Early cataract extraction and membrane excision may preserve some vision. An eye with leukocoria that is small is unlikely to harbor retinoblastoma. Likewise, retinoblastoma does not typically cause cataract.

56. **c.** The glands of Krause and Wolfring, which produce the basal tear secretion account for approximately 10% of total lacrimal secretory mass.

57. **a.** The actual count is closer to 3,000 cells/mm squared.

58. **b.** Topical administration of type E and type F prostaglandins, as well as arachidonic acid, causes miosis. High doses of prostaglandins will cause an increase in intraocular pressure. Low doses of some prostaglandins, in contrast, appear to lower intraocular pressure in some animal species. By blocking phospholipase, corticosteroids effectively inhibit both the lipoxygenase and cyclooxygenase pathways.

59. **d.** Carbonic anhydrase, although present in only trace amounts in the aqueous, has a high enough turnover that it is felt to be functionally significant. Hyaluronidase is present in aqueous and may participate in regulation of resistance to aqueous outflow. Lysozyme is present and provides antibacterial protection. Lactate dehydrogenase, not normally detectable in aqueous, may be a marker for retinoblastoma.

60. **b.** This is approximately one-third the concentration found in the earth's atmosphere and is entirely derived from anterior chamber blood flow.

61. **d.** Lens epithelial cells are located anteriorly underneath the lens capsule. Epithelial cells in a ring around the anterior lens, or the germinative zone, exhibit the highest level of DNA synthesis (the S-phase in the cell cycle). Newly formed cells migrate toward the lens equator, where they differentiate into lens fiber cells.

62. **b.** Crystallins are expressed in several other tissues besides the lens. Alpha crystallins are the largest, with molecular weights of over 500,000 Da. Beta crystallins are the most abundant, making up about 55% of the water-soluble protein. Gamma crystallins are the smallest.

63. **c.** The meibomian glands are most responsible for the lipid layer of the tear film.

64. **b.** The tear film contains IgA, IgG, IgD, IgM, and IgE. The other answers are true.

65. **c.** Aqueous humor is produced at a rate of approximately 2 µL/min.

66. **c.** Syneresis (i.e., vitreous liquefaction) is associated with a focal decrease in collagen concentration. More than half of the vitreous is usually liquid by the age of 80. Patients with Stickler's syndrome often undergo vitreous syneresis before the age of 30.

67. **a.** Both collagen and hyaluronic acid concentration are lower by 20% to 30% in myopic eyes (axial length >26 mm), compared to eyes with a normal axial length.

68. **c.** PVD is thought to decrease the likelihood of retinal detachment related to proliferative diabetic retinopathy. It prevents new vessels on optic disc/new vessels elsewhere (NVD/NVE) from growing on a vitreous scaffold. The PVD extends to the posterior border of the vitreous base. It does not go anterior to the base where the vitreous and retina are tightly adherent. PVD frequently occurs as an acute event. PVD can be induced surgically as well as occur naturally.

69. **c.** Cataract formation can occur after vitrectomy as a result of higher levels of oxygen present in the postvitrectomized eye. This higher oxygen tension may also lead to improvement in ischemic retinal disease after vitrectomy.

70. **b.** Vitamin A, stored hepatically, is transported in serum as all-trans retinol. Conversion between aldehyde and alcohol (and vice versa) occurs in the photoreceptors, whereas the trans-to-cis isomerization takes place in the RPE. There are typically three types of cones in normal retinas.

71. **d.** Photoreceptors are more active electrically (depolarized) in the dark. With light absorption, transducin (via PDE) lowers cGMP, which hyperpolarizes the cell and decreases synaptic exchange with bipolar cells.

72. **a.** The retina is primarily oxygen dependent (unlike the lens).

39

73. **a.** Adding a second drop will likely minimally increase systemic absorption and may also simply wash out the first drop—a normally dispensed 50 µL drop contains far more than the 10 µL of fluid normally found in the eye and cul-de-sac. Local anesthetic disrupts corneal epithelial barrier functions, enhancing local uptake. Blinking increases drainage of topical medications into the nasolacrimal drainage system and subsequently into the systemic vascular system.

74. **c.** pH extremes trigger reflex tearing, with subsequent dilution of the drug. Benzalkonium chloride, like local anesthetics, disrupts the corneal epithelium.

75. **a.** Miosis and induced myopia are generally problematic in younger patients. In the elderly, aggravation of cataractous visual loss may be important. Because cholinergic agonists cause forward displacement of the iris-lens diaphragm, angle closure can rarely result from their use. Headache may also occur.

76. **b.** Brimonidine and apraclonidine must be used with caution in patients taking MAO inhibitors/tricyclic antidepressant therapy.

77. **a.** Apraclonidine is a selective alpha-2 adrenergic agonist. Side effects of apraclonidine that have been reported include lid retraction, conjunctival blanching, mydriasis, lethargy, xerostomia, and allergic reactions. The first three are directly attributable to its adrenergic activity.

78. **c.** Beta-adrenergic agonists (e.g., epinephrine) are thought to decrease intraocular pressure, despite their tendency to increase aqueous humor production, by increasing uveoscleral outflow. Their use in the medical management of glaucoma has decreased considerably.

79. **c.** Dipivalyl epinephrine (Dipivefrin) is a prodrug of epinephrine. Epinephrine is released into the anterior chamber when the pivalyl groups are cleaved by corneal esterases.

80. **a.** Unlike a recent history of renal stones (fewer than 5 years earlier), a remote history of spontaneous nephrolithiasis is not thought to be a contraindication to CAI therapy. CAIs potentiate hepatic encephalopathy and the potassium-wasting effects of thiazides (hypokalemia is a side effect of CAIs). Sensitivity to digoxin is increased by hypokalemia. Psychiatric disturbances also may be exacerbated by CAIs. Patients with a sulfa allergy should not be given carbonic anhydrase inhibitors.

81. **d.** At the tissue level, glucocorticoids suppress early inflammatory responses such as local vascular congestion, edema, and hyperthermia as well as late inflammatory responses such as capillary and fibroblast proliferation and deposition of collagen. Glucocorticoids do not affect IgE immunoglobulin titers or the afferent limb of cell-mediated immunity, nor do they significantly deter epithelial healing (stromal healing and collagen synthesis, however, are affected).

82. **a.** Dexamethasone has the greatest relative potency. It is followed, in order of decreasing potency, by fluorometholone, prednisolone, medrysone, tetrahydrotriamcinolone, hydrocortisone.

83. **c.** Medrysone. The order of IOP elevation in decreasing order is as follows: dexamethasone, prednisolone, fluorometholone, hydrocortisone, tetrahydrotriamcinolone, medrysone.

84. **c.** Approximately 10% of patients with a history of a hypersensitivity reaction to penicillin will have cross-reactivity to the cephalosporins.

85. **d.** Sulfonamides indirectly inhibit bacterial DNA synthesis by blocking the synthesis of folic acid (folic acid is a cofactor in nucleic acid synthesis). Only aerobic bacteria are susceptible to aminoglycosides. Anaerobic organisms are resistant to aminoglycosides because the mechanism by which they are taken up by microorganisms is driven by aerobic metabolism.

86. **a.** Aminoglycosides cause these side effects, which are dose related when given systemically.

87. **b.** Gentamicin has been associated with macular infarction.

88. **b.** Vancomycin acts by the inhibition of cell wall synthesis. It is primarily active against gram-positive bacteria including methicillin-resistant strains of *Staphylococcus*, although plasmid-mediated resistance has resulted in Staphylococcal resistance. Because of increasing resistance to vancomycin, the CDC has recommended avoiding the use of empiric vancomycin in neutropenic patients unless clear evidence for a beta-lactam resistant gram-positive infection can be demonstrated.

89. **d.** Trifluridine and idoxuridine are thymidine analogs, whereas vidarabine is an adenine analog. All of these agents inhibit DNA synthesis and are effective in treating herpes simplex. Trifluridine is more effective than the other two. Cross-resistance to these agents has not yet been reported.

90. **c.** Note that the diameter of the anatomic fovea and that of the optic nerve head are roughly equal.

91. **b.** Each of the others can create significant conjunctival hyperemia or corneal epithelial toxicity.

92. **c.** Studies have shown that preoperative (72 hours) antibiotics reduces bacterial counts to a greater degree than 3 days of preoperative povidone-iodine. Adding povidone iodine at the time of surgery exerts a synergistic effect. Some studies have suggested that saline flushes actually increase bacterial colony counts.

93. **a.** Bradycardia is not a known side effect of the prostaglandin analogs.

94. **a.** The anterior lamellae consist of the skin, orbicularis, and associated fascial and vascular components. A vertical insufficiency of the anterior lamella can lead to congenital ectropion.

95. **d.** Sildenafil (Viagra) can cause mydriasis. All of the other answers have been reported to occur.

96. **c.** CPEO is inherited through maternal mitochondrial DNA. It involves progressive lid ptosis and paralysis of ocular muscles. In Kearns-Sayre syndrome, CPEO is associated with retinitis pigmentosa and heart block.

97. **d.** Duchenne muscular dystrophy is X-linked recessive. All of the other syndromes are associated with mitochondrial DNA mutations. NARP phenotype and Leigh's syndrome are related to the percentage of mutant mitochondrial DNA. They are associated with a base-pair mutation at position 8993 in the ATPase-6 gene.

98. **d.** Best disease is autosomal dominant, thus it has no carrier state. All of the other disorders have ocular findings in their carrier states.

99. **c.** Amacrine cells are located in the inner nuclear layer of the retina.

100. **a.** Müller cells traverse the entire retina. They are glial in nature and form the external limiting membrane. They may affect vitamin A cone metabolism.

101. **b.** There are 4 to 6 million RPE cells per eye. The RPE is a single layer of cuboidal cells. The ratio of photoreceptor cells to RPE cells is about 45 to 50:1. The RPE has no neural function.

102. **d.** The RPE is involved in the first three functions. Other functions of the RPE include adhesion of the retina, removal of waste products, and nutrient and ion transport.

103. **a.** Surfactants reduce the corneal epithelium barrier effect and thus allow increased topical drug delivery. High viscosity and lipid solubility increase topical penetration. Extremes of pH are not good for drug penetration.

104. **c.** Bronchospasm is associated with pilocarpine use. The other answers are true.

105. **a.** Pilocarpine can help in management of accommodative esotropia. Pilocarpine treatment does not replace laser iridotomy for chronic angle closure. The other answers are not correct.

106. **c.** Phosphoine iodide is an indirect-acting muscarinic.

107. **c.** Scopolamine is the longest acting of the group.

108. **d.** Cyclopentolate. The order from shortest to longest duration are as follows: phenylephrine 2.5% (3–5 hours), tropicamide (4–6 hours), cyclopentolate (2 days), homatropine (3 days), scopolamine (4–7 days), atropine (7–14 days).

109. **c.** Muscarinic antagonists may exacerbate angle closure.

110. **c.** Constipation is usually caused as a side effect, not diarrhea.

111. **a.** Cidofovir can be associated with hypotony and uveitis.

112. **b.** Fluoroquinolones have excellent intraocular penetration when given systemically. The other classes of medications do not penetrate the blood/ocular barrier well.

113. **a.** Other side effects include darkening of iris and periocular skin, conjunctival hyperemia, hypertrichosis of eyelashes, cystoid macular edema, and uveitis.

114. **d.** Procaine has the shortest duration of action. In order of decreasing duration: bupivacaine, lidocaine, mepivacaine, and then procaine.

115. **b.** Amphotericin B and natamycin are polyenes. Ketoconazole and miconazole are imidazoles. Fluconazole and itraconazole are triazoles.

116. **c.** Toxic epidermal necrolysis and Stevens-Johnson syndrome have been associated with sulfonamides.

117. **c.** Ocular findings in Down's syndrome include upslanting palpebral fissures, epicanthal folds, chronic blepharitis, strabismus, nystagmus, aberrant retinal vasculature, iris stromal hypoplasia, Brushfield spots, keratoconus, cataract, myopia, and optic atrophy. Other features include mental retardation, short height, hypotonia, brachycephaly, hypoplasia of fifth finger, wide spaced first and second toes, small ears, congenital hear defects, infertility, dental hypoplasia, palmar crease, shortened life span, and increased risk of Alzheimer's disease.

118. **a.** Both sexes are affected equally. The mutant gene generally does not cause the clinical disease (hence recessive). The ratio of normal to affected is 3:1. Consanguinity is a possible reason for this type of inheritance pattern.

119. **a.** Primary mode of action is listed below for several classes of medications.
Decrease aqueous humor formation: timolol, betaxolol, carteolol, levobunolol, apraclonidine, brimonidine.
Increase trabecular meshwork outflow: pilocarpine, epinephrine, dipivalyl epinephrine.
Increase uveoscleral outflow: latanoprost, travoprost, bimatoprost, apraclonidine, brimonidine.

120. **c.** Local anesthetics block smaller, unmyelinated fibers first. Clinically, sympathetic/parasympathetic fibers are blocked first and then the sensory fibers, followed by larger myelinated motor fibers.

CHAPTER 3

Optics

Questions

1. Which of the following regarding the wave properties of light is correct?
   a. Wavelength is determined by the distance between crests of the wave.
   b. The wavelength of visible light is between 200 and 500 nm.
   c. Frequency is the maximum value attained by the electric field.
   d. The speed of light in a vacuum is 6×10^8.

2. When light interacts with matter, individual quanta of energy (photons) are emitted or absorbed. Which of the following is not true regarding the particle or photon characteristics of light?
   a. The amount of energy (E) per photon is equal to Planck's constant multiplied by the frequency.
   b. A photon of red light has greater energy than a photon of blue light.
   c. The light emitted through fluorescence has a longer wavelength than the excitation light.
   d. Planck's constant is equal to 6.626×10^{-34} J/s.

3. Antireflection films prevent reflection of light by what mechanism?
   a. constructive interference.
   b. absorption of light photons.
   c. polarization.
   d. destructive interference.

4. The laser interferometer utilizes the principles of all of the following except
   a. constructive interference.
   b. destructive interference.
   c. high coherence.
   d. polarization.

5. The Haidinger brush phenomenon is due to which special characteristic of light transmission?
   a. interference.
   b. polarization.
   c. diffraction.
   d. scattering.

6. Which of the following concerning diffraction is not true?
   a. It is responsible for a limit on pinhole acuity of approximately 20/25.
   b. Diffraction is responsible for the blue color of the sky.
   c. It is a limiting factor for visual acuity with pupils smaller than about 2.5 mm.
   d. Long wavelengths are diffracted more than short wavelengths.

7. Why does the sky appear blue?
   a. Because blue light is scattered more than other light given its longer wavelength.
   b. Because blue light is scattered less than other light given its longer wavelength.
   c. Shorter wavelengths are scattered more.
   d. coherence.

8. The features of laser light that enhance its intensity include all of the following except
   a. polychromaticity.
   b. directionality.
   c. coherence.
   d. polarization.

9. Which of the following laser–tissue interactions are matched correctly?
   a. Photodisruption: selective absorption of light energy and conversion of energy to heat with thermally induced structural change in the target.
   b. Photocoagulation: uses pulsed lasers to ionize the target and rupture the surrounding tissues.
   c. Photoablation: high-powered ultraviolet light exceeds covalent bond strength of target protein precisely removing a submicron layer.
   d. Photodisruption: primary type of laser tissue interaction used in LASIK surgery.

10. In a simple thin lens system, the object is upright with a height of 5 cm, the image is inverted with a height of 10 cm, and the object is 2 cm from the center of the lens. What is the distance of the image from the center of the lens?
    a. 1 cm.
    b. 2 cm.
    c. 4 cm.
    d. 8 cm.

11. Which of the following concerning linear magnification is true?
    a. Magnification is equal to the ratio of object size to image size.
    b. A magnification value <0 implies inversion of the image relative to the object.
    c. Magnification is equal to the image vergence divided by the object vergence.
    d. A magnification value >-1, and <1 implies that the image is greater than the object.

12. All of the following concerning refraction of light at interfaces are true except
    a. Light will bend toward the surface normal as it enters a medium of higher index of refraction.
    b. The index of refraction of any given substance is greater for longer wavelengths.

c. Total internal reflection renders the anterior chamber angle invisible by a slit lamp.
d. Refractive index is the ratio of the speed of light in a vacuum to the speed of light in the medium.

13. You have gone fishing and see a fish in the water. You do not have a fishing rod. The only equipment that you have is a spear to catch the fish. Where do you throw the spear?
    a. in front of the fish.
    b. behind the fish.
    c. directly at the fish.
    d. It is not possible to hit the fish as it is a virtual image.

14. All of the following is true of total internal reflection except
    a. Total internal reflection occurs when light travels from a low-index medium to a high-index medium and the angle of incidence exceeds a certain critical angle.
    b. Total internal reflection makes it impossible to view the eye's anterior chamber angle without the use of a contact lens.
    c. The critical angle is the angle of incidence that produces a transmitted ray 90° to the surface normal.
    d. It may be possible to view the anterior chamber angle when the cornea is ectatic as in keratoconus.

15. What is the power of a +20 D lens under water?
    a. 6.2 D.
    b. 6.5 D.
    c. 7.3 D.
    d. 8.0 D.

16. Which is a true statement regarding vergence?
    a. If light rays converge to a point, the vergence is negative.
    b. Vergence is directly proportional to distance from the object point to the image point.
    c. As light travels away from an object point or toward an image point, its vergence stays the same.
    d. Vergence is the reciprocal of distance.

17. What is the vergence of an object 50 cm away from a lens? What is the vergence of an object 25 cm away from the lens?
    a. −4 D; −8 D.
    b. −2 D; −4 D.
    c. 2 D; 4 D.
    d. 4 D; 8 D.

18. What is the vergence of an image 50 cm away from a lens? What is the vergence of an image 100 cm away from the lens?
    a. −4 D; −2 D.
    b. −2 D; −1 D.
    c. 2 D; 1 D.
    d. 4 D; 2 D.

19. Consider an object 10 cm in front of a 5 D convex thin lens in air. What is the vergence after the light leaves the lens?
    a. −5 D.
    b. 5 D.
    c. 10 D.
    d. −10 D.

20. How far away is the image from the lens in question 19? Is the image virtual or real?
    a. 20 cm; real.
    b. 20 cm; virtual.
    c. 10 cm; real.
    d. 10 cm; virtual.

21. Consider an image is 50 cm in front of a 5 D convex thin lens in air. What is the vergence after the light leaves the lens?
    a. 1 D.
    b. −1 D.
    c. 3 D.
    d. −3 D.

22. How far away is the image from the lens in question 21? Is the image virtual or real?
    a. 11 cm; real.
    b. 11 cm; virtual.
    c. 33 cm; real.
    d. 33 cm; virtual.

23. Consider an object 25 cm in front of a 4 D concave thin lens in air. What is the vergence after the light leaves the lens?
    a. −8 D.
    b. 8 D.
    c. −2 D.
    d. 2 D.

24. How far away is the image from the lens in question 23? Is the image virtual or real?
    a. 12.5 cm; real.
    b. 12.5 cm; virtual.
    c. 50 cm; real.
    d. 50 cm; virtual.

25. Where will the image be formed for an object placed 25 cm in front of an 8 D convex lens that is separated from a 1 D concave lens by 50 cm?
    a. 20 cm to the left of the concave lens.
    b. 20 cm to the right of the concave lens.
    c. 30 cm to the left of the concave lens.
    d. 30 cm to the right of the concave lens.

26. An object is 25 cm to the left of a convex lens with a focal point of 10 cm. Is the image inverted or upright? Is the image to the left or right of the lens?
    a. inverted; left of the lens.
    b. upright; left of the lens.
    c. inverted; right of the lens.
    d. upright; right of the lens.

27. An object is 5 cm to the left of a convex lens with a focal point of 10 cm. Is the image inverted or upright? Is the image to the left or right of the lens?
    a. inverted; left of the lens.
    b. upright; left of the lens.
    c. inverted; right of the lens.
    d. upright; right of the lens.

28. An object is 25 cm to the left of a concave lens with a focal point of 10 cm. Is the image inverted or upright? Is the image to the left or right of the lens?
    a. inverted; left of the lens.
    b. upright; left of the lens.
    c. inverted; right of the lens.
    d. upright; right of the lens.

29. All of the following are true of a Galilean telescope except
    a. The Galilean telescope produces an upright image.
    b. The objective lens is positive and has a low power, whereas the eyepiece is negative and usually has a high power.
    c. The two lenses in the Galilean telescope are separated by the sum of the focal lengths.
    d. The Galilean telescope is often used as a low-vision aid or surgical loupes.

30. All of the following are true of Keplerian telescopes except
    a. The Keplerian telescope produces an inverted image.
    b. The two lenses in the system are separated by the sum of the focal lengths.
    c. The Keplerian telescope consists of a low-power objective and a high-power ocular, with both lenses being positive.
    d. In the Keplerian telescope, some of the light collected by the objective is lost.

31. What is the angular magnification of a Keplerian telescope whose eyepiece is +20 D and whose objective is +4 D.
    a. −5×.
    b. 5×.
    c. −10×.
    d. 10×.

32. An afocal telescope is constructed with −10 D and +4 D lenses. What is the distance between the lenses?
    a. 5 cm.
    b. 15 cm.
    c. 20 cm.
    d. 25 cm.

33. Which of the following is true in regard to ophthalmic prisms?
    a. The power in prism diopters is the number of centimeters light is displaced over a 100 cm distance.
    b. The image formed by a prism is virtual.

c. Images created by prisms are deviated toward the apex.
d. Prism power decreases as the distance from the optical center in a lens increases.

34. Which of the following is true regarding mirrors?
    a. Plane mirrors add negative vergence.
    b. Concave mirrors add plus vergence.
    c. Light rays reflected off of a convex mirror are convergent.
    d. Convex mirrors form real images to the left of the mirror.

35. All of the following are true regarding mirrors except
    a. Convex mirrors form virtual images on the opposite side of the object.
    b. The focal point of a convex mirror is to the left of the mirror.
    c. The focal length is equal to half the radius of curvature of the mirror.
    d. The reflecting power of a mirror is equal to the reciprocal of the focal length.

36. What is the reflecting power of a concave mirror whose radius of curvature is 50 cm?
    a. +2 D.
    b. −2 D.
    c. +4 D.
    d. −4 D.

37. What is the reflecting power of a convex mirror whose radius of curvature is 100 cm?
    a. +2 D.
    b. −2 D.
    c. +4 D.
    d. −4 D.

38. Consider an object 2 m to the left of a *concave* mirror with a radius of curvature of 100 cm. Where is the image?
    a. 33 cm to the left of the mirror.
    b. 33 cm to the right of the mirror.
    c. 66 cm to the left of the mirror.
    d. 66 cm to the right of the mirror.

39. Consider an object 2 m to the left of a *convex* mirror with radius of curvature of 100 cm. Where is the image?
    a. 20 cm to the left of the mirror.
    b. 20 cm to the right of the mirror.
    c. 40 cm to the left of the mirror.
    d. 40 cm to the right of the mirror.

40. If a man is 6 ft tall, what is the minimal length of a plane mirror for the man to see himself from head to toe?
    a. 1 ft.
    b. 3 ft.
    c. 6 ft.
    d. 12 ft.

41. If an object is 50 cm in front of a plane mirror, where is the image in relation to the mirror? Is the image virtual or real?
    a. 50 cm from the mirror; virtual.
    b. 50 cm from the mirror; real.
    c. 100 cm from the mirror; virtual.
    d. 100 cm from the mirror; real.

42. In the reduced schematic eye, what is the approximate focal length in air?
    a. 17 mm.
    b. 17 cm.
    c. 22 mm.
    d. 22 cm.

43. Using the dimensions from the reduced schematic eye, what is the image size on the retina of a Snellen letter that is 60 mm in height 20 ft (6,000 mm) from the cornea?
    a. 17 mm.
    b. 0.17 mm.
    c. 22 mm.
    d. 0.22 mm.

44. In a patient with astigmatism, all of the following are true of myopia and hyperopia except
    a. In simple myopic astigmatism, one focal line lies in front of the retina and the other is on the retina.
    b. In compound myopic astigmatism, both focal lines lie in front of the retina.

c. In simple hyperopic astigmatism, both focal lines lie behind the retina.
    d. In mixed astigmatism, one focal line lies in front of the retina and one lies behind the retina.

45. A patient wears a −10 D spectacle lens at a vertex distance of 20 mm for distance correction. What power contact lens will be required for proper distance correction?
    a. −8.25 D.
    b. −9.00 D.
    c. −12.50 D.
    d. −11.50 D.

46. A patient wears a spectacle correction of +10.0 D at vertex distance of 20 mm. Where should a +3.0 D lens be placed to correct this patient for distance?
    a. 10 cm in front of the eye.
    b. 25 cm in front of the eye.
    c. 33 cm in front of the eye.
    d. 35 cm in front of the eye.

47. A patient with a corneal scar is carefully refracted. Best corrected visual acuity is 20/40. With a pinhole over his correction, his acuity improves to 20/25. The best explanation for this is
    a. spherical aberration.
    b. myopic astigmatism.
    c. cataract.
    d. irregular astigmatism.

48. An examiner sits 50 cm from a patient being refracted by retinoscopy. With the streak oriented in the horizontal meridian (sweeping vertically), a +3.00 D sphere neutralizes the reflex; with the streak oriented in the vertical meridian (sweeping horizontally), a +5.00 D sphere neutralizes the reflex. What is the patient's final retinoscopic refraction?
    a. +3.00 +2.00 × 090.
    b. +3.00 +2.00 × 180.
    c. +1.00 +2.00 × 090.
    d. +1.00 +2.00 × 180.

49. The angular magnification of a retinal image afforded by direct ophthalmoscopy in an emmetrope is approximately
    a. 5×.
    b. 10×.
    c. 15×.
    d. 20×.

50. A 5-year-old child is noted to have a 20 prism diopter esotropia that increases to 45 prism diopters while reading at 20 cm. The patient's pupillary distance is 50 mm. With the child reading through his distance correction, a +3.00 D lens placed over each eye decreases the esotropia at near to 20 prism diopters. The patient's accommodative convergence to accommodation (AC/A) ratio, as determined by the gradient method, is
    a. 5:1.
    b. 8:1.
    c. 10:1.
    d. 15:1.

51. For the child described in the previous question, what would the AC/A ratio be, as determined by the heterophoria method?
    a. 5:1.
    b. 8:1.
    c. 10:1.
    d. 15:1.

52. A patient wearing new glasses comes in complaining of diplopia. The prescription is +3.00 −1.00 × 180 OD and −2.50 −1.00 × 90 OS with a +2.00 D add OU. You note a tropia present when the patient is reading at a comfortable distance. While reading, the visual axis is 2 cm nasal and 2 cm inferior to the distance optical center and 0.5 cm nasal and 1.2 cm above the optical center of the add in each lens. What is the induced prismatic effect for this patient?
    a. 3 prism diopters base up OD and 1 prism diopter base out OD.
    b. 3 prism diopters base up OD and 1 prism diopter base in OD.

c. 9 prism diopters base down OD and 1 prism diopters base in OD.
    d. 9 prism diopters base up OD and 1 prism diopter base out OD.

53. Image jump is most troublesome for bifocals of the
    a. round-top type.
    b. flat-top type.
    c. ribbon type.
    d. progressive type.

54. How far from a +24 D camera lens should an object be placed to be focused onto film 5 cm to the right of the lens?
    a. 25 cm to the left of the lens.
    b. 50 cm to the right of the lens.
    c. 50 cm to the left of the lens.
    d. 25 cm to the right of the lens.

55. A crystal ball with an opaque rear surface sits on a pedestal. Its internal radius of curvature is 50 cm. Its index of refraction is 3.00. What is the refractive power of the crystal ball?
    a. +2.00 D.
    b. +4.00 D.
    c. +8.00 D.
    d. +10.00 D.

56. Which of the following is a characteristic of handheld magnifiers?
    a. greater working distance.
    b. greater ease of use for patients with poor manual dexterity.
    c. smaller range of magnifying powers.
    d. wider field of view.

57. The main advantage of telescopic aids for near work is
    a. decreased convergence requirement.
    b. wider field of view.
    c. greater depth of focus.
    d. greater working distance.

58. Which of the following is true regarding accommodation and contact lenses?
    a. In a myopic patient, contact lenses decrease the accommodative demand compared to spectacles.
    b. In a hyperopic patient, contact lenses increase the accommodative demand compared to spectacles.
    c. In a myopic patient, contact lenses increase accommodative demand compared to spectacles.
    d. There is no difference noted in accommodation when wearing contact lenses.

59. A patient requesting rigid gas-permeable (RGP) contact lens has a best refraction in the right eye of −4.00 +1.25 × 90. Keratometry is 44.0 D at 90° and 42.5 D at 180°. The conversion to radius of curvature is 7.70 mm at 90°, 7.95 mm at 180°. The only posterior curve available is 7.80 mm. The contact lens power that should be prescribed for best vision is
    a. −2.00 D.
    b. −2.75 D.
    c. −3.00 D.
    d. −3.50 D.

60. Which of the following is true regarding rigid-gas permeable (RGP) contact lenses?
    a. Most lenses are made of PMMA.
    b. RGP lenses are useful in correcting astigmatism.
    c. RGP lenses generally have a shorter adaptation period compared to soft contact lenses.
    d. RGP lenses are easier to fit than soft contact lenses.

61. Which of the following is true regarding examination lenses?
    a. Goldmann fundus lens produces an inverted image.
    b. Images generated by the Goldmann contact lens are "real" images.
    c. The Hruby lens generates a virtual image.
    d. The Hruby lens generates an inverted image.

62. Goldmann applanation tonometry readings
    a. are not affected by corneal astigmatism.
    b. are not affected by scleral rigidity.
    c. are affected by surface tension of the tear film.
    d. are not affected by the corneal thickness.

63. Which one of the following concerning direct ophthalmoscopy is false?
    a. The linear magnification is 15×.
    b. The optic disc of a myopic eye appears larger than that of an emmetropic eye.
    c. The image is a virtual, upright image.
    d. The dial on a direct ophthalmoscope is intended to neutralize both the examiner's and patient's refractive error.

64. Which of the following regarding indirect ophthalmoscopy of an emmetropic eye is false?
    a. The image the examiner observes is a real, inverted image in the focal plane of the condensing lens.
    b. Conjugate planes include the patient's and the examiner's retinas and the patient's and examiner's pupils.
    c. If the examiner uses a 20 D condensing lens, the lateral magnification is approximately 3× and the axial magnification approximately 2.25×.
    d. A 30 D condensing lens provides greater magnification and a larger field of view than a 20 D condensing lens.

65. Which of the following concerning keratometry is false?
    a. Corneal curvature is measured by using the cornea's power as a convex mirror.
    b. A central image is doubled to negate the effect of eye movement.
    c. Conventional keratometry measures the curvature of the central 6 mm of the cornea.
    d. The refractive power of the average cornea equals 337.5 divided by its radius of curvature (in mm).

66. Which of the following is not a complication of ACIOLs?
    a. anterior uveitis.
    b. hyphema.
    c. chronic cystoid macular edema.
    d. inability to achieve good vision.

67. Which IOL calculation formula is most accurate for shorter eyes (<24.5 mm)?
    a. Holladay 1.
    b. SRK.
    c. Hoffer Q.
    d. SRK/T.

68. Which IOL calculation formula is most accurate for longer eyes (>26.0 mm)?
    a. Holladay 1.
    b. SRK.
    c. Hoffer Q.
    d. SRK/T.

69. Which of the following is false?
    a. A-scan ultrasound speed is higher in the lens and cornea than in the aqueous and vitreous.
    b. Axial length in staphylomatous eyes may be better measured with B-scan.
    c. Applanation A-scan measurements tend to give longer axial length readings.
    d. Immersion A-scan is more accurate than applanation A-scan.

70. A 60-year-old man with prior history of LASIK for myopia in both eyes presents to you for cataract evaluation. You perform your standard exam using refraction, potential acuity, axial length, and keratometry readings. Surgery is uncomplicated. That evening, you remember that you did not take into account the patient's prior refractive surgery into IOL calculations. What type of refractive error will the patient most likely have as a result?
    a. myopia.
    b. hyperopia.
    c. astigmatic error.
    d. none.

71. Which of the following refractive surgeries do not change the index of refraction of the cornea?
    a. LASIK.
    b. LASEK.
    c. RK.
    d. PRK.

72. Which of the below answers is true regarding IOL calculations in eyes with previous retinal surgery and silicone-oil implantation?
    a. A-scan velocity is faster in eyes with silicone oil versus vitreous.
    b. A-scan velocity is slower in eyes with silicone oil versus vitreous.
    c. Silicone oil acts as an intraocular positive lens when IOL's are placed.
    d. B-scan must be done to determine axial length.

73. Multifocal IOLs
    a. can induce monocular diplopia.
    b. improve night vision.
    c. improve contrast sensitivity.
    d. can contain only two zones of focus.

74. Which of the following is a third-order refractive aberration?
    a. tetrafoil.
    b. spherical aberration.
    c. vertical coma.
    d. secondary astigmatism.

75. What is true regarding the direct ophthalmoscope?
    a. A hyperopic eye has a higher magnification than an emmetropic eye.
    b. A myopic eye has a higher magnification than an emmetropic eye.
    c. An emmetropic schematic eye has a refractive power of about 80 D.
    d. Refractive status of an eye does not affect magnification when using a direct ophthalmoscope.

76. How can one improve fundus visualization using the indirect ophthalmoscope in a patient with small pupils?
    a. increasing the distance of the ophthalmoscope mirror and the observer.
    b. decreasing the distance between the ophthalmoscope eyepieces.
    c. moving closer to the patient's eyes.
    d. decreasing the observer's interpupillary distance.

77. Which of the following is true regarding the slit-lamp biomicroscope?
    a. The slit lamp contains both astronomical and Galilean telescope components.
    b. The slit lamp contains only astronomical components.
    c. The slit lamp contains only Galilean components.
    d. The slit lamp is a monocular viewing system.

78. The 78-D fundus lens when used in conjunction with the slit lamp produces an image that is
    a. virtual.
    b. real.
    c. minified.
    d. upright.

79. Which of the following is not a method used to accurately measure corneal thickness?
    a. optical focusing.
    b. optical doubling.
    c. slit-lamp measurement.
    d. ultrasound.

80. Which of the following is true regarding laser interferometry?
    a. It requires one clear area of the cataractous lens.
    b. The fringe spacing directly correlates with visual acuity.
    c. It is a good test for optic nerve function.
    d. It is based on the principle that cataractous lenses have some clear spaces.

81. Legal blindness as described by the World Health Organization (WHO) is defined as
    a. best-corrected vision of 20/100 or worse in the better eye.
    b. best-corrected vision of 20/200 or worse in the better eye.
    c. best-corrected vision of 20/70 or worse in the better eye.
    d. best-corrected vision of 20/400 or worse in the better eye.

82. Per WHO definition, what is the visual field limit of legal blindness in the better eye?
    a. 15°.
    b. 20°.
    c. 25°.
    d. 30°.

83. The Kestenbaum rule
    a. is used to measure horizontal deviation.
    b. is used to refract for distance vision.
    c. is used to determine the "add" needed for bifocals.
    d. is used to determine predicted prism needed for glasses.

84. What is true regarding stand magnifiers as low-vision aids?
    a. The stand magnifiers usually cause an unstable image.
    b. Maintaining lens working distance is difficult.
    c. They are useful for patients with limitation of hand dexterity.
    d. The magnifiers require no specific positioning of reading material.

85. What is the most favorable size for the pinhole in an occluder to provide the best vision?
    a. 1.0 mm.
    b. 1.2 mm.
    c. 1.5 mm.
    d. 1.7 mm.

3

■ Answers

1. **a.** Wavelength is determined by the distance between crests of the wave. Amplitude is the maximum value attained by the electric field as the wave propagates. Frequency is the number of wave crests that pass a fixed point per second. The visible light spectrum is normally defined as a wavelength between 400 and 700 nm. The speed of light in a vacuum (c) is 3×10^8. The wavelength of light (λ) is related to its frequency (v) by the equation, $\lambda v = c$.

2. **b.** The energy (E) per photon of light is equal to Planck's constant (h), 6.626×10^{-34} J/s, multiplied by the frequency (v). This is shown by the equation:

$$E = hv.$$

   Blue light is of higher frequency than red light and therefore has greater energy per photon. In general, light emitted through fluorescence has a longer wavelength than the excitation light. For example, when using fluorescein, a photon of blue light is absorbed by the fluorescein molecule, and this fluorescein molecule emits a photon that has a lower energy lying in the yellow-green spectrum of visible light.

3. **d.** Interference occurs when two light waves originating from the same source are brought together and most readily occurs when the light lies within a narrow band of wavelengths. Constructive interference occurs when the crests of the waves coincide. The energy of the electromagnetic fields is added together. Destructive interference occurs when the crest of one wave coincides with the trough of the other wave. The two electromagnetic fields cancel each other out.

4. **d.** Coherence describes the ability of two light beams, or different parts of the same beam, to produce interference. The laser interferometer uses the highly coherent light of the laser to create an interference pattern on the retina. The pattern seen by the patient consists of light and dark bands created by constructive and destructive interference, respectively.

5. **b.** The Haidinger brush phenomenon is useful in sensory testing of the fovea. The phenomenon is created by rotating a polarizer continuously in front of a uniform blue field. The normal subject will see a rotating figure that looks like a double-ended brush. The effect is created because Henle's layer of the macula (outer plexiform layer) is oriented in such a way as to polarize incoming light.

6. **b.** Because of diffractive effects, pinhole vision is rarely better than 20/25 even with an optimal pinhole aperture of 1.2 mm. Pupil sizes less than about 2.5 mm will create diffractive effects that limit acuity. Diffraction increases with the wavelength of incident light.

7. **c.** Scattering of light occurs at irregularities in the light path, such as with small particles in the atmosphere. The sky is blue because light of higher frequency/shorter wavelength is *scattered* more than light of lower frequency/longer wavelength.

8. **a.** Laser is an acronym for *L*ight *A*mplification by *S*timulated *E*mission of *R*adiation. A laser beam's high directionality, coherence, and linear polarization enhance its intensity. Laser light is *mono*chromatic (one precise wavelength).

9. **c.** *Photocoagulation* refers to the selective absorption of light energy and conversion of that energy to heat, with a subsequent thermally induced structural change. This is commonly used in retinal lasers. *Photodisruption* uses high-peak-power pulsed lasers to ionize the target and rupture the surrounding tissue. This is used to open tissues such as lens capsule, iris, and inflammatory membranes. *Photoablation* refers to ultraviolet light exceeding the covalent bond strength of corneal protein precisely removing a submicron layer of cornea without opacifying adjacent tissue. This is commonly used in refractive surgery.

10. **c.** The ratio of image height to corresponding object height is known as *transverse magnification*.

In optics, the term magnification refers to making images larger or smaller than the object. If an image is inverted, it is negative and if it is upright it is positive. Object and image distances are negative when they point to the left of the lens and positive when they point to the right. Object distance is measured from the anterior nodal point to the object, and image distance is measured from the posterior nodal point to the image. For a simple thin lens immersed in a uniform medium such as air, the nodal points overlap in the center of the lens. Therefore, the image distance and object distance are measured from the center of the lens. In this problem, we use the equation:

Transverse magnification = image height/object height = image distance/object distance

–10 cm/5 cm = image distance/–2 cm
Image distance = 4 cm to the right of the lens.

In this problem, 10 cm is negative because the image is inverted, and the distance of the object from the lens is negative because it is to the left of the lens. The image distance is positive. Therefore, it is to the right of the lens.

11. b. Magnification is equal to the ratio of *image size* to *object size* (i/o). Magnification <0, a negative value, implies an inverted image. Magnification <1 (or if negative, >−1) implies an image smaller than the object.

12. b. An imaginary line perpendicular to the optical interface is called the surface normal. Light will bend toward the surface normal as it enters a medium of higher index of refraction and away from the surface normal as it enters a medium of lower index of refraction. This can be shown by *Snell's law:*

$$n_i \sin \theta_i = n_t \sin \theta_t$$

where n_i is the refractive index of the medium, n_t is the refractive index of transmitted medium, θ_i is the angle of incidence, and θ_t is the angle of transmission.

The index of refraction for any medium is greater for shorter wavelengths. In any medium except for a vacuum, short wavelengths travel more slowly than long wavelengths. This is called *dispersion*. Chromatic dispersion in the human eye leads to *chromatic aberration*, where yellow wavelengths will be focused on the retina, blue light will be focused in front of the retina, and red light behind the retina. This chromatic aberration can be helpful in refraction when using the duochrome, or red-green, test. When the image is clearly focused on the retina, the green symbols will be focused in front of the retina and the red symbols behind the retina. Some clinicians use the RAM-GAP mnemonic (Red Add Minus, Green Add Plus) to help them with refraction.

13. a. It is true that the fish you see is a virtual image, but it is possible to hit the fish. Remember that the light coming from the fish is going from a medium of higher index of refraction (water) to a medium of lower index of refraction (air). Therefore, the light from the fish will be going away from the surface normal, which is perpendicular to the air–water interface. Because of this, the image of the virtual fish, which is what you see, will be behind the actual fish. You must aim in front of this virtual fish to hit the actual fish.

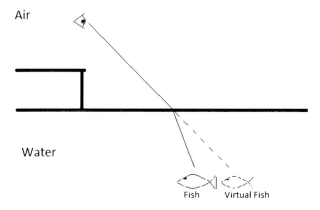

14. a. Total internal reflection occurs when light travels from a high-index medium to a low-index medium. The critical angle is the angle of incidence that produces a transmitted ray 90° to the surface normal. The critical angle θ_c can be calculated from *Snell's law* using the equation:

$$n_i \sin \theta_c = n_t \sin 90°$$

15. **c.** The power of a thin lens immersed in fluid can be calculated using the equation:

$$D_{air} / D_{fluid} = (n_{lens} - n_{air}) / (n_{lens} - n_{fluid})$$
$$+20 / D_{fluid} = (1.52 - 1.00) / (1.52 - 1.33)$$
$$D_{fluid} = 7.3 \text{ diopters.}$$

16. **d.** Vergence is the reciprocal of distance. Vergence is inversely proportional to distance from the object point or the image point. As light travels away from an object point or toward an image point, its vergence constantly changes. If an object point moves closer to the lens, the light is more divergent and when the object point is farther from the lens the light is less divergent. Similarly, if the lens is closer to an image point, light is more convergent and when the lens is farther from the image point, the light is less convergent.

17. **b.** Vergence is measured in diopters (D). Vergence is the reciprocal of the distance in meters: 1/distance in meters. Both answer choices are negative because the light rays are diverging from the object. The answers can be found by using the calculations: 1/0.5 m and 1/0.25 m. Therefore, the answers are −2 D and −4 D, respectively. As you can see by these calculations, the vergence is greater as the object moves closer to the lens.

18. **c.** Both answer choices are positive because the light rays are converging on to the image point. The answers can be found by using the calculations: 1/0.5 m and 1/1.0 m. Therefore, the answers are 2 D and 1 D, respectively. As you can see by these calculations, the vergence is less as the image point moves farther away from the lens.

19. **a.** In this problem, we must use the vergence formula:

$$U + D = V$$

U is the object vergence, D is the lens power, and V is the image vergence.

Remember that the light rays are diverging from the object, so the object vergence is negative.

The object vergence can be determined by taking the reciprocal of the distance in meters, which is 1/0.10 m. Thus, the object vergence is −10 D. Convex lenses add plus power and concave lenses add minus power. Therefore, the lens gives a power of +5 D.

In order to determine the vergence leaving the lens, we must use the equation, $U + D = V.$

$$-10 \text{ D} + (+5 \text{ D}) = V = -5 \text{ D.}$$

20. **b.** The vergence leaving the lens is −5 D. Because the vergence leaving the lens is negative, this means that the light leaving the lens is still diverging and does not converge to form an image to the right of the lens. Instead, imaginary lines from the diverging light rays leaving the lens can be drawn to form an image to the left of the lens. Because the image is to the left of the lens, and is not formed by the true light rays, the image is virtual. To find the distance of the image, we need to find the reciprocal of the vergence leaving the lens, which is (1/5 D) = 0.2 m = 20 cm to the left of the lens.

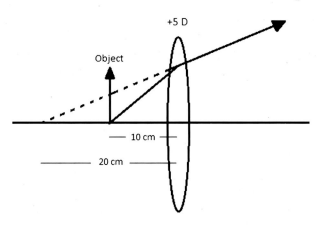

21. **c.** Again, in this problem we must use the vergence formula:

$$U + D = V$$

U is the object vergence, D is the lens power, and V is the image vergence.

Remember that the light rays are diverging from the object, so the object vergence is negative. The object vergence can be determined by taking the reciprocal of the distance in meters, which is 1/0.50 m. Therefore, the object vergence is −2 D. Convex lenses add plus power and concave lenses add minus power. Therefore, the lens gives a power of +5 D.

In order to determine the vergence leaving the lens, we must use the equation, $U + D = V$.

$$-2\,D + (+5\,D) = V = +3\,D.$$

22. c. The vergence leaving the lens is +3 D. Because the vergence leaving the lens is positive, this means that the light leaving the lens is now converging and will form an image to the right of the lens. Because the image is to the right of the lens, and is formed by the true light rays, the image is real. To find the distance of the image, we need to find the reciprocal of the vergence leaving the lens, which is (1/3 D) = 0.33 m = 33 cm to the right of the lens.

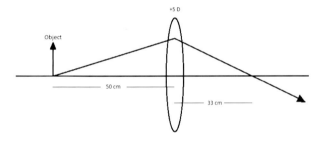

23. a. Remember that the light rays are diverging from the object, so the object vergence is negative. The object vergence can be determined by taking the reciprocal of the distance in meters, which is 1/0.25 m; the object vergence is −4 D. Convex lenses add plus power and concave lenses add minus power. Therefore, the lens gives a power of −4 D.

In order to determine the vergence leaving the lens, we must use the equation, $U + D = V$.

$$-4\,D + (-4\,D) = V = -8\,D.$$

24. b. The vergence leaving the lens is −8 D. Because the vergence leaving the lens is negative, this means that the light leaving the lens is still diverging and does not converge to form an image to the right of the lens. Instead, imaginary lines from the diverging light rays leaving the

lens can be drawn to form an image to the left of the lens. Because the image is to the left of the lens, and is not formed by the true light rays, the image is virtual. To find the distance of the image, we need to find the reciprocal of the vergence leaving the lens, which is (1/8 D) = 0.125 m = 12.5 cm to the left of the lens.

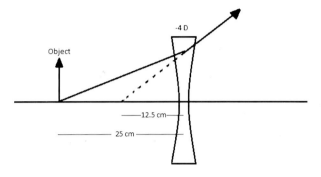

25. a. When solving a problem with multiple lenses, it is important to locate the first image. The position of this first image is then used to determine the vergence entering the second lens. For the first lens, we will use the equation:

$$U_1 + D_1 = V_1$$

U_1 is the object vergence, D_1 is the lens power, and V_1 is the image vergence for the first lens. Remember that the light rays are diverging from the object, so the object vergence is negative. The object vergence can be determined by taking the reciprocal of the distance in meters, which is 1/0.25 m. Therefore, the object vergence is −4 D. Convex lenses add plus power. Therefore, the lens gives a power of +8 D.

In order to find the vergence leaving the lens, we must use the equation, $U_1 + D_1 = V_1$
$-4\,D + (+8\,D) = V_1 = +4\,D$. The distance is the reciprocal of the vergence, which is 1/4 = 0.25 m = 25 cm.

The location of the image formed by the first lens becomes the object location of the second lens. Remember that the object distance used for the second lens must be the distance from the second lens, not the first lens. The total distance between the two lenses in this problem is 50 cm. The image formed is 25 cm to the right of the first lens. Thus, this image must be 25 cm to the left of the second lens.

For the second lens, we will use the equation:

$$U_2 + D_2 = V_2$$

U_2 is the object vergence, D_2 is the lens power, and V_2 is the image vergence for the second lens.

Remember that the light rays are diverging from the object, so the object vergence is again negative. The object vergence can be determined by taking the reciprocal of the distance in meters, which is $1/0.25$ m. Therefore, the object vergence is -4 D.

Concave lenses add minus power. Therefore, the lens gives a power of -1 D.

In order to find the vergence leaving the lens, we must use the equation, $U_2 + D_2 = V_2$
-4 D $+ (-1$ D$) = V_2 = -5$ D. The distance is the reciprocal of the vergence, which is $1/5 = 0.20$ m $= 20$ cm to the left of the second lens.

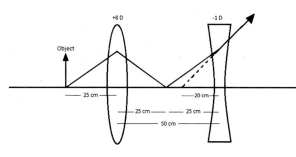

26. c. The image is inverted and to the right of the lens. Light coming from the anterior focal point (F_a) exits the lens and comes to a focus at plus optical infinity. Light coming from minus optical infinity images to the posterior focal point (F_p). Three rays can be drawn through a thin lens to locate a corresponding point in the image. Only two rays are needed. The first two rays can pass through F_a and F_p and the third ray, which is known as the central ray, pass through the nodal points. For a thin lens, the nodal points overlap at the optical center of the lens. For a convex lens, when the object lies at a distance from the lens greater than the focal point, the image is inverted, real, and to the

right of the lens. This can be shown through ray tracings.

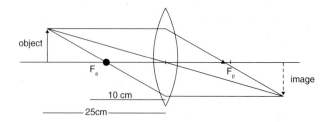

27. b. When the object distance from the lens is less than the focal point of a convex lens, the image is magnified, upright, and virtual, and is located to the left of the object and lens. This can be shown through ray tracings.

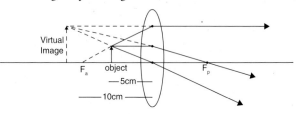

28. b. A ray of light directed through F_a will exit the lens parallel to the optical axis. A ray of light entering the lens parallel to the optical axis will pass through F_p. Using these same principles as used for the convex lens, three rays can be drawn through a concave lens to locate the corresponding image. No matter where a real object is placed in front of a minus lens, the resulting image is upright, minified, virtual, and to the left of the lens. This can be shown through ray tracings.

29. c. The lenses in a Galilean telescope are separated by the difference in focal lengths. Because the image produced by a Galilean telescope is upright, and the Galilean telescope is shorter than a Keplerian telescope, it makes it more ideal in surgical loupes and low vision aids.

30. d. In a Galilean telescope, some of the light is lost, not in a Keplerian telescope. Because of this, Keplerian telescopes use light much more efficiently than Galilean telescopes and as a result, are more ideal for astronomical observation.

31. **a.** The angular magnification (M_A) of both a Keplerian and Galilean telescope is equal to the power of the eyepiece (D_e) divided by the power of the objective (D_o). This is given by the equation:

$$M_A = -D_e / D_o$$

$M_A = -(+20)/(+4) = -5\times$. The negative sign indicates that the image is inverted, which is true of a Keplerian telescope.

32. **b.** In an afocal telescope, the lenses must be placed such that the secondary focal point of the objective lens coincides with the primary focal point of the eyepiece. If both lenses are positive, as in an astronomical or Keplerian telescope, the distance between the lenses is the sum of the focal lengths. If the eyepiece is negative, as in a Galilean telescope, the distance between the lenses is the difference between the focal lengths. In this Galilean telescope, $f_{objective} = 25$ cm, and $f_{eyepiece} = 10$ cm. The difference between the two, 15 cm, is the length of the device.

Loupe length = f₂ (objective) – f₁ (eyepiece)

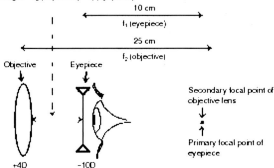

33. **a.** The image formed by a prism is real and images are deviated toward the base of a prism, not the apex. Prism power increases as the distance from the optical center in a lens increases. This prismatic effect becomes important clinically in patients with anisometropia in the reading position, where it can cause vertical misalignment of the visual axis.

34. **b.** Concave mirrors add plus vergence as the light rays reflected off of the mirror is convergent. Convex mirrors add minus vergence as the light

rays reflected off of the mirror is divergent. Plane mirrors add zero vergence.

35. **b.** The focal point of a convex mirror is to the right of the mirror and the focal point of a concave mirror is the left of the mirror.

36. **c.** Remember that a concave mirror adds positive vergence. The focal length (f) is equal to half of the radius of curvature (r) given by the equation: $f = r/2$. The radius and focal length are in meters. The focal length in this problem is $f = 0.50$ m/2 = 0.25 m.

The reflecting power of a mirror is given by the equation: $D_m = 1/f$.

The reflecting power of concave mirror in this problem is $D_m = 1/0.25$ m = +4 D.

37. **b.** The focal length is found by using the equation $f = r/2 = 1$ m/2 = 0.50 m to the right of the mirror. The reflecting power of a mirror is given by the equation $D_m = 1/f = -1/0.50 = -2$ D. Remember that a convex mirror adds minus vergence.

38. **c.** To find the image distance from the mirror, we can use the equation $U + D_m = V$. U is the object vergence, which in this problem is $U = -1/2$ m = -0.5 D. This is negative because light is diverging from the object. The focal length is

$$f = r/2 = 1.0 \text{ m}/2 = 0.50 \text{ m}.$$

The reflecting power of the mirror is $D_m = 1/f = 1/0.50$ m = +2 D. Remember that concave lenses give plus power. Now we need to find the vergence of the image rays (V) using the equation $U + D_m = V$.

-0.5 D + (+2 D) = V = +1.50 D. Using the image vergence, we can find the image distance from the mirror, which is 1/1.50 D = 0.66 m or 66 cm to the left of the mirror. The image formed is real.

39. **d.** To find the image distance from the mirror, we can use the equation $U + D_m = V$. U is the object vergence, which in this problem is $U = -1/2$ m = -0.5 D. The focal length is $f = r/2 = 1.0$ m/2 = 0.50 m. The reflecting power of the mirror is

$D_m = 1/f = 1/0.50$ m $= -2$ D. Remember that convex lenses give minus power. Now we need to find the vergence of the image rays (V) using the equation $U + D_m = V$.
-0.5 D $+ (-2$ D$) = V = -2.50$ D. Using the image vergence, we can find the image distance from the mirror, which is $1/-2.50$D $= 0.40$ m or 40 cm to the right of the mirror. The image is virtual.

40. b. The minimal length of a plane mirror needed to view the entire body from head to toe is half the height of the person.

41. a. Remember that a plane mirror adds no vergence, $D_m = 0$ D. To find the location of the object, we can use the equation $U + D_m = V$. $U = -1/0.50$ m $= -2$ D. The vergence of the rays forming the image is therefore -2 D $+ 0$ D $= V = -2$ D. The image location is $1/-2$ D $= 0.50$ m or 50 cm to the right of the mirror. The image is virtual.

42. a. It is important to know the dimensions of the reduced schematic eye. In this simplified version of the eye, the power of the eye is $+60$ D. The nodal point of the eye lies within the eye 5.6 mm posterior to the cornea. This distance is often insignificant in calculations and often ignored. Without taking into account this distance, the anterior focal length in air is 17 mm in front of the cornea, and the posterior focal point, which lies on the retina, is 17 mm posterior to the nodal point. The refractive index for air is taken to be 1.0 and the simplified refractive index for the eye is 1.33.

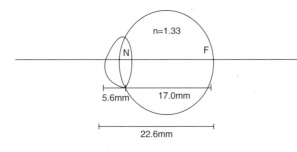

43. b. Similar triangles can be used to figure out the height of the image. Remember that the distance from the nodal point to the retina is 17 mm. To figure out the height of the image, we can use the equation:

Object height /Image height = Distance from nodal point to object /17 mm

60 mm/Image height = 6,000 mm/17 mm

Therefore, the image height is 0.17 mm.

44. c. In a patient with myopia, the eye possesses too much optical power for its axial length and the image is focused in front of the retina. In a patient with hyperopia, the eye does not possess enough optical power for its axial length and the image is focused behind the retina. In an astigmatic eye, there is no single focal point, but rather a set of two focal lines. In simple hyperopic astigmatism, one focal line lies on the retina and the other focal line lies behind the retina. In compound hyperopic astigmatism, both focal lines lie behind the retina.

45. a. The principle of neutralization of refractive errors is to create an image of an object at infinity at the eye's far point. With accommodation relaxed, the far point and the retina are conjugate. Thus, the corrective lens' secondary focal point must coincide with the eye's far point. Because this eye is corrected with a minus 10 D spectacle lens, this eye must be myopic. In a myopic eye, the far point lies somewhere in front of the eye. To find the secondary focal point of the spectacle lens, we take the reciprocal of the diopters, which is $1/10$ D $= 0.1$ m $= 10$ cm. The eye's far point must be 10 cm in front of the spectacle lens. Given a vertex distance of 2 cm, the far point must be 12 cm from the cornea. Thus, the proper contact lens must have its secondary focal point 12 cm or 0.12 m in front of the cornea. The power in the contact lens is found by taking the reciprocal of the secondary focal point: $1/0.12$ m $= -8.33$ D.

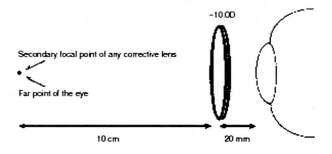

46. **b.** Again, the secondary focal point of a corrective lens must coincide with the eye's far point. The far point of a hyperope lies somewhere behind the retina. This eye's far point is 0.1 m (1/10 D) or 10 cm *behind* the spectacle plane. Given a 2 cm vertex distance, the far point is 8 cm behind the cornea. A +3.00 D lens must be placed with its secondary focal point at this same point. Because its secondary focal length is 0.33 m or 33 cm, it must be placed 25 cm in front of the cornea.

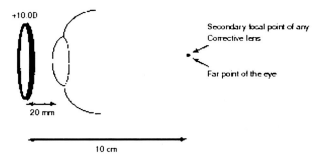

47. **d.** The corneal scar may be producing irregular astigmatism, which cannot be corrected by spherocylindrical spectacle lenses. The pinhole greatly minimizes nonaxial light rays, which require refraction to come into focus on the retina.

48. **c.** Remember that the working distance in this problem is 50 cm, so 2.00 D must be subtracted from the spherical portion, giving a net result of +1.00 +2.00 × 090.

49. **c.** The magnification of a simple plus lens is defined as the ratio of the angular size of the image produced by the lens to the angular size of the object viewed at 25 cm. The formula for angular magnification by a simple plus lens of power (*P*) is $M = P/4$. Because the average power of an emmetropic eye is +60 D, magnification $M = 60/4 = 15\times$.

50. **b.** Using the gradient method, AC/A (the ratio of prism diopters of accommodative convergence to diopters of accommodation) is calculated by placing plus lenses in front of each eye and determining the change in the deviation at near. This change,

divided by the power of the plus lens used (amount of weakened accommodation), gives the number of prism diopters of accommodative convergence per diopter of accommodation. In this case, $45 - 20 = 25$, divided by 3 is (approximately) 8:1.

Gradient method:

AC/A = [(deviation with lens – deviation without lens)/(lens power)].

In these calculations, esodeviations are positive and exodeviations are negative, by convention.

51. **c.** The heterophoria method makes use of similar reasoning, while taking into account the effect of interpupillary distance (PD), that is, larger PDs require greater convergence for fusion. Heterophoria method:

AC/A = [(deviation at near − deviation at distance)/(accommodation at near) + PD]

where PD = interpupillary distance in cm. The denominator represents the number of diopters of accommodation required for the near target (the reciprocal of the reading distance in meters). In this case, PD is 5 cm, the deviation at near is 45 prism diopters, and the deviation at distance is 20 D. Accommodation will be 5 D at 20 cm. Thus, AC/A = (45 − 20)/5 + 5 = 10:1.

52. **d.** Solving this problem is facilitated by preparing diagrams marked with the powers in the 90° and 180° meridians, the visual axes, and the optical axes for the distance corrections and adds. Image displacement in prism diopters is by Prentice's rule:

$$\Delta = hD$$

where *h* is in centimeters and *D* is the power of the lens in diopters.
This needs to be done for both the distance corrections and the adds separately. After this, the results are combined, first for each side, and then for a net effect on both eyes as shown in the figure at the top of the next page:

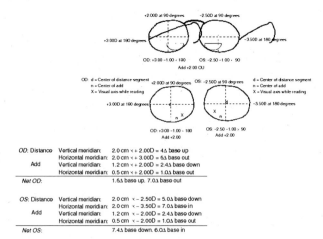

OD: Distance	Vertical meridian:	2.0 cm × +2.00D = 4Δ base up
	Horizontal meridian:	2.0 cm × +3.00D = 6Δ base out
Add	Vertical meridian:	1.2 cm × +2.00D = 2.4Δ base down
	Horizontal meridian:	0.5 cm × +2.00D = 1.0Δ base out
Net OD:		1.6Δ base up. 7.0Δ base out

OS: Distance	Vertical meridian:	2.0 cm × −2.50D = 5.0Δ base down
	Horizontal meridian:	2.0 cm × −3.50D = 7.0Δ base in
Add	Vertical meridian:	1.2 cm × −2.00D = 2.4Δ base down
	Horizontal meridian:	0.5 cm × −2.00D = 1.0Δ base out
Net OS:		7.4Δ base down. 6.0Δ base in

Note that when determining a net prismatic effect for two eyes, vertical prisms of different base orientation (base up plus base down) are additive, whereas horizontal prisms of same orientation (base in plus base in, or base out plus base out) are additive. For the net effect over one eye, prism of the same orientation are additive (e.g., base up plus base up, base in plus base in).

53. a. Image jump occurs at the segmentation line when the optical center of the add is not at its upper edge. A round top bifocal segment has its optical center farther from its upper edge than other types and therefore causes the greatest image jump. These are commonly used only for aphakic spectacles to minimize image displacement.

54. a. We can use the formula $U + D = V$. Because we know the power of the lens and the distance of the image from the lens, we can solve for U and therefore the distance from object to lens. $D = +24$ D and $V = 1/0.05$ m $= +20$ D (real image and converging light rays).

Thus, $U = V − D$, $U = 20−24 = −4$ D. Finally, to get the distance of the object from the lens, we must take the reciprocal of −4 D, which is 1/(−4 D) = −0.25 m or 25 cm to the left of the lens.

55. b. The refracting power of a spherical interface separating two media of different indices of refraction is given by

$D_s = (n_2 − n_1)/r$, where D_s = power of the surface, n_1 = refractive index of the first medium that the

light travels in, n_2 = refractive index of the second medium that the light travels in, and r = radius of curvature of surface in meters. $n_2 = 3.00$, $n_1 = 1.00$ (air), and $r = +0.5$ m. The sign of "r" is assigned by convention: r is positive if the center of curvature of the surface is on the opposite side of the origin of the incident light. If the center of curvature is on the same side of the interface as the origin of light, then r is negative. Thus, $D_s = (3−1)/+0.5 = +4.00$ D.

56. a. Hand–held magnifiers have a greater working distance (i.e., a greater eye to object distance). They are available in a range of powers from +3.00 to +68.00 D. However, they do have a smaller field of view than high adds and must be held in the hand.

57. d. Focal telescopes magnify without decreasing the working distance. Adds may be used to lessen the accommodative demand of these aids. However, they do have a small field of view and small depth of field, so the head must be positioned precisely.

58. c. Contact lenses also decrease the accommodative demand in a hyperopic patient.

59. d. When fitting rigid contact lenses, if there is greater than a 0.2 mm difference between the radii of the principal corneal meridians, then a lens of intermediate curvature, steeper than the flatter meridian by one-third to one-half the difference between meridians, can be used. This creates a positive tear film lens (add 0.25 D to every 0.05 mm difference in radius of curvature), so minus power must be added to the original power. The starting power is the *sphere* of the refraction written in minus cylinder form and corrected for vertex distance if necessary (powers greater than ±4.00 D). −4.00 +1.25 × 90 is equivalent to −2.75 +1.25 × 180 in positive cylinder form. A plus tear lens of +0.75 is created by the choice of 7.80 mm base curve (0.25 D for every 0.05 mm). Thus, −0.75 D must be added to −2.75 D. (Vertex distance is not important for powers <4.00 D.).

60. b. RGP lenses today tend to be made of silicone. They offer clearer vision and correct astigmatism. On the other hand, RGP lenses have a longer adaptation period and a greater difficulty of fit.

61. c. Both the Hruby lens (−55 D, planoconcave) and the Goldmann fundus contact lens (−64 D, planoconcave) essentially nullify the refractive power of the cornea and create an *upright, virtual* image of the fundus approximately 2 cm posterior to the lens.

62. c. Measurement of intraocular pressure (IOP) with applanation can be inaccurate if significant corneal astigmatism is present. An elliptical rather than a circular area will be applanated. Splitting the ellipse at a 43° angle to the major axis gives the best results. Alternatively, taking the mean of readings at 90° and 180° can reduce the error. With-the-rule cylinder causes underestimation (1 mm Hg/4 D) and against-the-rule cylinder causes overestimation of IOP. Forces of scleral rigidity and tear film surface tension cancel each other out.

63. a. The direct ophthalmoscope operates on the optical principle that light emanating from the retina of an emmetropic patient will be focused on the retina of an emmetropic observer. Lenses are used between the patient and observer to correct for nonemmetropic situations. In emmetropia, magnification obtained with the direct ophthalmoscope is approximately 15× because the patient's eye acts as a simple plus magnifier of power 60 D (*angular* magnification—$M = P/4$ or $60 D/4 = 15×$). In conditions of ametropia, the interposition of lenses creates a Galilean telescope. Therefore, if the patient is myopic, the retina appears more magnified, and if the patient is hyperopic or aphakic, it appears less magnified. Remember that in afocal systems, magnification must be considered in *angular* (not linear) terms.

64. d. A 30 D lens offers less magnification (2×) but a larger field of view than a 20 D lens. Although

axial magnification is the square of linear magnification, it must be reduced by a factor of 4 for indirect ophthalmoscopy because the patient's pupil is expanded by a factor of 4 for visualization by the examiner.

65. c. Conventional keratometry measures the curvature of only the central 3 mm of the cornea.

66. d. Good vision, including 20/20 vision, can be attained with proper ACIOL placement. Many complications related to ACIOL can be attributed to improper size of implant. These complications include uveitis, glaucoma, hyphema, dislocation of ACIOL, spinning of ACIOL, chronic CME, and Uveitis-Glaucoma-Hyphema (UGH) syndrome. Refractive error can also be a complication if not adjusted for during biometry should ACIOL placement be required.

67. c. The Hoffer Q formula is shown to be better for eyes with axial length <24.5 mm.

68. d. SRK/T is shown to be better for longer eyes. For eyes in between the two ranges, the Holladay 1 formula has been shown to be very accurate.

69. c. Applanation A-scan tends to give SHORTER axial length readings due to inadvertent indentation of the cornea during the procedure. Using immersion A-scan tends to be more accurate than applanation A-scan. Sound does indeed travel faster in the lens and cornea when compared to the aqueous and vitreous. In eyes with long axial length (>25.0 mm) B-scan and IOLMaster may be useful in determining an accurate axial length.

70. b. Refractive surgery for myopia flattens the central cornea. Most keratometers/corneal topographers miss this flattened central cornea. Keratometers take the readings from a 3.2 mm zone of the central cornea. Topography overestimates the power of the cornea. This can lead to a hyperopic error.

71. **c.** RK proportionately flattens both the anterior and posterior surface of the cornea. The index of refraction of the cornea is based on the association of the anterior and posterior curvature. PRK, LASIK, and LASEK change this ratio and thus the index of refraction of the cornea.

72. **b.** A-scan velocity through silicone oil is much slower than vitreous, 980 m/s (oil) and 1,532 m/s (vitreous). Silicone oil acts as a negative lens in the eye, thus IOL power usually needs to be increased to offset this action.

73. **a.** Disadvantages of multifocal IOLs include monocular diplopia, decrease in image clarity, decrease in contrast sensitivity, and decrease in night vision. Multifocal IOLs come in bifocal and multiple zone focus.

74. **c.** Vertical coma is a third-order refractive aberration. Others are listed below.
Second-order aberration: Astigmatism, Defocus
Third-order aberration: Trefoil, Horizontal coma
Fourth-order aberration: Tetrafoil, Secondary astigmatism, Spherical aberration.

75. **b.** The schematic emmetropic eye has about 60 D of power. The eye is a simple magnifier. At 25 cm, magnification = power/4 for the schematic eye. Therefore, the emmetropic schematic eye has a magnification of 15×. The more hyperopic the eye, the less magnification and the more myopic an eye the higher the magnification when using a direct ophthalmoscope.

76. **d.** Small pupils pose a challenge when using the indirect ophthalmoscope. The following can improve the ability to examine the fundus:
    1. Decreasing interpupillary distance.
    2. Decreasing the distance of the ophthalmoscope mirror and the observer.
    3. Increasing distance of eyepieces.
    4. Moving farther away from the patient.

77. **a.** The slit lamp optical components include astronomical telescope, inverting prism, Galilean telescope, objective lens, illumination system, and binocular viewing system. The astronomical component has two lenses that are both convex. The Galilean telescope has two lenses also, one convex and one concave.

78. **b.** The 60 D, 78 D, and 90 D lenses all produce images that are magnified, real, and inverted when examining the retina.

79. **c.** Optical focusing uses a specular microscope focused on the corneal endothelium. Optical doubling uses an image-doubling prism. Ultrasound and anterior segment ultrasound can be used also.

80. **d.** Laser interferometry is a good test for macular function. It is based on the principle that the cataractous lens has some clear spaces. For this test, one beam is optically split into two. This creates fringes on the retinal surface that can be appreciated. The fringes are not correlated to visual acuity.

81. **b.** The WHO defines legal blindness as best-corrected vision of 20/200 or worse in the better eye. The next question will address the second part of the requirement; visual field.

82. **b.** 20° or worse in the better eye. The combined definition is 20/200 or worse in the better eye or a visual field of 20° or worse in the better eye.

83. **c.** The Kestenbaum Rule is a starting point for determining the add needed for reading 1 M print. It is based on distance vision. For example, if a patient is 20/100, then take 100/20 = 5. This patient may benefit from a +5 D lens for viewing at 1/5 m. This is a good STARTING point for determining add.

84. **c.** The main advantage for stand magnifiers is the stability they can provide for patients with hand tremors or limitations of dexterity. These can provide a stable magnified image with little effort upon the patient. This allows the working distance to remain stable if the object is placed in a stable position.

85. b. 1.2 mm is the best size for a pinhole occluder. This allows a balance between diffraction and reducing inherent refractive error.

86. c. When testing near vision (Jaeger, Point type, or Reduced Snellen acuity), the conventional distance is usually 14 inches.

87. b. Visual evoked potential requires no response from the patient.

88. a. The Ferris-Bailey chart has five letters per line. Each space between letters is equal to the size of the letter on that specific line. Three line increases or decreases signify doubling or halving in the visual angle, respectively. This chart was used in the ETDRS and many subsequent studies.

89. d. Congenital glaucoma can cause acquired myopia due to increased axial length and increased corneal power. The others listed are causes of acquired hyperopia.

90. d. Posterior staphyloma causes acquired myopia since the eye wall is posterior to the point of focus. The other listed answers are causes of acquired hyperopia.

91. b. Sulfonamides can cause acquired myopia. Other medications that can cause acquired myopia include miotics, chlorthalidone, tetracycline, and carbonic anhydrase inhibitors. Acquired hyperopia can be caused by chloroquine, phenothiazines, benzodiazepines. Antihistamines may cause both acquired hyperopia and myopia.

92. c. Retinal disease may cause hyperopia and myopia but generally do not cause acquired astigmatism. Disorders that cause astigmatism are more anterior in nature.

93. d. Aphakic spectacles have several disadvantages. The lenses cause magnification, affect depth perception, cause a ring scotoma, and cause

pincushion distortion. The spectacles can also be heavy on the face and quite expensive.

94. b. The original SRK formula is $P = A - 2.5\,L - 0.9\,K$. This states that there is a 2.5 D/ 1 mm error for axial length and about a 1 to 1 diopter error for keratometry. Intraocular lens position is also important, and has about a 1 mm error = 1.0 D change in power ratio.

95. d. Pantoscopic tilt is used to decrease the amount of astigmatism of oblique incidence. This type of astigmatism is caused by tilting of a spherical lens. This adds the same power and cylinder as the original lens in the axis of the tilt. For example, tilting forward a +5 D lens will induce more plus spherical power AND plus cylinder power in the 180 axis. Most spectacles are tilted to give a compromised lens position for distance and near work.

96. d. CCTV is difficult for patients to use if they have manual dexterity issues. It is also not cheap or portable. It does, however, provide high levels of magnification for reading.

97. a. The Geneva lens clock measures radius of curvature of a spectacle lens. It usually is calibrated for crown glass.

98. c. The common pivot point or focus point is the most important feature of the slit lamp. It allows illumination and examination to be at the same point of focus.

99. d. Gradual steepening of the cornea throughout the waking hours leads to progressive myopia. Some patients require myopic correction as the day progress.

100. c. Applanation over a corneal scar will yield artificially high IOP measurements. All of the other answers listed will yield artificially *low* IOP measurements. Increased corneal thickness may also yield an artificially high IOP measurement during applanation.

CHAPTER 4

Ocular Pathology

■ Questions

1. Which of the following is true of a choristoma?
   a. There is hypotrophic, immature tissue present at a normal location.
   b. There is hyperplastic, mature tissue seen at a normal location.
   c. There is mature tissue at an abnormal location.
   d. A cavernous hemangioma is an example of a choristoma.

2. The most common intraconal orbital tumor is the
   a. meningioma.
   b. rhabdomyosarcoma.
   c. neurofibroma.
   d. cavernous hemangioma.

3. Which of the following is true regarding Russell bodies?
   a. Russell bodies result from production of erythropoetin.
   b. Russell bodies represent an aggregate of T cells.
   c. Russell bodies originate from plasma cells.
   d. Russell bodies occur only intracellularly.

4. All of the following are correct regarding corneal stromal wound healing except
   a. Keratin sulfate and chondroitin sulfate are the corneal glycosaminoglycans.
   b. Fibrovascular proliferation is a distinct aspect of the healing response.
   c. Normal wound healing depends on both the epithelium and endothelium.
   d. The subepithelial layer of the anterior, acellular stroma does not regenerate when incised.

5. Which of the following is true regarding anterior segment structures?
   a. The glycosaminoglycan found in sclera is chondroitin sulfate.
   b. Limbal wound healing involves scleral, episcleral, and corneal tissues.
   c. Iris stroma regenerates after injury, but iris melanocytes do not regenerate after injury.
   d. Retinal scars are produced by fibroblasts.

6. All of the following are correct regarding cyclodialysis except
   a. There is disinsertion of the longitudinal portion of the ciliary muscle from the scleral spur.
   b. Overproduction of aqueous humor and increased intraocular pressure are characteristic.
   c. There is free access of the aqueous humor to the suprachoroidal space.
   d. The condition is associated with a decreased blood supply to the ciliary body.

7. When obtaining a conjunctival biopsy for immunofluorescence studies in a patient suspected of having ocular cicatricial pemphigoid, what is the most appropriate solution to place the specimen?
   a. formalin.
   b. Zenker acetic fixative.
   c. glutaraldehyde.
   d. Michel fixative.

8. At approximately what rate does formalin diffuse through tissue?
   a. 0.5 mm/h.
   b. 1.0 mm/h.
   c. 2.0 mm/h.
   d. 5.5 mm/h.

9. A patient with lattice corneal dystrophy undergoes penetrating keratoplasty. All of the following tissue stains may be used to demonstrate the pathology in the corneal button specimen except
   a. thioflavin T.
   b. colloidal iron.
   c. crystal violet.
   d. Congo red.

10. What is the most helpful feature in distinguishing between a right and left eye specimen?
    a. the position of the vortex veins.
    b. the elliptical horizontal orientation of the cornea.
    c. the insertion of the inferior oblique muscle.
    d. the course of the long posterior ciliary artery and nerve.

11. Which of the following is true of traumatic angle recession?
    a. A fusiform appearance of the ciliary body is seen acutely.
    b. There is a plane of relative weakness between the oblique and circular muscle fibers of the ciliary body.
    c. The ciliary processes are anteriorly displaced.
    d. Damage to the ciliary body does not directly cause glaucoma.

12. All of the following are points of attachment of the uveal tract to the sclera except
    a. scleral spur.
    b. internal ostia of the vortex veins.
    c. peripapillary tissue.
    d. Schlemm's canal.

13. The definition of phthisis bulbi includes all of the following, except
    a. disorganization.
    b. atrophy.
    c. discomfort.
    d. shrinkage.

14. A patient suspected of having a schwannoma undergoes orbitotomy. What immunohistochemical stain is most appropriate to positively confirm the lesion is a schwannoma?
    a. HMB-45.
    b. S100.
    c. chromogranin.
    d. Her2Neu.

15. Which of the following is correct regarding the conjunctiva?
    a. The plica semilunaris is medial to the caruncle.
    b. The conjunctiva is formed of nonkeratinizing, stratified columnar epithelium and an underlying stroma.
    c. The palpebral conjunctiva lines a portion of the eyelids and contains lymphoid follicles in young individuals.
    d. Goblet cells are most numerous on the bulbar conjunctiva.

16. All of the following are true of dermolipomas, except
    a. The lesion is classified as a choristoma.
    b. There is often an absence of dermal adnexal structures within the lesion.
    c. The lesions tend to occur in the fornix at the inferotemporal quadrant.
    d. The lesion may extend into the orbit.

4

17. All of the following are correct regarding a pinguecula, except
   a. The stromal collagen in the lesion shows fragmentation.
   b. The stromal collagen in the lesion shows eosinophilic degeneration.
   c. There may be dysplasia of the overlying conjunctival epithelium.
   d. The lesion is caused by ultraviolet light.

18. All of the following are correct regarding a true conjunctival membrane, except
   a. The underlying epithelium is intact.
   b. Granulation tissue is present.
   c. Bleeding occurs when the membrane is removed.
   d. Fibrinopurulent exudates may occur.

19. Which of the following is correct regarding conjunctival amyloidosis?
   a. The condition is characterized by an eosinophilic, intracellular accumulation of hyaline-like material.
   b. The lesion usually reflects a systemic condition.
   c. There is an absence of dichroism when the specimen is stained with Congo red.
   d. The amyloid material collects within the substantia propria.

20. All of the following are true of hereditary benign intraepithelial dyskeratosis, except
   a. The condition has an autosomal dominant inheritance pattern.
   b. There may be lesions of the oral mucosa.
   c. The condition typically begins in the fourth to fifth decade of life.
   d. Dyskeratosis, acanthosis, and parakeratosis are characteristic.

21. All of the following may be helpful in characterizing a lymphoid lesion in a conjunctival biopsy, except
   a. flow cytometric analysis.
   b. polarization microscopy.
   c. immunoperoxidase staining.
   d. gene rearrangement studies.

22. What percentage of patients with primary acquired melanosis with atypia will progress to melanoma?
   a. 0%.
   b. 23%.
   c. 46%.
   d. 67%.

23. The corneal epithelium is composed of which of the following?
   a. stratified, squamous, nonkeratinizing epithelium.
   b. pseudostratified, columnar, nonkeratinizing epithelium.
   c. stratified, cuboidal, nonkeratinizing epithelium.
   d. bilayered, cuboidal, nonkeratinizing epithelium.

24. Which of the following anterior segment structures does not stain positively with the periodic acid-Schiff (PAS) stain?
   a. basement membrane of the corneal epithelium.
   b. Bowman's layer.
   c. Descemet's membrane.
   d. lens capsule.

25. The cornea is embryologically derived from which of the following?
   a. surface ectoderm.
   b. neural crest.
   c. mesoderm.
   d. surface ectoderm and neural crest.

26. All of the following are true of Descemet's membrane, except
   a. The membrane originates during fetal development.
   b. The membrane is composed of type IV collagen.
   c. The membrane gradually thins during adulthood.
   d. The membrane is produced by the corneal endothelium.

27. Which of the following is true of posterior keratoconus?
   a. Men are more often affected.
   b. Most cases are sporadic.
   c. Most cases are bilateral and nonprogressive.
   d. Descemet's membrane and the endothelium are usually absent in the area of the defect.

28. In comparing the two forms of congenital hereditary endothelial dystrophy, all of the following are correct, except
    a. The autosomal recessive form is more common.
    b. The autosomal dominant form appears later in life.
    c. The autosomal recessive form remains stable.
    d. The autosomal dominant form exhibits nystagmus.

29. Which of the following is correct regarding sclerocornea?
    a. Histologically, there is no differentiation between sclera and cornea.
    b. Women are more commonly affected.
    c. Most cases are unilateral.
    d. The condition is sporadic without a specific pattern of inheritance.

30. Which of the following organisms can be readily visualized using hematoxylin and eosin (H&E) stain preparations?
    a. *Actinomyces*.
    b. *Fusarium*.
    c. *Mucor*.
    d. *Acremonium*.

31. The photomicrograph (see image below) shows a corneal specimen. What is the most likely diagnosis for the patient?
    a. herpes simplex keratitis.
    b. *Aspergillus* infection.
    c. bullous keratopathy.
    d. *Acanthamoeba* infection.

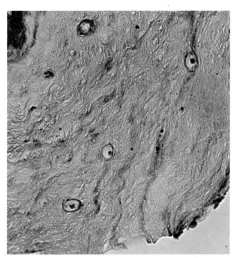

32. A patient with a corneal dystrophy undergoes penetrating keratoplasty. The corneal button is shown (see image, periodic acid-Schiff [PAS] stain, below). Which histologic stain would best demonstrate the patient's condition?
    a. Congo red.
    b. Alcian blue.
    c. Masson trichrome.
    d. hematoxylin and eosin.

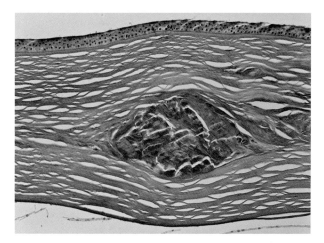

33. The corneal button of a patient is shown (see image, Alcian blue stain, below). Which of the following is true of the corneal dystrophy depicted?
    a. The condition is autosomal dominant.
    b. The lesions extend to the limbus.
    c. The accumulated material is birefringent.
    d. The abnormality has been mapped to chromosome 5q.

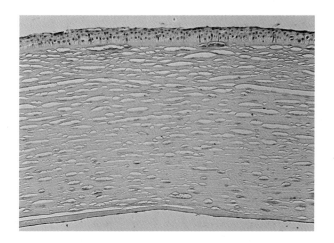

34. A lesion is removed from the limbus of a child (see image below). Which of the following is true?
    a. The epithelium is nonkeratining.
    b. The superotemporal quadrant is usually involved.
    c. There are associated congenital syndromes.
    d. There is an absence of skin adnexal structures.

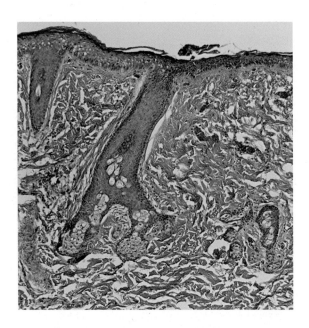

35. The corneal lesion shown had a golden-brown appearance clinically (see image below). What is the etiology of the histopathologic lesion in the figure?
    a. viral infection.
    b. ultraviolet light.
    c. chronic inflammation.
    d. topical anesthetic abuse.

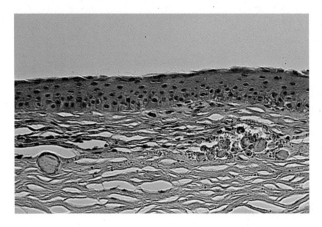

36. All of the following are potential causes of the histopathologic finding shown (see image below) of the posterior cornea, except
    a. pellucid marginal degeneration.
    b. endothelial dystrophy.
    c. terrien marginal degeneration.
    d. keratoconus.

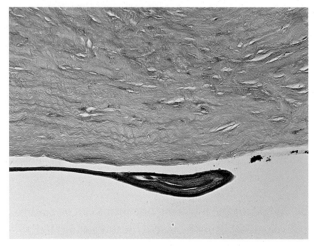

37. What material does the von Kossa stain shown in the photomicrograph confirm (see image below)?
    a. amyloid.
    b. calcium.
    c. iron.
    d. hemosiderin.

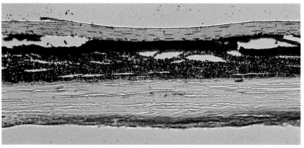

38. What is the diagnosis of the patient in question 37?
    a. pagetoid spread.
    b. keratoconus.
    c. Avellino dystrophy.
    d. band keratopathy.

39. The trabecular meshwork is derived from which of the following?
    a. endoderm.
    b. neural crest.
    c. mesoderm.
    d. surface ectoderm.

40. Which of the following is one of the structures that define the anterior chamber angle?
    a. ciliary body face.
    b. Schlemm's canal.
    c. iris pigment epithelium.
    d. external surface of the trabecular meshwork.

41. The photomicroph shows the corneal button of a patient that presented with a central opacity at birth (see image below). All of the following are typical of the condition, except
    a. absence of Descemet's membrane in the area of the defect.
    b. absence of the endothelium in the area of the defect.
    c. breaks in Bowman's layer.
    d. iridocorneal adhesions.

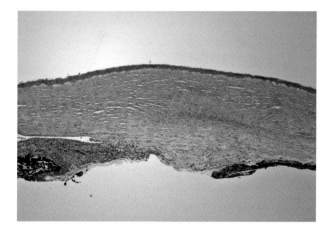

42. The condition of the patient in question 41 is characterized by which of the following?
    a. predominance of unilateral presentation.
    b. low risk of developing glaucoma.
    c. potential for improvement of corneal opacity.
    d. absence of associated syndromes.

43. The condition in the figure of question 41 is associated with all of the following, except
    a. persistent fetal vasculature.
    b. microphthalmia.
    c. aniridia.
    d. posterior polar cataract.

44. Abnormal proliferation of which of the following is a universal feature of all forms of the iridocorneal endothelial syndrome?
    a. trabecular meshwork.
    b. Descemet's membrane.
    c. corneal endothelium.
    d. iris stroma.

45. Which of the following is true regarding exfoliation (also known as pseudoexfoliation) syndrome?
    a. There is generalized depigmentation of the trabecular meshwork.
    b. There is splitting of the lens capsule.
    c. The accumulated material is PAS positive.
    d. The iris pigment epithelium is spared.

46. All of the following have been associated with exfoliation syndrome, except
    a. optic neuropathy.
    b. myocardial infarction.
    c. cerebrovascular events.
    d. orthostatic hypotension.

47. The sclera is derived from which of the following?
    a. surface ectoderm.
    b. mesoderm.
    c. neural crest.
    d. endoderm.

48. Which of the following is true of nanophthalmos?
    a. The eyes tend to have low to moderate myopia.
    b. The lens is of normal size.
    c. There is pathologic thinning of the sclera.
    d. The condition is typically unilateral.

49. The lens is derived from which of the following?
    a. surface ectoderm.
    b. endoderm.
    c. mesoderm.
    d. neural crest.

4

50. In patients with homocystinuria, the condition is caused by a defect in
    a. paired box gene 6 (PAX6).
    b. glutathione-S-transferase.
    c. cystathionine beta-synthase.
    d. lysine alpha-ketoglutarate reductase.

51. The condition of phacoantigenic endophthalmitis is mediated by which immunoglobulin?
    a. IgM.
    b. IgG.
    c. IgA.
    d. IgE.

52. All of the following statements about lens-induced uveitis and glaucoma are true, except:
    a. Phacoantigenic endophthalmitis is probably on the same spectrum as phacolytic glaucoma, simply being more severe.
    b. *Propionibacterium acnes* may be an important contributor to lens-induced uveitis, particularly in pseudophakic eyes.
    c. The classic pattern of inflammation in phacoantigenic endophthalmitis is the zonal granuloma centered about a site of injury to the lens.
    d. The stimulus for phacoantigenic uveitis appears to be lens cortical protein.

53. What is the average volume of the vitreous humor in adults?
    a. 10 mL.
    b. 8 mL.
    c. 4 mL.
    d. 2 mL.

54. The general characteristics of the secondary vitreous are which of the following?
    a. vascular and relatively cellular.
    b. avascular and relatively cellular.
    c. avascular and relatively acellular.
    d. vascular and relatively acellular.

55. All of the following may present as ocular inflammation (or pseudoinflammation), except
    a. non-Hodgkin's lymphoma.
    b. uveal melanoma.
    c. retinoblastoma.
    d. melanocytoma.

56. Which of the following is true regarding the phakomatous choristoma?
    a. The most frequent site of involvement is the eyelid.
    b. Phakomatous choristoma may be associated with ocular colobomata.
    c. There is frequently associated hyperpigmentation in phakomatous choristoma.
    d. Acquired forms of phakomatous choristoma have been reported.

57. All of the following are conditions that may be associated with granulomatous ocular inflammation, except
    a. sarcoidosis.
    b. rheumatoid arthritis.
    c. Behçet's disease.
    d. syphilis.

58. The earliest accumulations of cystoid macular edema (CME) fluid occur in the
    a. outer plexiform layer.
    b. nerve fiber layer.
    c. subretinal space.
    d. inner plexiform layer.

59. Due to variation in scleral thickness, at which of the following locations is globe rupture after blunt ocular trauma least likely to occur?
    a. in an arc at the limbus opposite the site of impact.
    b. at the insertion of the inferior oblique.
    c. at the equator of the globe.
    d. at the sclera immediately posterior to the lateral rectus insertion.

60. Which one of the following statements about retinal dialysis is false?
    a. Many patients with nontraumatic retinal dialysis will have a family history of retinal detachment.
    b. Most nontraumatic dialyses are superotemporal.
    c. Unlike typical retinal tears, the posterior vitreous is frequently attached in the setting of retinal dialysis.
    d. Retinal detachment caused by retinal dialysis is typically rapidly progressive.

61. All of the following are variations of the hyaloidolenticular vascular system, except
    a. persistent pupillary membrane.
    b. Mittendorf's dot.
    c. Bergmeister's papilla.
    d. persistent hyaloid artery.

62. The retinal circulation supplies all of the following layers, except
    a. inner plexiform layer.
    b. inner nuclear layer.
    c. ganglion cell layer.
    d. outer nuclear layer.

63. All of following are typical characteristics of the histopathology of diabetic eye disease, except
    a. lacy vacuolization of the iris pigment epithelium.
    b. thickening of the basement membrane of the ciliary epithelium.
    c. thinning of the corneal epithelial basement membrane.
    d. relative loss of pericytes.

64. Which of the following structures is the most sensitive to radiation?
    a. optic nerve.
    b. retina.
    c. lens.
    d. cornea.

65. Which of the following is true regarding the congenital tumor, phakomatous choristoma?
    a. It results from hyperplasia of the accessory lacrimal glands.
    b. Balloon cells are seen histologically.
    c. The upper eyelid is commonly affected.
    d. The material is PAS positive.

66. What is the etiology of the lesion shown in the photomicrograph (see image at the top of the right column)?
    a. ultraviolet light exposure.
    b. lipogranulomatous reaction.
    c. viral infection.
    d. hyperlipoproteinemic state.

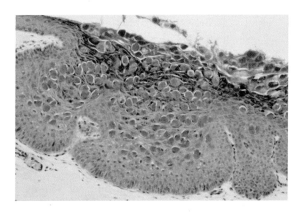

67. What clinical finding may commonly seen in the patient shown above?
    a. eyelid papules.
    b. follicular conjunctivitis.
    c. madarosis.
    d. meibomian gland inspissation.

68. The most common organisms for preseptal cellulitis in children are
    a. gram-positive rods.
    b. gram-positive cocci.
    c. gram-negative rods.
    d. gram-negative cocci.

69. Which of the following best characterizes the clear spaces shown in the photomicrograph (see image below)?
    a. The clear spaces result from fixation with neutral buffered formalin.
    b. The clear spaces result from processing the tissue for histology.
    c. The clear spaces are part of the cribriform pattern of a malignancy.
    d. The clear spaces represent accumulations of mucin.

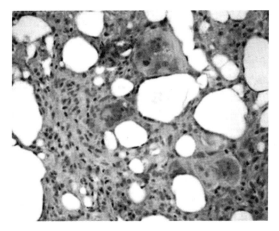

73

70. A biopsy is shown in the photomicrograph (see image below). What is the name of the sheet of configured protein in the condition?
   a. beta.
   b. lamda.
   c. alpha.
   d. kappa.

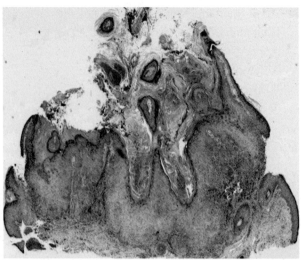

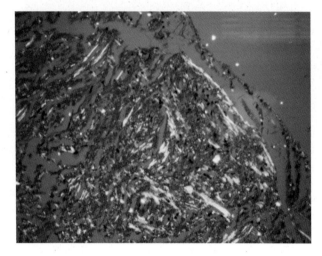

71. Which site of involvement has the highest association with a systemic disease process for the condition shown in question 70?
   a. eyelid.
   b. conjunctiva.
   c. orbit.
   d. lacrimal gland.

72. A 68-year-old patient presented with an eyelid lesion (see image at the top of the right column), which had grown over the last 6 weeks. Which of the following is true regarding this condition?
   a. Mitotic activity is often present at the superficial apices of the lesion.
   b. Perineural invasion is less likely than in squamous cell carcinoma.
   c. The central crater contains sebaceous material.
   d. Continued growth is likely over the next several months.

73. All of the following eyelid neoplasms are associated with systemic malignancies, except
   a. actinic keratoses.
   b. seborrheic keratoses.
   c. sebaceous adenomas.
   d. trichilemmomas.

74. What helpful diagnostic feature of squamous cell carcinoma is present throughout the photomicrograph (see image below)?
   a. keratin pearls.
   b. perineural invasion.
   c. separation artifact.
   d. intercellular bridges.

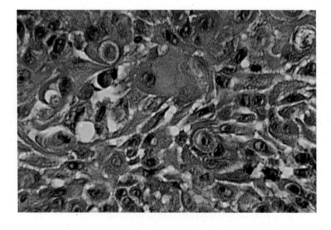

75. The photomicrograph shows a sagitally-oriented specimen depicting the orbit (right side of the figure) and superior half of the upper eyelid (left side of figure) (see image below). Which of the lettered anatomic sites (a–d) is incorrectly labeled?
   a. preaponeurotic fat pad.
   b. levator aponeurosis.
   c. upper eyelid tarsus.
   d. superior rectus muscle.

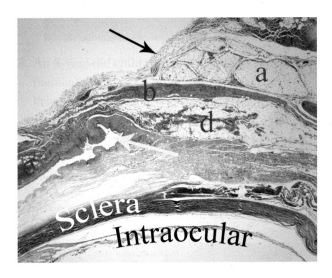

76. What structure does the black arrow mark in question 75?
   a. orbital septum.
   b. levator aponeurosis.
   c. levator muscle.
   d. superior transverse ligament.

77. What structure does the yellow arrow mark in the figure of question 75?
   a. plica semilunaris.
   b. caruncle.
   c. canaliculus.
   d. superior fornix.

78. A 74-year-old patient presents with a 1-year history of a growth along the upper eyelid margin. The photomicrographs show the results of the eyelid biopsy (see image at the top of the right column). What anatomic site is the origin of the lesion shown?
   a. meibomian glands of the tarsus.
   b. accessory lacrimal glands.
   c. basal layer of the epithelium.
   d. glands of Zeiss.

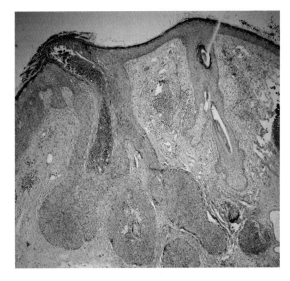

79. The biopsy results of a patient with a flat indurated eyelid plaque are shown (see image below). Which of the following is the treatment of choice for this lesion?
   a. Mohs micrographic surgery.
   b. exenteration.
   c. wide local excision.
   d. cryotherapy.

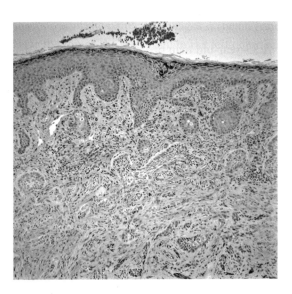

80. All of following are true, regarding the biopsy in the previous question (see image from question 79), except:
   a. The deep margin is positive.
   b. There is a desmoplastic reaction within the dermis.
   c. Separation artifact is present.
   d. Pagetoid spread is present.

97. The histopathology of a sulfur granule from a patient with purulent canalicular reflux is shown (see image, GMS stain, below). What would you use to treat this patient?
   a. metronidazole.
   b. penicillin G.
   c. valacyclovir.
   d. amphotericin B.

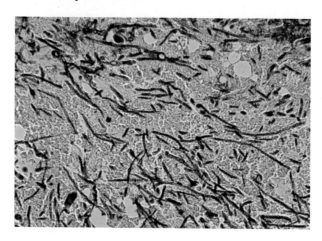

98. Which of the following is the most common ophthalmic site of metastasis for primary non-ocular tumors in children?
   a. orbit.
   b. choroid.
   c. retina.
   d. optic nerve.

99. Among patients younger than 5 years of age in the United States, which of the following is the most common presenting sign of retinoblastoma?
   a. hyphema.
   b. iris heterochromia.
   c. cataract.
   d. ocular inflammation.

100. The condition of a retinal capillary hemangioma (von Hippel's disease) is termed von Hippel's syndrome, when associated with which of the following?
   a. pancreatic cysts.
   b. renal cell carcinoma.
   c. cerebellar hemangioblastomas.
   d. pheochromocytomas.

Answers

1. **c.** Choice c is the definition of a choristoma. Dermoid cysts and dermolipomas are examples of choristomas. Choice b defines a hamartoma. Hemangiomas are a classic example of a hamartoma. Of note, Lisch nodules are iris hamartomas.

2. **d.** Cavernous hemangiomas are the most common benign neoplasm of the orbit in adults.

3. **c.** Russell bodies originate from plasma cells. Typically, Russell bodies are located intracellularly, but they can also occur extracellularly.

4. **b.** The cornea is avascular. Choice d refers to Bowman's layer, which does not regenerate when incised.

5. **b.** The limbal healing response involves are three tissue types seen at the limbus.

6. **b.** In cyclodialysis, there tends to be an underproduction of aqueous humor. Consequently, the intraocular pressure is decreased rather than increased. The other choices are correct.

7. **d.** Fresh tissue is needed for immunofluorescence (IF). While the Michel fixative is commonly referred to as a fixative, technically it is a transport medium, which does not fix the tissue and allows IF studies.

8. **b.** The formalin fixes the tissue at a rate of 1 mm/h. Thus an average globe with a radius of 12 mm needs at least 12 hours of fixation.

9. **b.** Colloidal iron stains mucopolysaccharides. Along with Alcian blue, the stain is useful in macular corneal dystrophy and Schnabel's cavernous optic atrophy. Thioflavin T, Crystal violet, and Congo red all stain amyloid, which is the substance seen in lattice corneal dystrophy.

10. **c.** Of the choices given, the insertion of the inferior oblique muscle is the only one specific for lateralizing a globe. The course of the long posterior ciliary artery and nerve and the oblong shape (in the horizontal meridian) of the cornea can facilitate differentiation of the horizontal and vertical axes of the globe, but not whether the eye is a right or left one.

11. **d.** Traumatic angle recession is an indirect indicator of potential damage to the trabecular meshwork. Recession of the angle itself does not directly cause glaucoma. The fusiform appearance of the ciliary body occurs over time and is a late finding. A plane of relative weakness exists between the longitudinal and circular muscles of the ciliary body. The ciliary processes are displaced posteriorly.

12. **d.** The uveal tract does not attach to the sclera in Schlemm's canal. The remaining three choices are the points of attachment of the uveal tract to the sclera.

13. **c.** Shrinkage, atrophy, and disorganization define phthisis bulbi. Pain or ocular discomfort may be a symptom of phthisis bulbi, but it is not a defining characteristic.

14. **b.** The S100 stain is markedly positive in schwannoma. HMB-45 reacts with melanocytic lesions and would only rarely react in the case of a schwannoma (e.g., a rare, pigmented schwannoma). Chromogranin stains neuroendocrine lesions, such as metastatic carcinoid, Merkel cell tumor, and small cell carcinoma. Her2Neu is positive in certain metastatic breast carcinomas.

15. **c.** Choice c is correct. The plica semilunaris is lateral to the caruncle. The conjunctival epithelium is stratified squamous. Goblet cells are most numerous in the plica and fornices.

16. **c.** Dermolipoma tends to occur in the superotemporal quadrant. The remaining choices are correct. Unlike a dermoid, dermolipomas often lack dermal adnexal structures.

4

17. **b.** The degeneration of the stromal collagen in a pinguecula is known as elastotic or basophilic degeneration. The other choices are correct. Histologically, the lesion is identical to a pterygium with the exception that a pterygium grows over the cornea and destroys Bowman's layer.

18. **a.** The underlying epithelium is absent in a true membrane. Because there is no underlying epithelium, clinically, once a true membrane is removed, bleeding occurs. The remaining choices are correct.

19. **d.** Amyloid collects within the substantia propria. The material is extracellular. Unlike in the orbit and eyelid, conjunctival amyloid usually reflects a localized process rather than a systemic condition. Less commonly, amyloid may occur in the setting of a chronic inflammatory condition, for example, trachoma, or a systemic condition, for example, multiple myeloma. When stained with Congo red, amyloid exhibits the properties of dichroism and birefringence.

20. **c.** Hereditary benign intraepithelial dyskeratosis (HBID) is an autosomal dominant condition. The rare condition was first described in a triracial population of Halifax County, North Carolina. The condition begins in early childhood. HBID is benign and does not undergo malignant transformation. Patients with HBID present with bilateral limbal conjunctival and oral mucosal plaques.

21. **b.** Polarization microscopy is useful for the assessment of amyloidosis and the detection of foreign material, but does not have a role in the evaluation of lymphoproliferative disease.

22. **c.** Nearly half of patients with primary acquired melanosis (PAM) with atypia will progress to melanoma. In contrast, PAM without atypia does not progress to melanoma.

23. **a.** The corneal epithelium is nonkeratinizing, stratified squamous epithelium and has a thickness of about four to six cells. Respiratory epithelium, such as that found in the nasolacrimal duct, is ciliated, pseudostratified, columnar.

24. **b.** Bowman's layer is the anterior, acellular aspect of the corneal stroma. It is not a true membrane and does not stain with PAS.

25. **d.** The cornea is both surface ectoderm and neural crest derived.

26. **c.** Descemet's membrane becomes gradually thicker as one ages.

27. **b.** Posterior keratoconus is typically sporadic, unilateral, and progressive. Women are more commonly affected. Descemet's membrane and the endothelium are typically intact.

28. **d.** The more common autosomal recessive form presents with nystagmus, whereas the autosomal dominant form does not.

29. **a.** Ninety percent of patients with sclerocornea are affected bilaterally. Men and women are equally affected. Half of cases are sporadic; half exhibit either a dominant or recessive pattern of inheritance.

30. **c.** *Mucor* is a relatively large nonseptate fungal organism. *Mucor* differs from the other three organisms in that *Mucor* is visible on H&E stain.

31. **d.** *Acanthamoeba* cysts are visible within the corneal stroma in the photomicrograph.

32. **a.** Unlike macular and granular dystrophies, lattice dystrophy stains positive with PAS (as seen in the image in question 32), Congo red, and crystal violet stains.

33. **b.** A photomicrograph of macular dystrophy is shown. Macular dystrophy involves the entire cornea, including up to the limbus. Macular dystrophy is autosomal recessive, while granular and lattice dystrophies are autosomal dominant.

Birefringent material collects in lattice dystrophy, but not macular. The genes for macular dystrophy and Avellino dystrophy are chromosomes 16q and 5q, respectively.

34. **c.** A corneal dermoid is covered by keratinizing stratified squamous epithelium and contains skin adnexal structures. A corneal dermoid is a choristoma and may be associated with congenital syndromes, for example, Goldenhar's syndrome. The superotemporal quadrant is the most frequent site of involvement for dermolipomas.

35. **b.** A photomicrograph of spheroidal degeneration (also known as actinic or Labrador keratopathy) is shown. The condition has a golden-brown appearance clinically and is caused by ultraviolet light exposure.

36. **b.** A discontinuity in Descemet's membrane is seen. Breaks in Descemet's membrane occur in choices a, c, and d, but not in endothelial dystrophy. The finding can also occur in obstetric forceps injury and congenital glaucoma.

37. **b.** Calcium stains positively with the von Kossa stain.

38. **d.** Calcium deposition in the corneal epithelial basement membrane and anterior stroma (including Bowman's' layer) is known as band keratopathy.

39. **b.** The trabecular meshwork arises from the neural crest.

40. **a.** The boundaries of the anterior chamber angle are the posterior cornea, the internal surface of the trabecular meshwork, the ciliary body face, and the anterior iris.

41. **c.** The corneal button of a patient with Peter's anomaly is shown. The abnormal posterior cornea and iris adhesions are seen. Bowman's layer is in the anterior cornea and is unaffected in Peter's anomaly.

42. **c.** The central opacity of Peter's anomaly may improve over time.

43. **d.** Peter's anomaly is associated with anterior cataracts (cortical or polar).

44. **c.** The corneal endothelium proliferates abnormally in all three forms of the iridocorneal endothelial syndrome.

45. **c.** The deposits stain positively with PAS and involve the anterior segment structures. There is increased pigment in the trabecular meshwork. Splitting of the lens capsule occurs in the rare true exfoliation syndrome, which is associated with exposure to infrared radiation, for example, glass blower's cataract.

46. **d.** Hypertension, rather than hypotension is associated with exfoliation syndrome. Choices a, b, and c have been associated with exfoliation syndrome.

47. **c.** The sclera arises from the neural crest.

48. **b.** In nanophthalmos, the eye is smaller than normal. The lens, however, may be either normal or enlarged. The condition is typically bilateral, results in hyperopia, is associated with glaucoma, and predisposed to uveal effusion (likely secondary to a thickened sclera).

49. **a.** The lens arises from the surface ectoderm.

50. **c.** Homocystinuria is an autosomal recessive condition with a defect in cystathionine beta-synthase. Homocystinuria is one of a number of systemic conditions associated with ectopia lentis. Classically, the lens is dislocated down (or inferonasal) in homocystinuria, whereas in Marfan's and Weill-Marchesani's syndromes, the lens is dislocated up and superotemporally (or temporal), respectively.

51. **b.** Phacoantigenic endophthalmitis is mediated by immunoglobulin G (IgG) directed against

globe just posterior to the word "Sclera" in the photomicrograph.

76. **a.** The black arrow shows the orbital septum, which is anterior to the preaponeurotic fat (structure "a").

77. **d.** The yellow arrow depicts the superior fornix.

78. **d.** Sebaceous carcinoma is seen arising from a gland of Zeiss. A normal pilosebaceous unit is seen to the right of the lesion.

79. **a.** A photomicrograph of the morpheaform (sclerosing) type of basal cell carcinoma is seen. Margin control with frozen sections or Mohs micrographic surgery is required.

80. **d.** Pagetoid spread is a characteristic of sebaceous carcinoma. Choices a–c are all present in the photomicrograph shown.

81. **b.** A photomicrograph of adenoid cystic carcinoma is shown. The tumor is unencapsulated and may arise de novo or from a pleomorphic adenoma. It is the basaloid pattern, rather than the cribriform pattern that carries a worse prognosis.

82. **b.** High and low magnification photomicrographs of a pleomorphic adenoma (benign mixed tumor [BMT]) are shown. BMT is the most common epithelial tumor of the lacrimal gland. Clinically, the tumor is more common in men (median age 35). The presentation is one of a painless lacrimal gland mass, which exhibits bony remodeling (rather than erosion) on CT imaging. The lesion can also occur in ectopic locations, accessory lacrimal gland sites, for example, Kraus or Wolfring, or in the salivary glands. Histologically, the lesion develops a capsule-like structure (pseudocapsule) from chronic compression of the surrounding tissue. The substance of the tumor is comprised of a mixture of epithelial and stromal components. The stroma may contain cartilage and bone. The epithelial aspect forms nests or tubules, which are lined by a bilayer of cells.

83. **b.** Please see discussion from previous question. In addition, inferonasal displacement is expected from a lacrimal gland mass. Complete removal, rather than incisional biopsy, is required to prevent tumor seeding.

84. **b.** A photomicroph of Lange's fold is seen. The fold is an expected finding and represents an artifact of fixation in the eyes of infants and children. Lange's fold is not present in unfixed eyes and does not occur in adult eyes.

85. **c.** MALT lymphomas arise from B cells and are generally CD5–, CD10–, and CD20+.

86. **d.** A photomicrograph of a medulloepithelioma (diktyoma) is shown. Medulloepithelioma is a rare, congenital tumor that arises from the nonpigmented ciliary epithelium. The tumor typically presents during the first decade of life. Clinically, the mass appears lightly pigmented or amelanotic. Ultrasound imaging may reveal large, highly reflective cysts posterior to the iris that are characteristic of the tumor. Histologically, the tumor secretes hyaluronic acid, which stain positively with Alcian blue. In addition, Homer Wright rosettes may be seen with light microscopy.

87. **d.** The photomicrograph shows Aspergillus organisms. Aspergillus are septate hyphae with a 45° angle branching pattern. The patient described has allergic aspergillosis sinusitis, which occurs in immunocompetent individuals. Peripheral eosinophilia occurs in patients with allergic aspergillosis sinusitis. CT imaging may show bony erosion or remodeling. The condition is treated with steroid therapy and potentially surgical debridement.

88. **c.** Choices a, b, and d are all encapsulated. Lymphangioma is unencapsulated.

89. **c.** A neurilemoma (schwannoma) is seen in the photomicrographs. The tumor arises from Schwann cells. Two histologic patterns are seen.

Figure (A) shows the Antoni A pattern, which has tightly configured spindle cells and palisading nuclei (may form Verocay bodies). Figure B shows the Antoni B pattern, which is characterized by myxoid appearance and loosely arranged cells. The areas of Antoni B correspond with tumor degeneration. Histologically, the lesion is markedly S100 positive with immunohistochemical staining. A schwannoma of the eighth cranial nerve is known as an acoustic neuroma and is associated with neurofibromatosis type 2. Sensory corpuscles are unrelated to schwannomas.

90. **d.** The botryoid variant originates from the embryonal type of rhabdomyosarcoma.

91. **a.** The patient has neurofibromatosis type 1 (NF1). NF2 (not NF1) is associated with posterior subcapsular cataracts. Choices b–d are associated with NF1. Lisch nodules are iris hamartomas. Orbital encephalocele may occur in the setting of dysplasia of the greater wing of the sphenoid bone. Optic nerve gliomas (and much less commonly meningiomas) also have associations with NF1.

92. **a.** A plexiform neurofibroma, which is composed of Schwann cells, axons, and endoneural fibroblasts, is shown. The tumor is unencapsulated. Plexiform neurofibromas occur in about 30% of patients with NF1 and are highly specific for NF1. Although widely described, in actuality, the bag-of-worms feel occurs infrequently.

93. **d.** The patient presents with a cavernous hemangioma. Pregnancy may accelerate the growth of the tumor.

94. **b.** There are no fluorescein angiographic signs that are pathognomonic for choroidal melanoma (or for any intraocular tumor, for that matter). Subretinal hemorrhage (most frequently from choroidal neovascularization) can be differentiated from melanoma by the absence of late hyperfluorescence characteristic of melanoma.

95. **a.** An optic nerve glioma is shown. In patients without neurofibromatosis, the tumor tends to remain confined to the optic nerve. In patients with neurofibromatosis, the tumor often proliferates in the subarachnoid space. Rosenthal fibers are not unique to optic nerve glioma.

96. **c.** The lesion shown is a xanthogranuloma. It is characterized by the presence of Touton's giant cells (shown in the image B in question 96). Patients with iris lesions secondary to juvenile xanthogranulomas are at risk for spontaneous hyphema and consequent secondary glaucoma.

97. **b.** Actinomyces is a gram-positive non–acid-fast anaerobic bacteria. The bacteria also stain positively with GMS. The bacteria form long, fine branching filaments. The organism can grow as a cluster, known as a sulfur granule. Appropriate treatment consists of removal of the canalicular concretions and antibiotic therapy. A number of antibiotics are effective in the treatment of actinomyces; however, metronidazole does not have any effect on the organism.

98. **a.** In adults, the choroid is the most common site of ocular/periocular metastasis. In children, however, the orbit is more commonly involved.

99. **d.** For children under 5 years of age, in the United States (in order of frequency), the three most common presenting signs of retinoblastoma are leukocoria (54%–62%), strabismus (18%–22%), and ocular inflammation (2%–10%). Choices a–c also occur, but are not in the top three.

100. **c.** Retinal capillary hemangiomatosis associated with cerebellar hemangioblastoma is termed von Hippel-Lindau syndrome. Other lesions, including renal cell carcinoma and pheochromocytoma, are associated but are not a part of the definition of the syndrome. Multiple retinal angiomas (without cerebellar tumors) are referred to as von Hippel's disease.

4

CHAPTER 5

Neuroophthalmology

Questions

1. A patient presents complaining of decreased vision in the left eye. His acuities are 20/20 in the right eye and 20/100 in the left eye. The examination is entirely unremarkable, and the diagnosis of factitious visual loss is considered. The test that would be most useful in establishing this diagnosis is
   a. optokinetic nystagmus testing.
   b. gently rocking a large mirror in front of the patient with the good eye occluded.
   c. introducing a prism base up in front of the left eye while the patient is reading binocularly.
   d. performing a fogging refraction.

2. Which one of the following concerning the visual evoked response (VER) is false?
   a. The VER is an electrical signal that must be extracted from the simultaneously generated electroencephalogram (EEG).
   b. The stimulus may consist of either a flash of white light or a pattern, presented either transiently or continuously via pattern reversal.
   c. The two critical parameters used for functional evaluation include the height of the first positive or upward wave (amplitude) and the amount of time between stimulus presentation and the appearance of this wave (latency).
   d. Uses of the flash VER include visual acuity assessment in preverbal children, assessment of optic nerve function in suspected multiple sclerosis, and reliable establishment of factitious visual loss.

3. Which of the following is true of cancer-associated retinopathy (CAR)?
   a. ERG findings are typically normal.
   b. The underlying tumor expresses an antigen that is homologous to a 23-kd retinal photoreceptor protein identified as the calcium-binding protein recoverin.
   c. The underlying cancer is typically breast cancer.
   d. Vision loss is stationary.

4. Which of the following is true of melanoma-associated retinopathy (MAR)?
   a. This syndrome primarily involves the rods.
   b. ERG is typically normal.
   c. Treatment is effective for MAR.
   d. MAR is a common syndrome in patients diagnosed with melanoma.

5. Which of the following concerning magnetic resonance imaging (MRI) is true?
   a. Long repetition times (TR) and long echo times (TE) are used to generate T1-weighted images.
   b. On a T1-weighted image, vitreous is dark, and on a T2-weighted image, vitreous is bright.
   c. Air and cortical bone give a bright (hyperintense) signal on MRI.
   d. T1-weighted images tend to show pathology well, whereas T2-weighted images tend to show anatomy well.

6. Which one of the following concerning the intracranial portion of the optic nerve is false?
   a. It is typically 10 to 17 mm in length.
   b. It enters the intracranial cavity medial to the internal carotid artery.
   c. There is generally some redundancy within the intracranial optic nerve.
   d. Once it enters the intracranial cavity, the optic nerve no longer has a sheath.

7. Which of the following concerning the optic chiasm is true?
   a. As many fibers cross as do not cross.
   b. The posterior portion of the chiasm has a high density of macular fibers.
   c. The chiasm typically lies 1 mm above the anterior pituitary gland.
   d. The superior fibers are the first to cross.

8. Which of the following retrochiasmal locations can induce a monocular visual field defect with a single lesion alone?
   a. lateral geniculate body.
   b. parietal lobe.
   c. temporal lobe.
   d. occipital lobe.

9. The lateral geniculate body is divided into six layers and they are segregated depending on which eye the axons originate. Which layers of the lateral geniculate receive axons from the ipsilateral eye versus the contralateral eye?
   a. The contralateral eye terminates in layers 1, 2, and 3; the ipsilateral eye terminates in layers 4, 5, and 6.
   b. The contralateral eye terminates in layers 1, 3, and 6; the ipsilateral eye terminates in layers 2, 4, and 5.
   c. The contralateral eye terminates in layers 1, 4, and 6; the ipsilateral eye terminates in layers 2, 3, and 5.
   d. The contraleral eye terminates in layer 2, 3, and 5; the ipsilateral eye terminates in layers 1, 4, and 6.

10. Which of the following features is consistent with a temporal lobe lesion?
    a. unformed visual hallucinations.
    b. optokinetic nystagmus (OKN) abnormalities.
    c. formed visual hallucinations.
    d. high congruity of visual field deficits.

11. Which of the following features is not consistent with a parietal lobe lesion?
    a. agnosia.
    b. right–left confusion.
    c. OKN abnormalities.
    d. homonymous hemianopia denser superiorly.

12. Which of the following features is not consistent with an occipital lobe lesion?
    a. OKN abnormalities.
    b. unformed hallucinations.
    c. macular sparing.
    d. sparing of the temporal crescent.

13. The cause of optic disc edema is
    a. swollen peripapillary myelinated nerve fiber layer.
    b. extracellular fluid accumulation.
    c. interruption of axonal transport.
    d. breakdown of the blood retinal barrier.

14. Which of the following concerning papilledema is true?
    a. Loss of venous pulsations is a particularly specific finding.
    b. Symptoms accompanying papilledema may include visual loss and transient obscurations of vision.
    c. The most typical visual field finding in chronic papilledema is an enlarged blind spot.
    d. Papilledema is more commonly unilateral.

15. Which of the following are universal findings in patients with pseudotumor cerebri?
    a. papilledema.
    b. abnormal cerebrospinal fluid composition.
    c. normal neurologic examination.
    d. increased intracranial pressure.

5

16. Indication for treatment of pseudotumor cerebri includes which of the following?
    a. papilledema.
    b. obesity.
    c. visual field loss.
    d. optic disc drusen.

17. Pseudotumor cerebri, also known as idiopathic intracranial hypertension (IIH), can be associated with the use of all of the exogenous substances except
    a. acetylsalicylic acid.
    b. nalidixic acid.
    c. tetracycline.
    d. vitamin A.

18. The most common cause of permanent visual loss in patients with cavernous sinus–dural fistulae is
    a. neovascular glaucoma.
    b. corneal exposure.
    c. open-angle glaucoma.
    d. choroidal effusions.

19. All of following concerning giant cell arteritis are true except:
    a. It is exceedingly rare in patients <50 years old and is more common in females.
    b. Forty percent of untreated patients will develop some form of permanent visual loss.
    c. Ninety-five percent of untreated patients will have contralateral involvement of the other eye, within days to weeks.
    d. Visual loss is typically mild with visual acuity being better than 20/100 in 60% of the patients.

20. A 63-year-old male walks in with complaints of sudden onset of blurring of vision in his right eye. His visual acuity when checked is 20/30 in that eye. The patient's history includes hypertension and diabetes. The patient currently has no other systemic symptoms. A photo of his right optic nerve and his visual field is shown at the top of the next column (images A and B). His left optic nerve is normal with a cup/disc ratio of 0.1. What is his most likely diagnosis?
    a. arteritic anterior ischemic optic neuropathy (AAION).
    b. nonarteritic anterior ischemic optic neuropathy (NAION).

c. myelinated nerve fiber layer.
d. optic disc drusen.

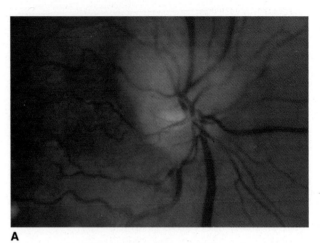

A

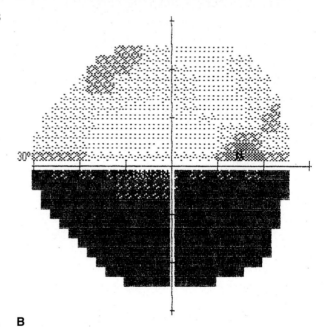

B

21. Which one of the following concerning the patient in question 20 is not true?
    a. Visual loss is generally less severe than in the arteritic variety.
    b. The condition most frequently associated with it is hypertension.
    c. Fluorescein angiography is usually not of benefit in differentiating optic neuritis from this condition.
    d. There is approximately a 15% chance of subsequent occurrence in the contralateral eye within 5 years.

22. Treatment for the condition in question 20 is
    a. observation.
    b. corticosteroids.
    c. immunomodulators.
    d. hyperbaric oxygen.

23. Approximately what percentage of patients with optic neuritis (and no lesions observed on MRI at the time of the attack) will develop multiple sclerosis (MS) at 15-year follow-up?
    a. 1%.
    b. 5%.
    c. 10%.
    d. 25%.

24. What percentage of patients with severe MS will, on autopsy examination, have demyelinated lesions of the optic nerves?
    a. 10%.
    b. 25%.
    c. 50%.
    d. more than 90%.

25. Which of the following concerning optic nerve glioma is true?
    a. Optic nerve glioma is more frequently seen in children than adults.
    b. The vast majority of patients will have associated neurofibromatosis.
    c. Optociliary shunt vessels of the disc occur more commonly with optic nerve gliomas than with meningiomas of the optic nerve.
    d. These tumors are more likely to be aggressively malignant in children than in adults.

26. Which of the following concerning optic nerve meningiomas is true?
    a. It primarily affects children.
    b. The majority of patients will have associated neurofibromatosis.
    c. On computed tomography (CT) scanning, affected optic nerves have a "kinked" appearance.

d. These tumors are more likely to be aggressively malignant in children than in adults.

27. All of the following are true regarding autosomal dominant optic atrophy except:
    a. The most common hereditary optic neuropathy.
    b. Dominant optic atrophy is usually slowly progressive throughout life.
    c. Presentation typically occurs in the first decade of life.
    d. At detection, visual acuity loss is usually moderate, in the range of 20/50 to 20/70.

28. Which of the following concerning Leber's hereditary optic neuropathy (LHON) is false?
    a. All offspring of a female carrier are either affected or carriers.
    b. Ten percent of female carriers will be affected.
    c. LHON is generally unilateral with vision loss occurring only in the affected eye.
    d. A small percentage of patients will enjoy partial recovery late in their course.

29. LHON mitochondrial DNA mutation occurs most frequently at which position of the mitochondrial DNA?
    a. 11778.
    b. 3460.
    c. 14484.
    d. 8280.

30. A 23-year-old man presents complaining of sudden loss of vision in his right eye. His acuities are 20/200 in the right eye and 20/20 in the left eye. Examination is normal with exception of a swollen optic nerve, dilated retinal veins, and scattered dense retinal hemorrhages. The factor that most convincingly argues against the diagnosis of papillophlebitis is the patient's
    a. age.
    b. sex.
    c. visual acuity.
    d. retinal hemorrhages.

48. The finding that all three types of Duane's syndrome share is
   a. a deficit of abduction.
   b. a deficit of adduction.
   c. globe retraction with adduction.
   d. esotropia.

49. Which one of the following concerning oculomotor apraxia is false?
   a. Pursuits are generally affected more than saccades.
   b. Horizontal movements are generally affected much more than vertical movements.
   c. In the acquired form, blinks are frequently used to break fixation.
   d. In the congenital form, children frequently use compensatory exaggerated head turns to refixate.

50. The saccadic movement that is often affected in progressive supranuclear palsy (PSP) is
   a. upward.
   b. downward.
   c. leftward.
   d. rightward.

51. Hypertropia associated with ipsilateral adduction weakness is most suggestive of
   a. decompensated congenital fourth nerve palsy.
   b. dorsal midbrain syndrome.
   c. "One-and-a-half" syndrome.
   d. skew deviation with internuclear ophthalmoplegia (INO).

52. The dorsal midbrain syndrome is associated with all of the following except
   a. upward gaze paresis.
   b. paradoxic OKN.
   c. light-near dissociation.
   d. lid retraction.

53. Which of the following would not normally be found in congenital nystagmus?
   a. oscillopsia.
   b. amplitude increased by distance fixation.
   c. paradoxic OKN.
   d. amplitude dampened by convergence.

54. A 43-year-old man presents complaining of persistent red eye in the right eye (seen in the image below), present ever since a car accident 6 weeks earlier. Besides redness, he has noted intermittent horizontal diplopia without pain. The results of his examination are normal, except for 4 mm of proptosis on the right, a mild deficit in abduction, and prominent conjunctival vessels. His left eye is entirely normal. What is the most likely diagnosis?
   a. carotid cavernous sinus fistula.
   b. dural sinus fistula.
   c. cavernous sinus thrombosis.
   d. viral conjunctivitis.

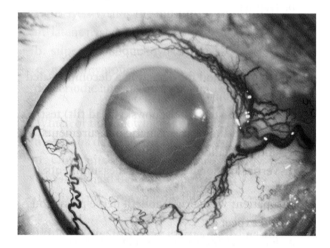

55. Which of the following ocular motor disorders is most associated with malignancy?
   a. square-wave jerks.
   b. opsoclonus.
   c. dysmetria.
   d. ocular bobbing.

56. Monocular nystagmus in a toddler raises the specter of
   a. optic nerve meningioma.
   b. craniopharyngioma.
   c. rhabdomyosarcoma.
   d. chiasmal glioma.

57. According to Alexander's law, in which position should upbeat nystagmus be most prominent?
   a. upgaze.
   b. downgaze.
   c. left gaze.
   d. right gaze.

58. Which pattern of nystagmus is most commonly found in patients with large tumors in the parasellar region?
    a. upbeat nystagmus.
    b. vestibular nystagmus.
    c. downbeat nystagmus.
    d. see-saw nystagmus.

59. Which visual field defect is most likely to be associated with see-saw nystagmus?
    a. central scotoma.
    b. bitemporal hemianopia.
    c. incongruous hemianopia.
    d. congruous hemianopia.

60. Which of the following eye movements is not matched correctly with its corresponding site of origin?
    a. Vestibular ocular reflex—Brainstem.
    b. Saccades—Contralateral frontal lobe.
    c. Pursuit—Ipsilateral parietal lobe.
    d. Vergence—Brainstem.

61. Which one of the following concerning the facial nerve is false?
    a. The sensory innervation of the anterior two-thirds of the tongue terminates in the nucleus solitarius, and the motor innervation to the lacrimal gland arises, in part, from the superior salivatory nucleus.
    b. The first branch of the facial nerve is the greater superficial petrosal nerve, which synapses in the geniculate ganglion.
    c. Within the fallopian canal, the facial nerve gives off a motor branch to the stapedius muscle and sensory branches for the skin behind the ear.
    d. Nerves from the chorda tympani synapse in the geniculate ganglion, carrying sensory innervation to the tongue and motor innovation to the salivary glands.

62. Which of the following concerning Marcus Gun jaw-winking syndrome is false?
    a. It is an example of aberrant regeneration.
    b. The patient can present with ptosis.
    c. The eyelid can elevate upon opening of the mouth.
    d. It is a synkinetic movement of the eyelid associated with jaw movement.

63. A 26-year-old female presents to your office with blurred vision for 3 days in her left eye. Fundus examination reveals disc edema with a macular star. She has no medical problems including diabetes or hypertension. You astutely diagnose her has having neuroretinitis. What is the most likely cause?
    a. underlying hypertension.
    b. underlying diabetes.
    c. *Bartonella henselae*.
    d. multiple sclerosis.

64. Which of the following cranial nerves is most frequently involved cranial nerve in sarcoidosis?
    a. CN II.
    b. CN III.
    c. CN VII.
    d. CN VIII.

65. Which of the following is true regarding hemifacial spasm?
    a. It is bilateral.
    b. Most commonly occurs because of compression of the seventh nerve root by an aberrant vessel.
    c. Functional neuroimaging suggests that it may be caused by basal ganglia dysfunction.
    d. It is a benign condition, so neuroimaging is not needed once it is diagnosed.

66. Facial myokymia in a child is frequently associated with
    a. chiasmal glioma.
    b. spasmus nutans.
    c. cerebellar hemangioblastoma.
    d. pontine glioma.

67. Which of the following is false regarding essential blepharospasm?
    a. Onset typically occurs after age 65.
    b. Causes of reflex blepharospasm, for example, dry eyes or ocular irritation should be ruled out.
    c. It is a bilateral condition.
    d. Treatment of choice is injection of botulinum toxin into the orbicularis muscle.

5

5

68. Which of the following regarding the pupillary reflex is true?
    a. The pupil pathway terminates in pretectal nuclei after passing, without synapsing, through the lateral geniculate body (LGB).
    b. The decussation at the chiasm is responsible for a normal consensual pupillary response.
    c. Sympathetic pupillary fibers originate in the superior cervical ganglion, travel in the cranial vault with the internal carotid artery, and enter the orbit with the ophthalmic artery through the optic foramen.
    d. The pathway for accommodative miosis enters the Edinger-Westphal nucleus anterior to the pathway for light-induced miosis.

69. Which of the following statements concerning these conditions with light-near dissociation is true?
    a. A key finding in the diagnosis of Argyll Robertson pupils is the presence of mydriasis.
    b. Argyll Robertson pupils react to light, but do not have a near response.
    c. The most common etiology of the dorsal midbrain syndrome in a child under 10 years of age is a pineal gland tumor.
    d. The most common etiology for the dorsal midbrain syndrome in a patient over the age of 60 is multiple sclerosis (MS).

70. Which one of the following concerning Adie's tonic pupil is false?
    a. The majority of affected patients will have unilateral involvement.
    b. Patients may have accommodative symptoms or photophobia.
    c. Pupillary constriction in response to pilocarpine 1% is conclusive evidence of denervation hypersensitivity.
    d. The differential diagnosis of a tonic pupil includes herpes zoster, syphilis, and giant cell arteritis.

71. Which of the following concerning Horner's syndrome is true?
    a. The distribution of anhidrosis does not help in localizing the lesion.
    b. Cocaine 4% will dilate the pupil of the patient with Horner's syndrome, whereas it will leave a normal pupil unchanged.
    c. The evaluation of a patient whose miotic pupil does not dilate with topical cocaine, but does dilate with topical hydroxyamphetamine consists, in part, of chest x-ray and careful neurologic examination.
    d. Horner's syndrome with coincident ipsilateral headache is benign and requires no further neuroimaging.

72. Which of the following statements regarding the condition shown below is false?
    a. The successful use of photodynamic therapy (PDT) to treat this condition has been reported.
    b. Vitreous hemorrhage can occur spontaneously in this condition.
    c. Patients with no other medical history presenting with a similar fundus should undergo neuroimaging.
    d. An orbital bruit can be heard in patients with this condition.

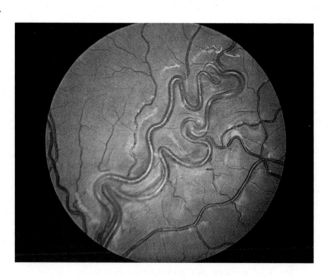

73. Which of the following statements regarding the condition shown below is false?
   a. The condition is unilateral.
   b. Retinal vessels originating from the periphery of the disc is a classic finding.
   c. Visual acuity is often good.
   d. The patient may have an RAPD.

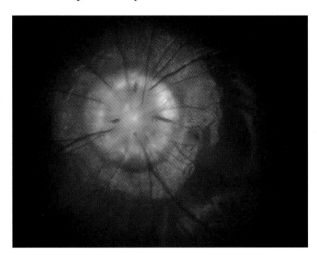

74. A patient with the lesion shown in the pathology slide below most likely has
   a. choroidal melanoma.
   b. medulloepithelioma.
   c. congenital hypertrophy of the retinal pigment epithelium.
   d. melanocytoma.

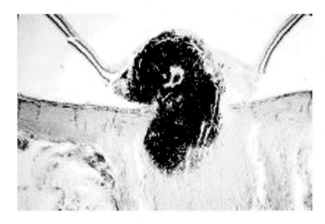

75. Pheochromocytoma may be seen in patients with
   a. Sturge-Weber syndrome.
   b. tuberous sclerosis.
   c. von Hippel-Lindau disease.
   d. ataxia–telangiectasia.

76. A 23-year-old male was found to have to have the retinal abnormality found below. This is a
   a. retinal cavernous hemangioma.
   b. racemose angioma.
   c. retinal capillary hemangioma.
   d. astrocytic hamartoma.

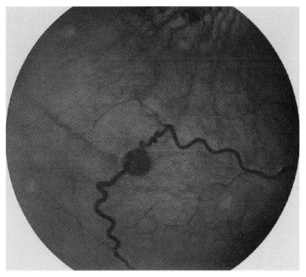

77. The lesion above is associated with which phakomatoses?
   a. Sturge-Weber syndrome.
   b. von Hippel-Lindau disease.
   c. tuberous sclerosis.
   d. ataxia–telangiectasia.

78. The next step following examination of the patient in question 76 would be
   a. observation.
   b. radiation therapy.
   c. prompt referral of the patient for a thorough systemic investigation.
   d. prescription of epileptic medications.

79. A 42-year-old male's retinal findings are seen at the top of the next page. What is the diagnosis?
   a. retinal cavernous hemangioma.
   b. racemose angioma.
   c. retinal capillary hemangioma.
   d. astrocytic hamartoma.

5

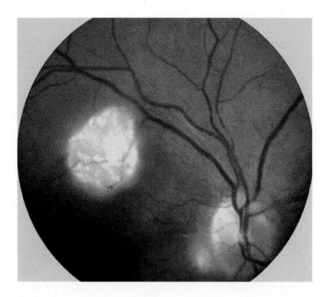

5

80. The lesion shown in question 79 is more commonly associated with which phakomatoses?
   a. Sturge-Weber syndrome.
   b. von Hippel-Lindau disease.
   c. tuberous sclerosis.
   d. ataxia–telangiectasia.

81. The next step following examination of the patient in question 79 would be
   a. observation.
   b. laser therapy.
   c. I-125 plaque therapy.
   d. chemotherapy.

82. Glaucoma is associated with which phakomatoses?
   a. von Hippel-Lindau disease.
   b. tuberous sclerosis.
   c. Sturge-Weber syndrome.
   d. ataxia–telangiectasia.

83. Chronic sinopulmonary infections may be seen as part of
   a. neurofibromatosis.
   b. tuberous sclerosis.
   c. angiomatosis retinae.
   d. ataxia–telangiectasia.

84. All of the following can have chronic progressive external ophthalmoplegia (CPEO) except
   a. myotonic dystrophy.
   b. oculopharyngeal dystrophy.

c. thyroid eye disease.
   d. Kearns-Sayre syndrome.

85. Which one of the following concerning Kearns-Sayre syndrome is false?
   a. The complete syndrome has an onset of symptoms or signs before age 20 years.
   b. The pigmentary retinopathy is generally associated with good visual function throughout life.
   c. The progressive external ophthalmoplegia associated with the syndrome typically presents as diplopia.
   d. Heart block develops late in the course of the syndrome.

86. Which of the following statements is false regarding monocular diplopia?
   a. There are no genetic syndromes associated with monocular diplopia.
   b. It can be caused by retinal pathologies.
   c. It can be caused by lenticonus.
   d. It can be caused by high astigmatism.

87. The most common sign of Graves' ophthalmopathy is
   a. lid retraction.
   b. conjunctival injection over the horizontal rectus muscles.
   c. esotropia.
   d. proptosis.

88. The most frequently involved extraocular muscle in Graves' ophthalmopathy is the
   a. inferior rectus.
   b. lateral rectus.
   c. superior rectus.
   d. medial rectus.

89. A patient with a history of bilateral occipital lobe infarcts adamantly states that he can see quite well and confabulates visual images. He most likely suffers from
   a. Anton's syndrome.
   b. palinopsia.
   c. Charles Bonnet's syndrome.
   d. blindsight.

90. What percentage of patients with myasthenia gravis (MG) present with ocular findings only?
    a. 10%.
    b. 25%.
    c. 50%.
    d. 75%.

91. What percentage of patients with myasthenia gravis will develop Graves' disease?
    a. 5%.
    b. 10%.
    c. 15%.
    d. 20%.

92. What percentage of patients with myasthenia gravis have thymomas visible on CT?
    a. 1%.
    b. 10%.
    c. 25%.
    d. 50%.

93. For a patient to be reassured that systemic disease is unlikely, ocular myasthenia should remain localized for what length of time?
    a. 6 months.
    b. 1 year.
    c. 2 years.
    d. 5 years.

94. Animal studies show that irreversible ischemic retinal damage occurs after what duration of retinal vascular occlusion?
    a. 30 minutes.
    b. 90 to 100 minutes.
    c. 3 hours.
    d. 6 hours.

95. Typical symptoms in vertebrobasilar insufficiency include all of the following except
    a. ataxia.
    b. hemiparesis.
    c. vertigo.
    d. monocular blurring or loss of vision.

96. A 29-year-old woman presents to an ophthalmologist complaining of pain on eye movements and blurry vision in her right eye. Review of systems documents a 3-week history of paresthesias in the right lower leg approximately 6 months prior to the onset of her visual disturbance. The patient reports that she noticed her visual disturbance develop over the 2 or 3 days prior to presentation. Examination discloses a visual acuity of 20/60 in the right eye and 20/20 in the left eye. She is able to interpret correctly 4 of 11 Ishihara plates with her right eye and 10 of 11 plates with her left eye. Visual fields disclose a central scotoma in the right eye and are normal for the left eye. There is no afferent pupillary defect (APD) noted. Which one of the following is most likely true?
    a. The patient probably has an acute maculopathy.
    b. The patient probably has factitious visual loss.
    c. The patient probably had a similar episode affect her left eye sometime in the past.
    d. Oral steroid therapy is indicated.

97. Which of the following diseases have been observed in association with Coats' disease?
    a. facioscapulohumeral muscular dystrophy.
    b. myotonic dystrophy.
    c. cerebral angiitis.
    d. chronic progressive external ophthalmoplegia.

98. A 14-year-old girl is brought to the ophthalmologist by her parents after complaining that "the page swims when I try to read." The examination is normal with the exception of pronounced downbeat nystagmus. A careful review of systems documents the presence of intermittent headaches in the occipital region, which are intensified with anger or sudden head movement. The patient denies any use of prescription or illicit drugs, including alcohol. Which of the following CT scans (in the left column at the top of the next page) is most likely depicts her condition?

99

5

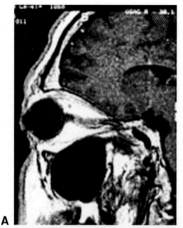

A

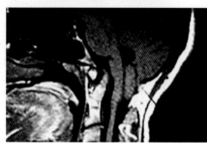

B

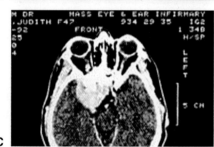

C

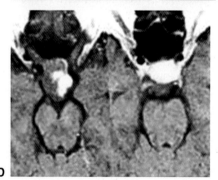

D

100. A 9-year-old boy presents to the ophthalmologist complaining that he has lost his position on the school basketball team because he cannot see the basket. He notes occasional morning headaches but denies any nausea or vomiting. Examination reveals visual acuity of 20/40 in the right eye and 20/25 in the left eye. The patient has marked symmetric weakness of upgaze bilaterally. His pupils are 7 mm and poorly reactive to light with better reaction to a near target. There is approximately 2 mm of superior scleral show bilaterally. Fundus examination suggests optic atrophy in both eyes. Review of systems documents increased consumption of water with frequent urination at night. The most likely diagnosis is
   a. pinealoma.
   b. cerebellar astrocytoma.
   c. chiasmal glioma.
   d. hereditary optic atrophy.

101. After neuroimaging, an important step in diagnostic evaluation of the patient in question 100 would be
   a. visual evoked responses (VERs).
   b. EEG.
   c. Farnsworth D–15 color vision testing.
   d. lumbar puncture.

102. Which of the following concerning optic neuritis in childhood is true?
   a. It is more commonly bilateral than unilateral.
   b. The visual prognosis is almost always very poor.
   c. The pathophysiology is believed to be ischemia of the optic nerve.
   d. Enlargement of optic nerves on neuroimaging implies another, more ominous, diagnosis.

99. Modalities likely to relieve the patient's reading difficulties successfully include
   a. clonazepam (Klonopin).
   b. carbamazepine (Tegretol).
   c. bifocals.
   d. psychotherapy.

103. Posterior ischemic optic neuropathy (PION) typically occurs in what setting?
   a. post radiation therapy.
   b. post spinal surgery.
   c. 1 to 2 weeks after viral infection.
   d. raised intracranial pressure.

104. In a patient complaining of headache and transient visual obscurations whose examination reveals bilateral disc edema, the first diagnostic intervention to be undertaken is
    a. lumbar puncture.
    b. measurement of sedimentation rate.
    c. CT scanning.
    d. measurement of blood pressure.

105. Which of the following disorders is clearly associated with optic nerve drusen?
    a. migraines.
    b. pseudotumor cerebri.
    c. giant cell arteritis.
    d. retinitis pigmentosa.

106. Which histopathologic variety of meningioma is most commonly seen within the orbit?
    a. angioblastic.
    b. meningothelial.
    c. fibroblastic.
    d. pilocytic.

107. Optociliary shunt vessels are most commonly seen in what condition?
    a. optic nerve sheath meningioma.
    b. optic glioma.
    c. carotid occlusive disease.
    d. central retinal artery occlusion.

108. Important blood tests in the evaluation of patient with bilateral optic atrophy and cecocentral scotomas include all of the following except
    a. serum B12 level.
    b. fluorescent treponemal antibody-absorption test (FTA-Abs).
    c. serum folate level.
    d. serum cyanide level.

109. A 58-year-old gentleman appears in your office with bilateral blurry vision. He appears disheveled and gaunt. He has been unemployed for 1 year and smells of alcohol. The patient's visual acuity was 20/200 in both eyes with no RAPD. Images A and B at the top of the right column are the patient's visual fields. What is the most likely diagnosis?
    a. NAION.
    b. dominant optic atrophy.

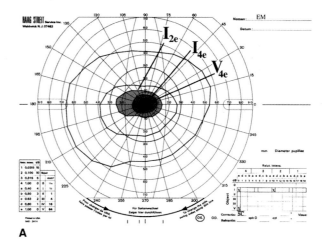

A

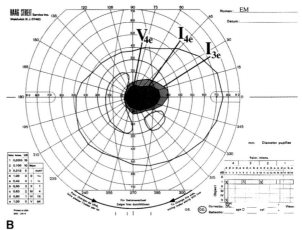

B

    c. toxic/nutritional optic neuropathy.
    d. nonorganic vision loss.

110. The most common fundus finding in a patient with acute traumatic optic neuropathy is
    a. disc edema.
    b. disc pallor.
    c. choroidal ruptures.
    d. unremarkable fundus.

111. Which of the following concerning diabetic papillopathy is true?
    a. It is typically painful.
    b. Development of the disorder seems to be independent of the degree of blood sugar control.
    c. The papillopathy is generally followed by the development of florid neovascularization.
    d. Visual loss is generally severe.

112. Modalities useful in the treatment of optic neuropathy secondary to thyroid eye disease include all of the following except
    a. subtotal thyroidectomy.
    b. orbital radiation.
    c. corticosteroid therapy.
    d. orbital decompression surgery.

113. Bromocriptine treatment may be indicated in the management of a patient with a pituitary tumor that is secreting
    a. prolactin.
    b. growth hormone.
    c. thyrotropin.
    d. nonsecreting.

114. The development of sudden severe headache with accompanying acute visual loss is a well-recognized complication of
    a. meningioma.
    b. intracavernous carotid artery aneurysm.
    c. pituitary adenoma.
    d. hypothalamic glioma.

115. Which one of the following nerves supplies the cornea?
    a. frontal nerve.
    b. lacrimal nerve.
    c. nasociliary nerve.
    d. supraorbital nerve.

116. Which feature is necessary to conclude a motility disturbance is a skew deviation?
    a. a horizontal component.
    b. comitance in all gaze directions.
    c. pattern of motility inconsistent with a single muscle or nerve dysfunction.
    d. other obvious brainstem abnormalities.

117. Brainstem nuclei critical for the generation of normal vertical eye movements includes which of the following?
    a. paramedian pontine reticular formation.
    b. the rostral interstitial nucleus of the medial longitudinal fasciculus.
    c. the abducens nucleus.
    d. the inferior olivary nucleus.

118. What finding in a child with isolated abduction deficit most strongly argues for the diagnosis of Duane's retraction syndrome rather than congenital sixth nerve palsy?
    a. inability to fully abduct the eye volitionally.
    b. involvement of the left eye.
    c. orthotropia in primary gaze.
    d. normal adduction.

119. Which of the following features is found in all cases of internuclear ophthalmoplegia (INO)?
    a. ipsilateral adduction slowing or weakness.
    b. exotropia.
    c. contralateral adduction nystagmus.
    d. skew deviation.

120. A feature frequently found coincidentally with bilateral internuclear ophthalmoplegia (INO) is
    a. rotary nystagmus.
    b. vertical nystagmus.
    c. convergence–retraction nystagmus.
    d. see-saw nystagmus.

121. A brainstem lesion that involves the medial longitudinal fasciculus as well as the ipsilateral abducens nucleus will most likely cause
    a. internuclear ophthalmoplegia with skew.
    b. Foville's syndrome.
    c. Walleyed bilateral internuclear ophthalmoplegia (WEBINO).
    d. "One-and-a-half" syndrome.

122. A lesion that involves both medial longitudinal fasciculi near their junctions with the third nerve nuclei may cause
    a. "One-and-a-half" syndrome.
    b. Walleyed bilateral internuclear ophthalmoplegia (WEBINO).
    c. Fisher's syndrome.
    d. internuclear ophthalmoplegia with skew.

123. A variant of Guillain-Barré syndrome that only involves only the brainstem and cranial nerves is known as
    a. internuclear ophthalmoplegia skew.
    b. Foville's syndrome.
    c. Miller-Fisher syndrome.
    d. "One-and-a-half" syndrome.

124. The clinical distinction between a cavernous sinus syndrome and an orbital apex syndrome is best made by the dysfunction of which cranial nerve?
    a. CN II.
    b. CN III.
    c. CN V.
    d. CN VI.

125. Potential complications of carotid-cavernous fistulae include all of the following except
    a. retinal neovascularization.
    b. retinal vasculitis.
    c. glaucomatous optic nerve damage.
    d. corneal ulceration.

126. A 59-year-old man presents to the emergency room complaining of sudden-onset oscillopsia and diplopia. Examination reveals an alcohol smell on his breath, normal acuity, bilateral abduction deficits, and coarse binocular nystagmus. Appropriate intervention should include
    a. intravenous glucose.
    b. intravenous naloxone.
    c. intravenous chlordiazepoxide.
    d. intravenous thiamine.

127. Which of the following optic disc lesions are distinguished by autofluorescence?
    a. myelinated nerve fibers.
    b. optic nerve neovascularization.
    c. optic nerve pits.
    d. astrocytic hamartoma.

128. The approximate prevalence of giant cell arteritis in Scandinavians is one in
    a. 10.
    b. 100.
    c. 1,000.
    d. 10,000.

129. The approximate prevalence of polymyalgia rheumatica (PMR) in the population over the age of 50 is one in
    a. 20.
    b. 200.
    c. 2,000.
    d. 20,000.

130. Clinical characteristics that may be seen with chiasmal compression include all of the following except
    a. congruous homonymous hemifield defect.
    b. postfixation blindness.
    c. temporal color desaturation.
    d. diplopia.

131. Afferent pupillary fibers from the optic tract exit at
    a. the lateral geniculate body.
    b. the pretectal olivary nuclei.
    c. the occipital cortex.
    d. the medial longitudinal fasciculus.

132. A woman with known multiple sclerosis (MS) presents to an ophthalmologist complaining of "a tiny blind spot in my right eye." Examination discloses a right afferent pupillary defect and slight ocular tenderness in the right eye. The examiner attempts to confirm diagnostic suspicions by eliciting the Pulfrich phenomenon. To do this, the examiner
    a. asks the patient to glance quickly back and forth horizontally and report any photopsias.
    b. asks the patient to climb briskly several flights of stairs and report any visual loss.
    c. asks the patient to watch the pendulum on the grandfather clock across the room and report any three-dimensional movement.
    d. spins the examining chair while the patient fixates her outstretched thumb, watching for any nystagmus.

133. The test that best correlates with the pathophysiology underlying the Pulfrich phenomenon is
    a. electrooculography (EOG).
    b. visual evoked response (VER).
    c. electroretinography (ERG).
    d. calorics and electronystagmography.

5

5

134. A 23-year-old male presents to his ophthalmologist complaining that colors do not seem as bright as they used to appear. His acuities are 20/20 in the right eye and 20/200 in the left eye. He is able to name 10 of 12 color plates correctly with the right eye, but only one of 12 with the left. Visual fields show a cecocentral scotoma in the left eye only. His color photo of his left optic nerve is shown below. A fluorescein angiogram did not show any leakage or staining of his left optic nerve. Which of the following is not true?
   a. The right eye is likely to be similarly affected within the next several months.
   b. Diagnostic evaluation must include electrocardiography.
   c. He should be counseled to avoid tobacco and heavy alcohol consumption.
   d. He should be counseled to expect no improvement in the left eye over time.

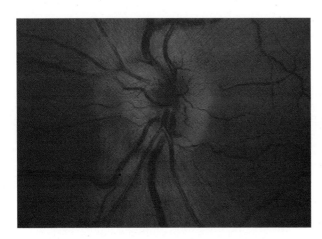

135. Each of the following regarding the disorder in question 134 is true, except
   a. The patient's brothers are more likely to be similarly affected than his sisters.
   b. Other than siblings, similarly affected family members are far more likely to be maternally related than paternally related.
   c. The disease is frequently associated with abnormalities of the X chromosome.
   d. Unfortunately, no specific test exists to confirm the suspected diagnosis.

136. A 42-year-old woman presents to her ophthalmologist complaining of double vision. Her eye movements are shown in the figures below (images A-D). Figure A shows her in primary position. Figure B shows her immediately after being requested to look to her right. Figure C shows her immediately after being asked to look to her left. Figure D shows her approximately 10 to 15 seconds after being requested to look to her left. Each of the following is true regarding her case except
   a. She may have intermittent nystagmus.
   b. The responsible lesion is on the left side of her brainstem.
   c. There may be a history of recent closed head trauma.
   d. The right eye may adduct normally with convergence.

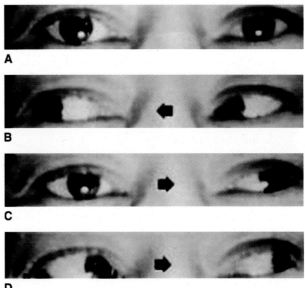

137. The patient in question 136 may demonstrate nystagmus while looking in which field of gaze, as depicted by the figures in that question?
   a. Figure A.
   b. Figure B.
   c. Figure C.
   d. The patient will have nystagmus in all of the above fields.

138. A 63-year-old man presents with the pupillary findings shown in Figure A (below). Figure B shows his pupils after bilateral installation of 4% cocaine. Figure C shows his pupils after bilateral installation of 1% hydroxyamphetamine. Each of the following regarding his situation is true except:

   a. His anisocoria is worse in low ambient illumination.

   b. No workup is necessary if the findings can be shown to be longstanding.

   c. Associated findings might include unilateral hypotony or a mild anterior chamber reaction.

   d. One potential etiology might be occult lung cancer.

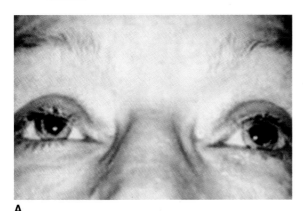

A

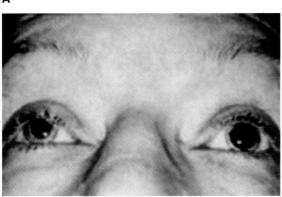

B

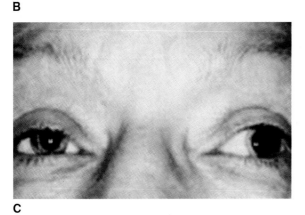

C

139. If the patient in question 138 presents with acute headache, the workup must include urgent

   a. cranial MRI.

   b. carotid angiography.

   c. lumbar puncture.

   d. chest CT.

140. A 23-year-old obese woman is seen for routine ophthalmologic examination. The examination is entirely normal with the exception of bilaterally elevated discs with indistinct margins. The right optic nerve is shown in the color photo below (top). The second figure (bottom of page) is a preinjection photo from fluorescein angiography. Which one of the following regarding this patient is true?

   a. The condition depicted is typically associated with mild to moderate visual loss.

   b. There may be an associated arcuate field defect.

   c. The clinical and histologic findings reflect axoplasmic stasis and congestion.

   d. The filters on the fluorescein camera are of poor quality.

5

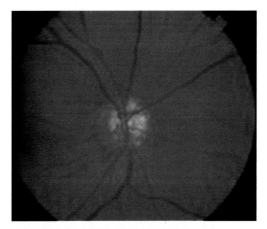

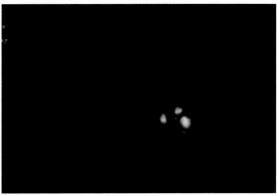

105

141. Select the CT scan that is most likely to create the visual field disturbance shown in the figures below.

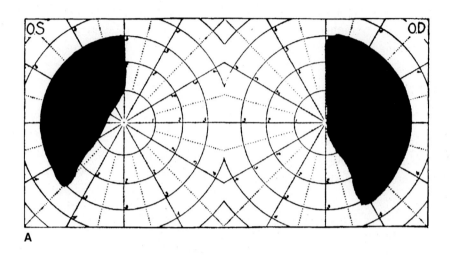

A

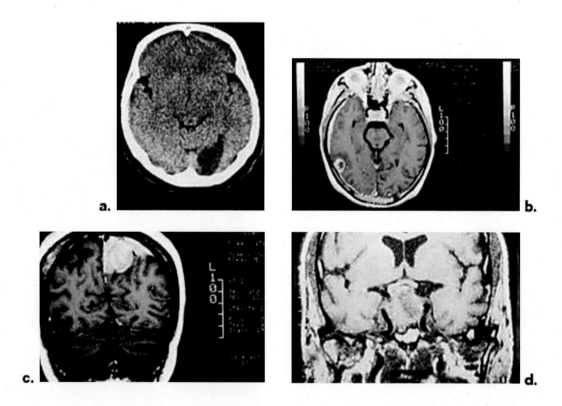

a.

b.

c.

d.

142. Which one of the following abnormalities might be expected in a young child with bilaterally poor vision and the CT scan shown below?
    a. precocious puberty.
    b. ash-leaf macules.
    c. panhypopituitarism.
    d. pheochromocytoma.

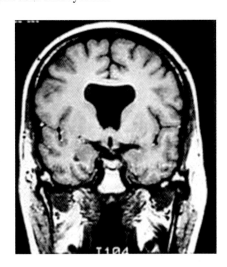

143. A unilateral brainstem lesion at the level of the central nervous system shown below is most likely to produce which one of the following neurologic deficits?
    a. corneal hypesthesia.
    b. third nerve palsy and contralateral hemiplegia.
    c. combined abducens and facial palsies.
    d. "One-and-a-half" syndrome.

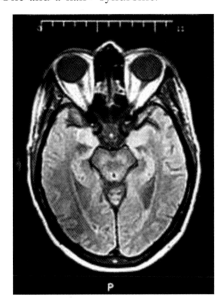

144. Which of the following would be the best choice for treatment of acute, severe migraine headache?
    a. sumatriptan.
    b. acetaminophen.
    c. methysergide.
    d. propranolol.

145. Which of the following would be the best initial choice for prophylaxis of acute, severe migraine headache?
    a. sumatriptan.
    b. acetaminophen.
    c. methysergide.
    d. propranolol.

146. Which one of the following regarding the Ischemic Optic Neuropathy Decompression Trial (IONDT) is false?
    a. Spontaneous improvement of vision was seen in over 40% of control (nonsurgical) cases.
    b. Patients in both the surgical and the nonsurgical groups were equally likely to gain three or more lines of visual acuity.
    c. Patients in both the surgical and the nonsurgical groups were equally likely to lose three or more lines of visual acuity.
    d. The study represented the first randomized controlled prospective clinical trial of optic nerve sheath decompression (ONSD) for AION.

147. Which one of the following regarding pseudotumor cerebri is true?
    a. Headache is the sine qua non of the disease (i.e., it is a universal symptom among patients with the disorder).
    b. Neurologic abnormalities, including abducens palsy, are common.
    c. Opening pressure and CSF protein levels are typically elevated.
    d. Many cases are probably on the basis of decreased reabsorption of CSF.

5

148. Which one of the following autoantibodies are most commonly found in patients with generalized myasthenia gravis (MG)?
    a. binding antibodies to acetylcholine receptors.
    b. blocking antibodies to acetylcholinesterase.
    c. blocking antibodies to acetylcholine receptors.
    d. blocking antibodies to acetylcholine.

149. Relative to generalized myasthenia, ocular myasthenia is
    a. more commonly associated with Graves' disease.
    b. more responsive to anticholinesterase drugs.
    c. more responsive to steroids.
    d. completely localized to ocular or bulbar involvement.

150. Which of the following medications is most clearly associated with drug-induced myasthenia?
    a. warfarin.
    b. D-penicillamine.
    c. diltiazem.
    d. ranitidine.

5

Answers

1. **d.** Although optokinetic nystagmus, the rocking mirror test, and the base-up prism test can help discover factitious monocular blindness, they are not sensitive enough to diagnose factitious visual deficit at the 20/100 level. For such mild visual deficits, a fogging refraction, stereo acuity, and red–green glasses may be useful in diagnosing factitious visual loss.

2. **d.** A pattern VER (as opposed to a flash VER) is required for visual acuity assessment in preverbal children. Although the VER is useful in establishing factitious visual loss, its reliability is limited by the fact that patients can produce false readings by using accommodation to fog their vision. Abnormalities in VER latency and amplitude have been reported in various maculopathies and retinopathies and thus cannot distinguish optic neuropathy from retinal disorders with complete reliability.

3. **b.** Cancer-associated retinopathy (CAR) presents with photopsias, nyctalopia, impaired dark adaptation, dimming, ring scotoma, and peripheral or central visual field loss. The underlying malignancy is usually small cell carcinoma of the lung, although other lung tumors and breast, uterine, and cervical malignancies have been reported. ERG is typically markedly reduced in amplitude. Deterioration is progressive, with eventual bilateral involvement and severe visual loss. The retinal arterioles become attenuated, the RPE thinned and mottled, and the optic discs atrophic.

4. **a.** Melanoma-associated retinopathy (MAR) is an extremely rare syndrome that primarily involves rods. Symptoms include photopsia, nyctalopia, and bilateral peripheral visual loss. Visual symptoms typically develop in the setting of previously diagnosed melanoma, and investigation of visual loss often reveals metastasis. The fundus may be normal, or may show RPE irregularity, retinal arteriolar attenuation, and optic disc pallor. There is no treatment that has been proven effective.

5. **b.** MRI is based on applying a radiofrequency pulse to tissue within a strong magnetic field and measuring the change in tissue's nuclear spin and magnetic vector. The longitudinal relaxation time is termed T1. Fat is bright and water is dark on T1-weighted images. In contrast, fat is dark, and water is bright on T2-weighted images. Some tissues such as cortical bone, rapidly flowing fluid (blood), and air give no signal at all on MRI. T1-weighted images are optimal for demonstrating anatomy. T2-weighted images maximize the differences in tissue water content and state. Therefore, T2-weighted images are the most sensitive to inflammatory, ischemic, or neoplastic alterations in tissue.

6. **c.** Although there is some redundancy of the optic nerve within the orbit, the intracranial optic nerve has little "slack." The dimensional characteristics of the optic nerve can be remembered with the mnemonic phone number 125-1017, which stands for the lengths of the intraocular (1), intraorbital (25), intracanalicular (10), and intracranial (17) portions of the optic nerve.

7. **b.** Fifty-three percent of the retinal ganglion cells cross in the chiasm (this difference is occasionally important clinically). The macular fibers constitute a large portion of the optic chiasm and most decussate in the posterior chiasm. The chiasm lies approximately 1 cm (not 1 mm) above the anterior pituitary gland. The inferior nasal retinal fibers cross in the anterior chiasm and were thought to loop anteriorly in the contralateral optic nerve before traveling posteriorly—leading to the term Wilbrand's knee. It is now thought that Wilbrand's knee may be an artifact.

8. **d.** The temporal 30° of a binocular visual field is perceived by the nasal-most retina of the ipsilateral eye only. These "temporal crescents" are represented in the most anterior portion of the occipital lobe. Thus, a lesion in this area will produce a monocular visual field defect in the far

5

temporal periphery of the contralateral eye, the so-called temporal crescent syndrome. For example, a right anterior occipital lobe lesion would produce a far temporal field defect in the left eye. Similarly, a right posterior occipital lobe lesion may spare the far temporal field in the left eye.

9. **c.** The retinal ganglion cell terminals are segregated by eye. The ipsilateral ganglion cells synapse in layers 2, 3, and 5, whereas the contralateral ganglion cells synapse in layers 1, 4, and 6.

10. **c.** OKN abnormalities indicate lesions of the parietooccipital (slow-phase pursuit abnormalities) or the frontal lobe (fast-phase recovery abnormalities). High congruity of visual field deficits indicates a lesion in the occipital lobe. Formed visual hallucinations, partial complex seizures, and olfactory hallucinations may be seen with temporal lobe lesions. Unformed hallucinations are common with disorders of the occipital lobe. Inferior nerve fibers from the superior retina course anteriorly in Meyer's loop; thus lesions affecting Meyer's loop will result in pie-in-the-sky defects contralateral to the lesion.

11. **d.** Parietal lobe lesions are associated with agnosia and right–left confusion. A parietal lobe lesion will also affect slow-phase pursuit movements toward the ipsilateral side. Unlike temporal lobe lesions, which produce hemianopias that are denser superiorly, parietal lobe lesions produce hemianopias that are denser inferiorly.

12. **a.** Formed hallucinations occur with temporal lobe pathology. Depending on the location of the occipital lobe lesion, the temporal crescent, the representation of which is located in the most anterior visual cortex, may be either spared (more common) or affected. Although OKN asymmetry may rarely occur with occipital lesions, this finding is generally indicative of a parietal locus of disease.

13. **c.** Key events in the development of true disc edema include cessation of axonal transport with swelling of axons. The increase in disc volume is due to enlargement of axons, rather than increased extracellular fluid, as seen in edema of other tissues. Breakdown of the blood–retinal barrier does occur, detected as leakage on fluorescein angiography, but this is not important in the development of disc edema.

14. **b.** Although loss of spontaneous venous pulsations is an early sign of papilledema, remember that about 20% of normal patients lack venous pulsations. Transient obscurations of vision (TOV) often accompany papilledema and are episodes of unilateral or bilateral visual loss lasting only a few seconds. The most typical visual field finding in acute papilledema is an enlarged blind spot. Although rare, unilateral papilledema may occur. For example, if contralateral optic atrophy exists, papilledema may be detectable only in the viable disc.

15. **d.** Pseudotumor cerebri is characterized by increased intracranial pressure on lumbar puncture, normal neuroimaging studies (although the ventricles may be small), and normal cerebrospinal fluid (CSF). Papilledema need not be present for the diagnosis. Although the neurologic examination is usually normal, sixth nerve palsy may occur with increased intracranial pressure of any etiology.

16. **c.** Obesity is not an indication for treatment, although weight loss (even as little as 6% of total body weight) often improves the condition. Most cases of pseudopapilledema are due to the presence of optic disc drusen.

17. **a.** Acetylsalicylic acid or aspirin is not associated with pseudotumor cerebri. Pseudotumor cerebri can be associated with the use of vitamin A, tetracycline, nalidixic acid, cyclosporine, oral contraceptives, as well as the use of or withdrawal from corticosteroids.

18. **c.** Studies have documented that up to 80% with cavernous sinus–dural fistulae will develop

ocular hypertension. Twenty-five percent will develop optic disc cupping and 20% visual field defects. Any entity that raises episcleral venous pressure can cause secondary open-angle glaucoma.

19. **d.** Visual loss is typically severe. Visual acuity is less than 20/200 in over 60% of patients.

20. **b.** The most likely diagnosis in this vaculopathic patient is NAION. Risk factors for NAION include hypertension, diabetes, smoking, hyper-lipidemia, and crowding of the contralateral disc ("Disc at risk"). Altitudinal visual field loss is also more common in patients with NAION.

21. **c.** NAION is far more common than AAION, approximately 95% vs. 5%, and patients have a lower mean age at diagnosis than patients with AAION, 60 years versus 70 years. It usually occurs in a younger age group, and may resemble optic neuritis. Ways to differentiate NAION from optic neuritis include (a) lack of pain with eye movement; (b) the age group affected; (c) delayed optic disc filling present in 75% of NAION cases (whereas filling should be normal in optic neuritis). The role of aspirin in reducing the incidence of fellow eye involvement after the initial episode is unclear.

22. **a.** There is no proven therapy for NAION.

23. **d.** The 15-year data from the optic neuritis treat-ment trial (ONTT) demonstrate a risk for MS of 25% in patients with zero lesions on MRI versus 72% with at least one lesion, with the highest rate of conversion within the first 5 years. Visual recovery to a level of 20/40 or better occurs in 92% of patients with optic neuritis.

24. **d.** In a retrospective review of autopsy findings, nearly 100% of patients dying of MS had some degree of optic nerve demyelination.

25. **a.** Ninety percent of optic gliomas occur in the first two decades of life. The most common

presenting findings are proptosis, visual loss, optic disc pallor, disc edema, and strabismus. The number of patients with optic nerve glioma that have associated neurofibromatosis (NF-1) ranges from 14% to 60%. Optociliary shunt vessels are less commonly seen with optic gliomas than with optic nerve meningiomas. Malignant gliomas of the visual pathways, although rare, occur more frequently in middle-aged adults than in children. Survival averages 6 to 12 months after diagnosis.

26. **d.** In contrast to optic nerve gliomas, meningio-mas occur primarily in adults, and are three times more common in women. Although persons with NF-1 have a higher incidence of meningiomas than the general population, only a minority of people with meningiomas have NF-1. With contrast CT scanning, the peripheral part of the involved optic nerve may show enhancement, resulting in the "railroad track" or "tram track" sign. "Kinking" is specific for optic nerve glioma.

27. **b.** Dominant (Kjer) optic neuropathy (DOA) manifests between age 5 and 10 years. Visual loss may progress until the midteens, at which point it usually stabilizes. Color defects are almost universally present, and tritanopia (which can be detected with the Farnsworth-100 hue testing) is suggestive of DOA. Inheritance is naturally auto-somal dominant, and DOA is linked to the OPA1 gene on chromosome 3.

28. **c.** LHON typically affects males age 10 to 30 years. The syndrome presents with acute, severe vision loss (<20/200), which is initially mon-ocular, but then sequentially affects the fellow eye. Classic fundus findings include hyperemia of the optic disc, peripapillary telangiectasia, and tortuosity of the medium-sized retinal arterioles. The incidence of spontaneous partial recov-ery of vision has been reported to be as high as 10%. LHON exhibits mitochondrial inheritance (inheritance from the mother).

29. **a.** LHON is related to a mitochondrial DNA mutation, most frequently at the 11778 position,

and less commonly at the 3460 or 14484 location. The corresponding single base-pair nucleotide substitution results in impaired mitochondrial adenosine triphosphate production, which tends to affect highly energy-dependent tissues, such as the optic nerve.

30. **c.** Patients with "papillophlebitis" have normal or near normal visual acuity. An RAPD is absent, color vision is normal, and visual field testing shows enlargement of the blind spot. Fundus examination shows marked retinal venous engorgement associated with hyperemic optic disc edema. Retinal hemorrhages extending to the equatorial region are common. It may be a form of incomplete CRVO, and usually resolves spontaneously within 12 months.

31. **c.** Optic disc drusen are refractile, often calcified nodules located on the optic nerve head. In childhood, optic disc drusen tend to be buried, but they become more visible over the years. When visible, optic drusen appear as round, whitish yellow refractile bodies.

32. **b.** Optic disc drusen occur almost exclusively in whites. They are bilateral in 75% to 86% of cases.

33. **a.** Morning glory disc anomaly is a funnel-shaped staphylomatous excavation of the optic nerve and peripapillary retina. It is more common in females and is most often unilateral. White glial tissue is present on the central disc surface. The characteristic feature is the emanation of retinal vessels from the periphery of the disc. Visual acuity is often 20/200 or worse, and an RAPD and a visual field defect are present. Serous retinal detachments can occur in 30% of cases. Transsphenoidal basal encephaloceles may be present.

34. **b.** Superior oblique myokymia is a disorder that produces paroxysmal, monocular, high frequency bursts of contraction of the superior oblique muscle. They usually produce vertical or torsional oscillopsia.

35. **a.** Optics pits are depressions of the optic disc surface that is often gray or white. They are most often located temporally, and can be associated with a mild visual field defect. Optic pits are unilateral but can be bilateral in 15% of cases. Serous detachment of the macula develops in 25% to 75% of cases.

36. **a.** The optic neuritis treatment trial (ONTT) demonstrated that corticosteroid therapy had no long-term beneficial effect for vision. Intravenous methylprednisolone for 3 days followed by 11 days of oral prednisone accelerated recovery by 1 to 2 weeks. Oral prednisone as the initiating therapy was associated with an increased recurrence rate. Intravenous therapy demonstrated a reduction in the rate of development of clinical MS in the subgroup of patients with MRI scans showing two or more lesions at year two, but by year 3, this protective effect was lost. The value of intravenous corticosteroids to reduce the long-term risk of MS is unproven.

37. **d.** The most common location for a cerebral aneurysm with third nerve palsy is the junction of posterior communicating artery and internal carotid artery.

38. **a.** Third nerve aberrant regeneration never occurs with diabetic oculomotor neuropathy. Aberrant regeneration of the third nerve implies another etiology, such as aneurysm, tumor, inflammation, or trauma. Other classic findings of aberrant regeneration include persistent vertical gaze limitation secondary to simultaneous contraction of superior and inferior recti, and pupillary miosis with elevation, adduction, or depression.

39. **b.** The long intracranial course of the trochlear nerve leaves it especially susceptible to damage from closed head trauma. This occurs due to contrecoup injury from the free tentorial edge. Ischemic damage, usually due to diabetes mellitus, is second, and idiopathic palsies are third. Hydrocephalus, vascular loops, or tumor can compress the trochlear nerve as well.

40. d. The three-step test is useful for diagnosis but does not differentiate between congenital and acquired trochlear nerve palsy. Large vertical fusional amplitudes (greater than five prism diopters) and facial asymmetry from childhood head tilting suggest a decompensated congenital lesion.

41. b. The three steps of the Parks-Bielschowsky three-step test in order are (a) find the side of the hypertropia; (b) determine if the hypertropia is greater on left or right gaze; (c) determine if the hypertropia is greater on left or right head tilt. A right fourth nerve palsy shows a right hyperdeviation in primary position that worsens on left gaze and right head tilt. The opposite is true of a left fourth nerve palsy.

42. c. Nasopharyngeal carcinoma can involve numerous cranial nerves because of its proximity to the prepontine basal cistern. Most frequently, the trigeminal nerve is involved, causing facial hypesthesia or facial pain. The abducens nerve is the second most common. The hallmark of nasopharyngeal carcinoma is its propensity to involve multiple cranial nerves noncontiguously. Nasopharyngeal carcinoma is common in Chinese men. The least differentiated forms are also known as Schmincke's and Regaud's tumors.

43. b. An ischemic mononeuropathy is the most common cause of isolated sixth nerve palsy. At the onset of isolated sixth nerve palsy in a vasculopathic patient, neuroimaging is not required. Ocular motility typically resolves within 3 months. If improvement has not occurred after 3 months, a cranial MRI is mandatory. Impaired abduction in patients under 50 requires special attention because few cases are due to an ischemic neuropathy. Younger patients should undergo appropriate neuroimaging.

44. a. Neuromyotonia is a rare cause of episodic diplopia. Prior skull-base radiation therapy, typically for a neoplasm such as a meningioma is the most common historical feature. Months to years post-radiation, patients experience episodic diplopia lasting typically 30 to 60 seconds. Neuromyotonia may affect the oculomotor, trochlear, or abducens nerve.

45. c. Charles Bonnet's syndrome is the triad of visual hallucinations, ocular pathology causing bilateral visual deterioration, and preserved cognitive status. Hallucinations may be simple or highly organized and complex. Patients with visual allesthesia see their environment rotated, flipped, or inverted.

46. b. The hallmark of ophthalmoplegia secondary to a lesion of the cavernous sinus is multiple, ipsilateral ocular motor nerve dysfunction with some combination of third, fourth, fifth, and sixth cranial nerves and sympathetic fibers. If only one oculomotor nerve is involved, it is usually the sixth nerve, which is the only ocular motor nerve not protected within the dural wall of the cavernous sinus. Within the cavernous sinus, sympathetic branches of the paracarotid plexus joins the sixth nerve briefly. Occasionally, an intracavernous lesion can produce sixth nerve palsy with postganglionic Horner's syndrome, producing pupillary miosis. Lesions of the cerebellopontine angle may involve the sixth cranial nerve as well as involve cranial nerves V, VII, and VIII. Chronic inflammation of the petrous bone may cause ipsilateral abducens palsy and facial pain called Gradenigo's syndrome.

47. d. Tolosa-Hunt syndrome is an idiopathic, sterile inflammation that primarily affects the cavernous sinus. The pain in patients with Tolosa-Hunt syndrome typically responds rapidly and dramatically to corticosteroid therapy. Tolosa-Hunt syndrome is a diagnosis of exclusion.

48. c. Duane's syndrome may be secondary to hypoplasia or aplasia of the abducens nucleus, with lateral rectus innervation via the oculomotor nerve. It has various presentations, but retraction of the adducted globe appears most consistently. The three types of Duane's syndrome are distinguished by the relative ability to adduct or abduct:

5

68. **d.** The afferent pupillomotor fibers exit the optic tracts just before the lateral geniculate body (LGB); they do not pass through the LGB. Although postganglionic pupillomotor fibers in the sympathetic pathway do arise from the superior cervical ganglion, the sympathetic pathway leading to these fibers is thought to originate in the posterior hypothalamus. In addition, postganglionic sympathetic fibers enter the orbit with the ophthalmic division of the trigeminal nerve through the superior orbital fissure. The consensual pupillary response is seen because of decussation at the pretectal nuclei. Were the chiasm split in half, consensual responses would be preserved.

69. **c.** Argyll Robertson pupils are miotic, irregular, do not react to light, but have a normal near response. This is a rare finding in some patients with tertiary syphilis. In the light-near dissociation of Parinaud's dorsal midbrain syndrome, the pupils are larger. In young children, the most common cause of this syndrome is a tumor in the region of the pineal gland. In young adults, head trauma and multiple sclerosis are frequently seen. In patients over 60, stroke is most commonly to blame.

70. **c.** Patients with normal pupils will respond to pilocarpine 1%. Thus, a weaker preparation (0.10%) is recommended that can demonstrate denervation supersensitivity. Features of an Adie tonic pupil include sluggish, segmental vermiform response to light with better response to the near reaction. The majority of patients (80%) will have unilateral pupillary involvement. After many months or years, an Adie's pupil will become miotic.

71. **c.** Horner's syndrome includes ipsilateral ptosis, miosis, and anhidrosis. Ptosis is secondary to lack of Müller's muscle function. The distribution of anhidrosis depends on the location of the lesion. Interruption of the central or preganglionic neuron causes anhidrosis of the ipsilateral face. Lesions that are postganglionic, distal to the superior cervical ganglion, result in anhidrosis limited to the ipsilateral forehead. 4% cocaine is used to diagnose Horner's syndrome. A normal pupil will dilate, but a Horner's pupil will dilate poorly. Hydroxyamphetamine is used to localize the lesion. In postganglionic Horner's syndrome, the eye will dilate poorly if at all in response to hydroxyamphetamine, whereas a preganglionic and normal pupil will dilate. Painful Horner's syndrome may be caused by many disorders (neck trauma, migraine, cluster headaches), but spontaneous dissection of the common carotid artery must be ruled out with angiography or MRI/MRA.

72. **a.** The fundus photograph demonstrates a retinal racemose angioma. Wyburn-Mason syndrome is a sporadic condition, characterized by a retinal racemose angioma with ipsilateral intracranial arteriovenous malformation (AVM). Patients with Wyburn-Mason syndrome can have orbital AVMs as well (and consequent ocular bruits). PDT is not used to treat Wyburn-Mason syndrome. However, it has been used to treat another vascular lesion of the retina, the retinal capillary hemangioma. PDT can be used for a retinal capillary hemangioma often when the patient is symptomatic from an exudative retinal detachment caused by this lesion.

73. **c.** The fundus photograph demonstrates a morning glory disc anomaly, a unilateral condition usually accompanied with severe visual loss. It can also cause RAPD. The other answers are correct.

74. **d.** Optic nerve head melanocytomas are dark brown lesions on the optic nerve head, which are typically benign, but can rarely undergo malignant transformation. They can produce relative APDs and visual field defects and should be followed to document growth.

75. **c.** Pheochromocytomas produce, secrete, and store catecholamines. They are most often derived from the adrenal medulla but may arise in any of the sympathetic ganglia. Two phakomatoses, neurofibromatosis, and von Hippel-Lindau disease, are associated with the tumor.

76. **c.** A retinal capillary hemangioma is a spherical orange-red tumor fed by a dilated, tortuous retinal artery and drained by an engorged vein. Racemose angiomas are retinal arteriovenous communications without intervening capillary bed and are associated with Wyburn-Mason syndrome. Retinal cavernous hemangioma is characterized by the formation of grapelike clusters of thin-walled saccular angiomatous lesions.

77. **b.** Retinal capillary hemangioma is associated with von Hippel-Lindau disease.

78. **c.** Cerebellar, brainstem, or spinal cord hemangioblastomas can occur in these patients. These patients may also have pheochromocytomas or renal cell carcinoma.

79. **d.** Astrocytic hamartomas can appear as a whitish-yellow mass ("mulberry lesion").

80. **c.** Astrocytic hamartomas can be seen in tuberous sclerosis and neurofibromatosis, but is more commonly seen in tuberous sclerosis.

81. **a.** The vast majority of patients with astrocytic hamartomas are asymptomatic and do not require treatment.

82. **c.** Unilateral congenital glaucoma is seen in 30% to 70% of patients with Sturge-Weber syndrome and is usually associated with angioma of the upper lid.

83. **d.** Patients with ataxia–telangiectasia may have associated thymic hypoplasia, defective T-cell function, and IgA (secretory immunoglobulin) deficiency, with severe respiratory infections.

84. **c.** Many systemic syndromes such as myotonic dystrophy, oculopharyngeal dystrophy, and Kearns-Sayre syndrome include CPEO, which is a nondescriptive term for chronically progressive loss of eye movements. Oculopharyngeal dystrophy is classically seen in patients of French-Canadian ancestry. They typically present with progressive dysphagia followed by proximal muscle weakness and ptosis. Patients with myotonic dystrophy may have ptosis, pigmentary retinopathy, polychromatic ("Christmas tree") cataracts, and thinning of the temporalis and masseter muscles ("hatchet face"). Patients with thyroid eye disease may have a restrictive ophthalmoplegia.

85. **c.** Four signs constitute complete Kearns-Sayre syndrome: (a) progressive external ophthalmoplegia; (b) mild pigmentary retinal degeneration; (c) onset before age 20; and (d) heart block, potentially lethal and among the last signs to develop. Some studies indicate that elevated CSF protein correlates with the presence of heart block.

86. **a.** There are several genetic syndromes associated with monocular diplopia due to lens subluxation. These include Marfan's syndrome, Ehlers-Danlos syndrome and Weill-Marchesani syndrome. All of the other answers are potential causes for monocular diplopia.

87. **a.** Conjunctival injection, strabismus, and proptosis are seen in thyroid eye disease. Lid retraction is the most common sign.

88. **a.** The most frequently involved muscle in dysthyroid orbitopathy is the inferior rectus. The medial rectus is the second most frequently affected muscle and may simulate a sixth nerve palsy. One mnemonic for this is "I M Stuart Little" (inferior, medial, superior, lateral) in order of their involvement.

89. **a.** This is a classic description of Anton's syndrome.

90. **c.** Although 75% of all myasthenics will have eye findings at presentation, only 33% to 50% will have ocular myasthenia only. A higher percentage (90%) of patients with MG will develop ocular symptoms during the course of the disease. Ptosis is the most common.

91. **a.** A tiny fraction of patients with MG will develop Graves' disease as well.

5

92. b. Radiologic investigation is mandatory for all myasthenics in order to discover thymic enlargement. Thymectomy may be curative in this setting.

93. c. If ocular signs remain isolated for more than 2 years, the disease is likely to remain clinically ocular; though, late conversion to generalize MG is possible.

94. b. Studies of central retinal artery ligation in rhesus monkeys established this value (Hayreh).

95. d. Transient monocular blindness is the hallmark of carotid (anterior) disease. Vertebrobasilar insufficiency typically causes binocular visual blurring or oculomotor symptoms. Other symptoms of vertebrobasilar insufficiency include transient dysarthria, drop attacks, photopsias, and hemi-sensory defects.

96. c. The patient's ocular signs and symptoms clinically suggest the diagnosis of demyelinative optic neuritis. With a history of paresthesias in her right leg, the diagnosis of multiple sclerosis should be entertained. An afferent pupillary defect almost invariably occurs in the acute phase. This patient most likely had a subclinical contra-lateral episode of optic neuritis in the past and therefore no detectable APD. APDs are always relative, that is, comparing one optic nerve to the contralateral nerve. In the Optic Neuritis Treatment Trial, oral steroid therapy showed to offer no improvement in long-term prognosis and had a higher rate of subsequent optic neuritis recurrence.

97. a. The etiology of Coats' disease is unknown, and there does not appear to be any genetic, familiar, racial, or ethnic predisposition. However, Coats'-type retinal vascular changes have been noted in patients with facioscapulohumeral muscular dystrophy, Turner's syndrome, Senior-Loken syndrome, and one variant of the epidermal nevus syndrome. In addition, Coats'-like retinopathy has been noted in up to 3.6% of patients with retinitis pigmentosa.

98. b. Downbeat nystagmus in primary position is localized to the craniocervical junction (or certain intoxications). This patient's clinical symptoms of intermittent occipital headaches with sudden head movements or anger suggest the diagnosis of Arnold-Chiari malformation. Arnold-Chiari malformation is one of the most common causes of downbeat nystagmus.

99. a. Clonazepam, baclofen, gabapentin, base-out prisms, memantine, and 3,4-diaminopyridine have been used in the treatment of downbeat nystagmus.

100. a. This patient appears to have Parinaud's dorsal midbrain syndrome, which may include the following findings: pupillary light-near dissociation, lid retraction (Collier's sign), upgaze paresis, convergence–retraction nystagmus, fixation instability, small-amplitude skew deviation, and papilledema (if ventricular outflow has been compromised). The most common cause in this age group would be a pinealoma. Other causes include stroke, hydrocephalus, and multiple sclerosis.

101. d. After neuroimaging has been obtained, a lumbar puncture would be an important step in the diagnostic evaluation of this patient because pinealoma classically sheds cells into the CSF.

102. a. Optic neuritis in childhood is more commonly bilateral. Visual loss can be severe, although intravenous corticosteroids can improve visual function. Diffuse enlargement of the optic nerve on CT scan may be seen in this condition, mimicking a neoplasm of the optic nerve sheath. The demyelination typically follows a viral illness or vaccination by ten to 14 days.

103. b. Posterior ischemic optic neuropathy (PION) occurs in three distinct settings: perioperative, arteric, or nonarteric. There has been increasing reports associated with spinal surgery. Risk factors for this condition include being in the prone position during surgery, significant blood loss, and long anesthesia time. Vision loss in perioperative PION is often bilateral and severe.

104. **d.** Bilateral disc edema and headache may be caused by several things, but hypertension should be first on the list to be excluded because it is easy to do so and important to identify. After checking blood pressure, neuroimaging should be obtained.

105. **d.** Optic disc drusen may be associated with retinitis pigmentosa and with pseudoxanthoma elasticum.

106. **b.** Meningothelial (syncytial) meningioma is the most common histopathologic type of meningioma seen within the orbit. "Pilocytic" describes the cell type of gliomas of the visual pathways.

107. **a.** Optociliary shunt vessels are vessels that shunt retinal venous outflow to the choroidal circulation. They occur in approximately 30% of patients with optic nerve sheath meningiomas but are nonspecific. They can also occur in patients with sphenoid wing meningioma, optic glioma, CRVO, and chronic papilledema.

108. **d.** The most common etiologies of bilateral central or cecocentral scotomas include hereditary optic neuropathy and nutritional optic neuropathy (vitamin B12 and folate deficiency), drug toxicity, tobacco-alcohol amblyopia, and infiltrative disorders such as syphilis and tuberculosis. Cyanide levels are not helpful in suspected tobacco-alcohol amblyopia.

109. **c.** Optic neuropathy from toxic exposure or nutritional deficiency is characterized by gradual, progressive, bilaterally symmetric, painless visual loss affecting central vision and causing central or cecocentral scotomata. Ethanol abuse probably is associated with optic neuropathy in that it may contribute to malnutrition. Medications can also cause a toxic optic neuropathy. Most commonly implicated medications include ethambutol,

isoniazid, chloramphenicol, hydroxyquinolones, penicillamine, cisplatin, and vincristine.

110. **d.** Although disc edema, disc hemorrhages, and choroidal rupture may be seen in acute traumatic optic neuropathy, the most common finding is a normal fundus. Disc pallor would be unusual in the acute setting, but present in all cases after several weeks (4–8 weeks.)

111. **b.** The development of diabetic papillopathy appears to be independent of serum glucose levels. Diabetic papillopathy is classically seen in young adults with type 1 diabetes with moderate to severe retinopathy (although it can be seen in type 2 patients as well). It is painless, and associated visual loss is generally mild. The distinction of diabetic papillopathy as an entity unique from AION remains controversial. The disorder generally resolves spontaneously.

112. **a.** Thyroid optic neuropathy is considered to be a compressive optic neuropathy due to enlargement of extraocular muscles at the orbital apex. Treatment of thyroid optic neuropathy may include orbital radiation (usually 1,500–2,500 rad over a 10-day period) and orbital decompression, which provides the most potential for decompression of the optic nerve. Systemic corticosteroids are thought to be effective only in the acute congestive phase and not in the fibrotic period. Thus, if no response is noted within 3 weeks, systemic steroids should be tapered and another modality should be considered. Although a subtotal thyroidectomy may provide primary treatment of dysthyroid state, it will have no effect on the eye findings (except, perhaps, lid retraction).

113. **a.** Bromocriptine has been shown to be effective primarily in the management of prolactin-secreting pituitary tumors and is less effective or ineffective with other types of pituitary tumors.

114. **c.** The symptoms presented in this question are indicative of pituitary apoplexy (Sheehan's

syndrome), in which there is a hemorrhage into a pituitary tumor. A sudden severe headache is a common presenting symptom; other manifestations depend on the direction of the expansion of pituitary gland. Acute painful visual loss is uncommon with the other disorders.

115. **c.** The nasociliary nerve is a division of CN V1 and supplies the cornea.

116. **c.** A skew deviation is a motility disturbance with a vertical component that does not have a pattern consistent with a discrete muscle underaction or nerve palsy. They are generally due to supranuclear or vestibuloocular dysfunction and generally reflect brainstem disease. They are typically comitant, but not always.

117. **b.** Although transient changes in vertical eye movements and slowing of vertical saccades can result from lesions of the paramedian pontine reticular formation, nuclei critical for the initiation of vertical eye movements are the rostral interstitial nucleus of the medial longitudinal fasciculus (riMLF) and the interstitial nucleus of Cajal (INC).

118. **c.** Medial rectus contracture is distinctly uncommon in Duane's syndrome. In congenital sixth nerve palsy, it is quite common and results in esotropia in primary position. Although the left eye is more commonly involved in Duane's syndrome, this does not help in distinguishing from congenital sixth nerve palsy.

119. **a.** Disruption of the medial longitudinal fasciculus (MLF), which carries projections of interneurons from the contralateral sixth nerve nucleus to the ipsilateral medial rectus subnucleus, results in ipsilateral absence or slowing of adduction and contralateral abduction nystagmus. This combination of findings is termed internuclear ophthalmoplegia. Vertical nystagmus and skew deviations are frequently found in association with internuclear ophthalmoplegia but are not universal.

120. **b.** A bilateral INO produces bilateral adduction lag, bilateral abducting nystagmus, and vertical, gaze-evoked nystagmus that is best appreciated in upgaze. The two most common causes of INO are demyelination and stroke. In adolescents and younger adults, INO is typically caused by demyelination. In older adults, microvascular disease is the most common cause.

121. **d.** A lesion that disrupts both the abducens nucleus or pontine paramedian reticular formation and the ipsilateral MLF will result in the combination of an ipsilateral gaze palsy and internuclear ophthalmoplegia. This combination has been termed the "one-and-a-half" syndrome. The only horizontal eye movement that remains is contralateral abduction.

122. **b.** A large-angle exodeviation can occasionally occur in association with a bilateral INO, resulting in a syndrome called "wall-eyed" bilateral INO.

123. **d.** Miller-Fisher syndrome is generally considered a variant of Guillain-Barré syndrome that results in ophthalmoplegia, ataxia, and areflexia. Serum IgG autoantibodies and elevated CSF protein may be present. Complete recovery is common.

124. **a.** The presence of optic nerve dysfunction, manifested by decreased vision, an afferent pupillary defect, and/or dyschromatopsia, distinguishes an orbital apex syndrome from a cavernous sinus syndrome because the optic nerve passes through the optic canal and does not enter the cavernous sinus.

125. **b.** Iris and posterior segment neovascularization and rapidly progressive cataract may all be seen as complications of the ischemic oculopathy that these fistulae generate. These fistulae often produce elevated intraocular pressure and proptosis. Corneal exposure due to proptosis is another potential complication of carotid–cavernous fistula.

126. **d.** Acute thiamine deficiency (Wernicke's encephalopathy) can result in central scotomas as well as ophthalmoplegia, primarily affecting cranial nerves III and VI. It can be precipitated in nutritionally depleted alcoholics given intravenous glucose alone, due to sudden consumption of systemic thiamine stores.

127. **d.** Autofluorescence is produced when certain tissues/material are stimulated with monochromatic blue light and emit in the yellow-green range, as fluorescein does. The two optic nerve lesions that may autofluoresce are astrocytic hamartomas and drusen. Large accumulations of lipofuscin also may autofluoresce. To demonstrate this, fundus photographs should be obtained through the standard fluorescein setup, but without fluorescein injection. Lesions will appear bright, as if they had absorbed fluorescein, even though none was injected. Note that this is not the same as a "red-free" photographs (which are produced with a green filter that does not provide sufficient blue light to stimulate autofluorescence).

128. **b.** Based on autopsy studies, the prevalence of GCA has been estimated to be 1.1% of the Scandinavian population. People born in Northern European countries appear to have higher rates of giant cell arteritis. People of Scandinavian origin are particularly at risk.

129. **b.** PMR is a surprisingly common disorder. Patients with PMR are at higher risk for developing GCA.

130. **a.** The classic field abnormality associated with optic chiasmal disorders is a bitemporal hemianopia, not a homonymous hemianopia, which is seen with retrochiasmal lesions. Postfixation blindness is a necessary concomitant of bitemporal hemianopia. Objects behind the point of fixation are in the temporal hemifield of each eye. With loss of these fields, nothing beyond the point of fixation is visible. Reds and greens often appear "washed out" in the temporal

hemifield of affected patients. "Hemifield slip" refers to the diplopia these patients may also notice. By mechanisms that are not entirely understood, binocular input at the vertical midline seems necessary for motor fusion. When a substantial portion of the vertical midline is not overlapped by both visual fields, there may be loss of motor fusion with resultant diplopia.

131. **b.** Pupillary fibers from the optic tract exit before reaching the lateral geniculate body and exit into the pretectal olivary nuclei.

132. **c.** The Pulfrich phenomenon probably reflects delayed conduction in the demyelinated nerve. Oscillating objects perceived by the affected eye appear to be behind the image seen with the healthy eye, simulating three-dimensional movement where there is only movement within one plane.

133. **b.** The delayed implicit time is the electrophysiologic correlate of the bizarre perception known as the Pulfrich phenomenon.

134. **d.** The examination reveals pseudo-disc edema: the disc appears elevated with blurred, indistinct disc margins with dilated, telangiectatic peripapillary capillaries but no dye leakage on angiography. This constellation is pathognomonic for Leber's hereditary optic neuropathy (LHON). The disease is typically asynchronous and bilateral. Many patients have asymptomatic, but important electrocardiographic abnormalities, most commonly a preexcitation syndrome. It is theorized that the added metabolic burden of tobacco and alcohol use may exacerbate the defect in oxidative metabolism caused by the defects in mitochondrial and nuclear DNA. A small percentage of patients can have partial recovery of vision.

135. **d.** As is now well understood, the primary genetic defect underlying LHON resides in the mitochondrial DNA of every somatic cell. This defect is inherited strictly from the cytoplasm

5

of the maternal egg. As paternal sperm carry no mitochondria, the disease is maternally inherited. There is clearly a gender predilection, with 80% to 90% of affected individuals being men. Fifty percent of affected individuals will have a point mutation at position 11778 of the mitochondrial DNA, resulting in impaired ATP production. No treatment has been proven effective

136. b. The right eye's adduction is clearly slowed, indicating a right internuclear ophthalmoplegia (INO). The lesion is always on the same side of the brainstem as the eye with impaired adduction. Thus, her lesion is on the right side of her brainstem. Some patients with myasthenia gravis (MG) will present with a pseudo-INO virtually indistinguishable from a true INO. Any other associated motility disorders, particularly ptosis or fatigability of adduction, should prompt a Tensilon test. Traumatic INO has a good prognosis for recovery. If convergent adduction is preserved, the term "posterior" INO has been used, historically. Anterior INO implies a more rostral lesion, more likely to impair convergent as well as saccadic adduction.

137. c. Patients with INO typically show "abduction nystagmus" of the contralateral eye. Thus, a patient with a right INO may have nystagmus when looking to the left.

138. d. Anisocoria aggravated by cocaine implies Horner's syndrome. Cocaine blocks reuptake of catecholamines at the synapse. In Horner's syndrome, the catecholamine level at sympathetic synapses (iris dilator) is lower, so the mydriasis normally caused by cocaine is lessened. Hydroxyamphetamine stimulates release of catecholamines from the presynaptic neuron at the effector junction. If hydroxyamphetamine fails to dilate the abnormal, miotic pupil (in this case, the right pupil), the lesion must be postganglionic. In Horner's syndrome, the miotic pupil is the abnormal one, due to relative lack of sympathetic stimulation. In the acute phase, the affected eye may be injected (lack of sympathetic vasodilation), hypotonous (reduced aqueous

secretion), and mildly inflamed (breakdown of the blood–ocular barrier). So-called Pancoast's tumor, a primary pulmonary carcinoma of either upper lobe, may compress the second order sympathetic neurons, causing preganglionic Horner's syndrome.

139. b. Painful Horner's is an acute dissection of the internal carotid artery until proven otherwise. The diagnosis of exclusion then becomes migraine if the angiogram is normal.

140. b. Bilaterally elevated discs with indistinct margins raise the possibility of papilledema, particularly in an obese young woman (pseudotumor cerebri). The photo demonstrates two findings arguing against this diagnosis. First, the vessels are clearly visible, with no obscuration of their borders. This is a sensitive finding in true papilledema. Second, two or three tiny excrescences with a crystalline appearance within the neural rim are visible. The figure reveals either auto- or pseudofluorescence (hyperfluorescence despite no injection of fluorescein). The clinical findings are consistent with a lesion known to be associated with autofluorescence, optic nerve drusen. Typically, visual acuity is normal, although there may be associated field defects. Axoplasmic stasis is a feature of true papilledema, rather than pseudopapilledema, which is present here. Autofluorescence is well described for both optic nerve drusen and astrocytic hamartomas of the optic nerve head. Both lesions may appear quite similar clinically. A distinguishing feature is the hypervascularity of astrocytomas, best revealed with fluorescein angiography.

141. d. The visual fields reflect a bitemporal hemianopia. This indicates chiasmal compression. Although this may occur with severe hydrocephalus of any cause, the primary lesion is usually parasellar. In this case, there is a huge pituitary tumor, probably nonsecreting; the chiasm can be seen riding on top of this impressive mass. Option (a) is a large occipital infarct, (b) is a parietal lobe metastasis, and (c) is a meningioma of the falx cerebri.

142. **c.** The CT scan reveals absence of the septum pellucidum, a thin layer of serous connective tissue separating the two lateral ventricles. This is clearly associated with bilateral optic nerve hypoplasia and hypothalamic–pituitary disturbances, typically underfunctioning. Precocious puberty may be a part of polyostotic fibrous dysplasia (Albright's syndrome). Ash-leaf macules and pheochromocytoma may be seen in various phakomatoses (tuberous sclerosis, neurofibromatosis, and von Hippel-Lindau syndromes).

143. **b.** This MRI image demonstrates central nervous system anatomy at the level of the midbrain. A unilateral brainstem lesion here could result in numerous defects. Weber's syndrome refers to an intramedullary CN III lesion within the substance of the cerebral peduncle where descending fibers of the corticospinal tract run. This results in third nerve palsy and contralateral hemiplegia (the motor fibers within the corticospinal tract decussate at the caudal medulla, distal to the lesion of Weber's syndrome).

144. **a.** Sumatriptan is a serotonin antagonist available orally, via injection, or as a nasal spray. The "-triptan" antimigraine drugs are used for symptomatic relief of migraines, but are contraindicated in patients with basilar artery migraine. They can produce MI and should be used with caution in patients with severe hypertension or coronary artery disease.

145. **d.** Methysergide is an ergot alkaloid with numerous potential side effects. Prophylaxis can be achieved with the use of beta-blockers, calcium channel blockers, tricyclic antidepressants, selective serotonin reuptake inhibitors, sodium valproate, topiramate.

146. **c.** Patients in the surgical group were significantly more likely to lose at least three lines of acuity. There is no proven therapy for NAION.

147. **d.** Pseudotumor cerebri typically (not universally) presents with visual loss and headaches. Neurologic abnormalities are usually absent, except for occasional abducens paralysis. Although the opening pressure is elevated, CSF protein levels are either normal or low.

148. **a.** Binding antibodies to acetylcholine receptors are found in 90% of patients with generalized MG.

149. **d.** Ocular myasthenia has only ocular involvement without any systemic manifestations.

150. **b.** The disease is indistinguishable from MG, with an onset averaging 6 months after initiation of therapy. Approximately 80% of patients will remit completely within 6 to 8 months of cessation.

5

123

CHAPTER 6

Oculoplastics

■ Questions

1. A patient is referred for a postoperative evaluation of a 1.2 g gold weight implanted in the left upper eyelid for facial nerve palsy. The patient is shown below in attempted closure of the eye. The complication depicted may be avoided by which of the following?
   a. Using a 0.8 g gold weight implant.
   b. Using a 1.8 g gold weight implant.
   c. Inserting the weight under the orbicularis muscle.
   d. Meticulous suture closure of the skin.

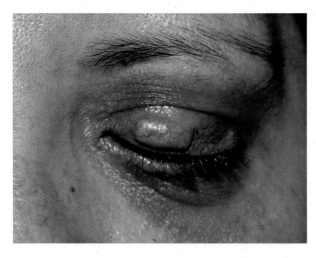

2. A patient is (shown in the right column) in attempted closure of his eyes. The surgical management of the patient's condition includes all of the following, except
   a. gold weight implantation.
   b. lower eyelid repair.

   c. blepharoplasty.
   d. brow lifting.

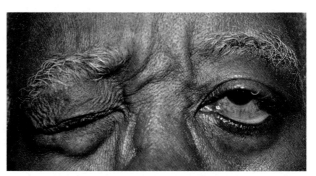

3. A patient with eyelid ptosis, suspected of having myasthenia gravis, undergoes pharmacologic testing with edrophonium chloride (Tensilon). All of the following are potential side effects of edrophonium testing, except
   a. respiratory arrest.
   b. tachycardia.
   c. vomiting.
   d. syncopy.

4. Which of the following is the most appropriate imaging study for a patient diagnosed with myasthenia gravis (MG)?
   a. MRI scan of the brain.
   b. B-scan ultrasonography.
   c. CT scan of the chest.
   d. carotid Doppler ultrasonography.

124

5. The patient developed the lesion shown below on the left lower eyelid over the last month. All of the following are true of this condition, except:
   a. The central crater is filled with sebaceous material.
   b. There is an increased incidence in immunosuppressed individuals.
   c. Complete surgical excision is advised.
   d. The lesion may involute over the next 3 to 6 months.

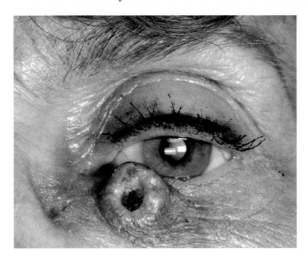

6. An 11-year-old patient photographed below presents with a variable position of the left upper eyelid. The observed changes occur with opening and closing of the mouth. The condition is most commonly due to synkinesis of which two cranial nerves?
   a. oculomotor and trigeminal.
   b. abducens and oculomotor.
   c. facial and oculomotor.
   d. trochlear and abducens.

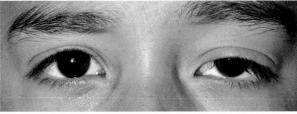

A

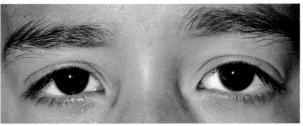

B

7. Eyelid synkinesis can occur in all of the following, except
   a. congenital neurogenic blepharoptosis.
   b. ocular myasthenia gravis.
   c. aberrant nerve regeneration.
   d. duane retraction syndrome.

8. A 74-year-old patient had noticed eyelid drooping, which had worsened over the last several years (photographed below). The levator function was 15 mm bilaterally and the extraocular motility was full in both eyes. The patient is seen preoperatively and postoperatively after having undergone ptosis repair. Which of the following is characteristic of this patient's ptotic eyelids?
   a. eyelid lag.
   b. supratarsal thickening.
   c. difficulty reading.
   d. unrelated to cataract surgery.

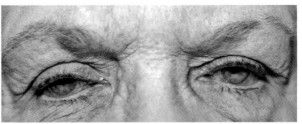

A

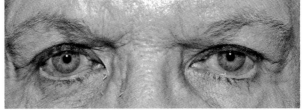

B

9. The patient in the figures at the top of the next page is noted to have developed axial proptosis and downward displacement of the left eye over the last 2 weeks. After complete examination, the next most appropriate step is to proceed with which of the following?
   a. observation.
   b. chemotherapy.
   c. bone marrow biopsy.
   d. anterior orbitotomy for biopsy.

6

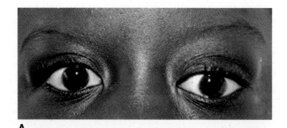

A

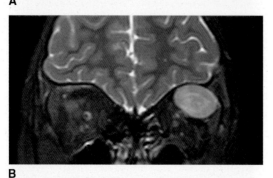

B

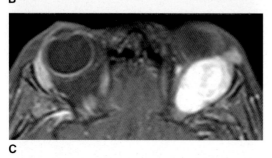

C

10. The gross examination of tissue following a patient's surgery is shown below. With regard to the type of surgery performed, all of the following tumors may appropriately be addressed by the type of surgery shown, except
    a. sebaceous carcinoma with deep orbital invasion.
    b. primary orbital rhabdomyosarcoma.
    c. extraocular extension of melanoma without systemic metastasis.
    d. orbital phycomycosis.

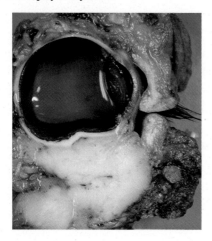

11. In comparison to benign mixed tumor, all of the following clinical features are more characteristic of adenoid cystic carcinoma, except
    a. progression over weeks to months.
    b. presence of bone erosion.
    c. hypesthesia in temporal region.
    d. older age.

12. In comparison to benign mixed tumor, all of the following clinical features are more characteristic of lymphoid tumors of the lacrimal gland, except
    a. bony remodeling.
    b. absence of globe ptosis.
    c. more anterior location.
    d. soft to palpation.

13. Where is the peripheral arterial arcade in the upper eyelid located?
    a. between the levator aponeurosis and Müller's muscle.
    b. along the anterior surface of the tarsus.
    c. 2 mm superior to the eyelid margin.
    d. between the orbicularis oculi muscle and levator aponeurosis.

14. Distention of the lacrimal sac superior to the medial canthal tendon is suggestive of which of the following?
    a. primary acquired nasolacrimal duct obstruction.
    b. canaliculitis.
    c. tumor.
    d. dacryolithiasis.

15. As the bony nasolacrimal canal runs inferiorly it initially curves
    a. medial and anterior.
    b. lateral and posterior.
    c. medial and posterior.
    d. lateral and anterior.

16. The patient shown below was referred in consultation for a malposition of the right lower eyelid. Six years prior, the patient had a basal cell carcinoma of the inferonasal right lower eyelid removed. The postexcision defect had been repaired with a full thickness skin graft to the medial half of the eyelid. Appropriate surgical management for the patient's current right lower eyelid condition includes all of the following, except
    a. incision and relaxation of vertical traction.
    b. horizontal eyelid tightening.
    c. eyelid retractor repair.
    d. vertical lengthening of anterior lamella.

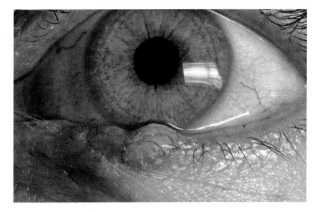

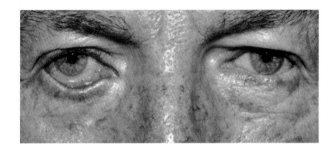

17. Which one of the following disorders typically produces downward and lateral displacement of the globe?
    a. malignant mixed tumor of the lacrimal gland.
    b. squamous cell carcinoma of the maxillary sinus.
    c. frontal sinus mucocele.
    d. optic nerve sheath meningioma.

18. All of the following disorders typically present with a rapid onset, except
    a. benign mixed tumor of the lacrimal gland.
    b. ruptured dermoid cyst.
    c. rhabdomyosarcoma.
    d. orbital cellulitis.

19. A 42-year-old patient presents with a left lower eyelid lesion shown in the image at the top of the right column. What is the most appropriate initial step in the management of this patient's condition?
    a. incision and curettage.
    b. observation.
    c. full-thickness excisional biopsy.
    d. incisional biopsy.

20. Compared with botulinum toxin type A, all of the following are true regarding botulinum toxin type B, except
    a. more injection discomfort.
    b. greater diffusion of the toxin.
    c. quicker onset of effect.
    d. longer duration of action.

21. All of the following favor the diagnosis of benign essential blepharospasm over hemifacial spasm, except
    a. absence of abnormal movements during sleep.
    b. no involvement of lower facial muscles along with orbicularis muscle.
    c. synchronous contractures of involved muscles.
    d. lack of response to neurosurgical decompression of the facial nerve.

22. A 49-year-old patient presents with bilateral upper eyelid ptosis as demonstrated in the photograph below. The patient has been using rigid gas permeable contact lenses for years. The levator function is 16 mm bilaterally and the extraocular motility is full in both eyes. What is the most likely etiology of her condition?
    a. involutional attenuation.
    b. repetitive eyelid traction.
    c. levator muscle dysgenesis.
    d. diffuse muscular disease.

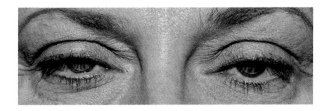

6

127

23. The most common cause of unilateral proptosis in children is
    a. thyroid ophthalmopathy.
    b. rhabdomyosarcoma.
    c. orbital pseudotumor.
    d. orbital cellulitis.

24. The most common location for an orbital meningocele is the
    a. supraorbital notch.
    b. lateral canthus.
    c. lacrimal gland fossa.
    d. medial canthus.

25. The patient represented in the photograph below is referred for evaluation of right eye proptosis, chemosis, and tortuous conjunctival vessels, which extend to the limbus. In addition, the right eye has limitation of right lateral gaze and an audible cranial bruit. The patient has a history of severe head trauma. Subsequent CT scan confirms the absence of a mass and shows a dilated superior ophthalmic vein. All of the following are true of the patient's condition, except
    a. elevated orbital venous pressure.
    b. direct high-flow fistula.
    c. low thyroid stimulating hormone.
    d. extraocular muscle enlargement.

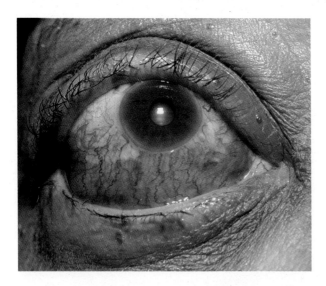

26. A 73-year-old woman presents to the ophthalmologist complaining of mild redness and irritation of her left eye for approximately 2 months.

She denies any head trauma. Visual acuity is normal bilaterally. There is 3 mm of proptosis on the left with mild tortuosity of the retinal vasculature of the left eye. Intraocular pressure is 12 mm Hg in the right eye and 30 mm Hg in the left eye. Arterialization of the orbit is most likely caused by a disturbance in the
    a. central retinal artery.
    b. branches of the middle meningeal artery.
    c. common carotid artery.
    d. intracavernous internal carotid artery.

27. The most common orbital or eyelid finding in the craniosynostosis syndromes is
    a. ankyloblepharon.
    b. blepharophimosis and ptosis.
    c. V-pattern exotropia.
    d. hypertelorism and proptosis.

28. The most common risk factor for the development of preseptal cellulitis is
    a. recent upper respiratory infection.
    b. recent skin trauma.
    c. recent orbital fracture.
    d. sinusitis.

29. A 58-year-old woman presents with a 6-week history of left upper eyelid ptosis as demonstrated in image A at the top of the next page. With lifting of her eyelid she experiences diplopia and has poor extraocular motility of the left eye. Her past medical history is significant for estrogen-receptor–positive breast cancer treated 6 years ago. Orbital imaging (images B and C at the top of the next page) shows a mass of the orbital apex and subsequent biopsy shows an estrogen-receptor–negative breast cancer. Which of the following is true of breast cancer metastatic to the orbit?
    a. the majority of orbital metastases in women originate from breast cancer.
    b. this patient will likely benefit from hormone therapy.
    c. bone metastasis is more common than extraocular muscle involvement.
    d. enophthalmos is an expected finding in this patient.

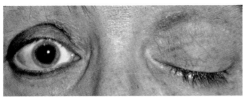

A

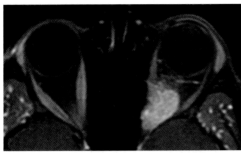

B

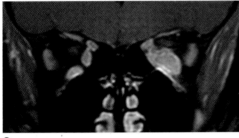

C

30. The position of the patient's *right* upper eyelid in question 29 is best explained by
   a. coexistent hyperthyroidism.
   b. right facial nerve palsy.
   c. left upper eyelid ptosis.
   d. metastatic infiltration of right superior rectus/ levator muscle complex.

31. An infant presents with ptosis of the right upper eyelid as pictured below. Which of the following best describes the type of blepharoptosis?
   a. aponeurotic.
   b. mechanical.
   c. neurogenic.
   d. myogenic.

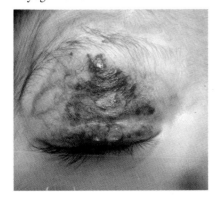

32. With varying frequency, all of the following are used in the treatment of the condition in the previous question, except
   a. dextromethorphan.
   b. propranolol.
   c. clobetasol propionate.
   d. interferon-α.

33. Which of the following can be associated with multiple large capillary hemangiomas?
   a. thrombocytosis.
   b. leukocytosis.
   c. thrombocytopenia.
   d. leukocytopenia.

34. A patient with suspected orbital cellulitis suddenly worsens with a virtually frozen globe, without a measurable increase in proptosis. Corneal sensation is likewise diminished, but visual acuity remains grossly intact. The most likely explanation for these events is
   a. cavernous sinus thrombosis.
   b. orbital compartment syndrome.
   c. meningitis secondary to orbital cellulitis.
   d. orbital apex syndrome.

35. A sensitive finding in direct naso-orbital-ethmoid fracture is
   a. telecanthus.
   b. hypoglobus.
   c. infraorbital hypesthesia.
   d. epistaxis.

36. All of the following findings are consistent with an isolated inferior orbital wall fracture and soft issue entrapment except
   a. subcutaneous emphysema.
   b. infraorbital hypesthesia.
   c. limitation in ocular motility in all fields of gaze.
   d. hypoglobus.

37. A 5-year-old boy fell while riding his bicycle. A CT scan performed in the emergency room is shown at the top of the next page. Which of the following is characteristic of the injury shown in this patient?
   a. Fractures of the orbital floor or medial wall are more common.
   b. The injury tends to occur in adults.
   c. The patient likely fell from a height greater than that of his bicycle.
   d. An upper eyelid hematoma is an expected finding.

6

129

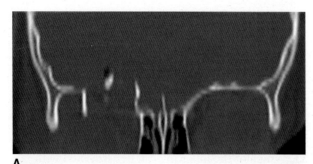

A

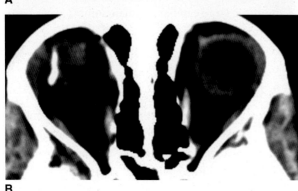

B

38. All of the following are recognized causes of enophthalmos, except
    a. silent sinus syndrome.
    b. orbital varix.
    c. medial wall orbital fracture.
    d. malar hypoplasia.

39. The nevus flammeus, which may be mistaken for a capillary hemangioma, is seen as a part of what systemic disorder?
    a. neurofibromatosis.
    b. Treacher Collins' syndrome.
    c. von Hippel's disease.
    d. Sturge-Weber syndrome.

40. Greater than 90% of periocular capillary hemangiomas manifest by
    a. 4 to 8 weeks of age.
    b. 6 to 8 months of age.
    c. 12 to 18 months of age.
    d. 3 to 4 years of age.

41. Most capillary hemangiomas reach their peak size at approximately what age?
    a. 2 to 3 months.
    b. 6 to 12 months.
    c. 12 to 24 months.
    d. 3 to 5 years.

42. The key clinical feature distinguishing between nevus flammeus and capillary hemangioma is
    a. lesion color.
    b. presence or absence of blanching with pressure.
    c. area of skin affected.
    d. extent of skin thickening.

43. Which one of the following most accurately reflects the relative percentages of patients with thyroid eye disease (Graves' patient percentages)?
    a. 96% hyperthyroidism, 1% autoimmune thyroiditis, 3% euthyroid.
    b. 93% hyperthyroidism, 1% autoimmune thyroiditis, 6% euthyroid.
    c. 90% hyperthyroidism, 1% hypothyroidism, 3% autoimmune thyroiditis, 6% euthyroid.
    d. 87% hyperthyroidism, 3% hypothyroidism, 5% autoimmune thyroiditis, 5% euthyroid.

44. Which one of the following signs is considered classic for CT scanning in Graves' ophthalmopathy?
    a. kinking of extraocular muscles.
    b. nodular muscle enlargement.
    c. fusiform muscle enlargement with sparing of tendons.
    d. solitary muscle enlargement.

45. After eyelid retraction, what is the expected order of eyelid findings in patients with Graves' ophthalmopathy (in order from most frequent to least frequent)?
    a. von Graefe's sign > lid lag > lagophthalmos.
    b. lagophthalmos > von Graefe's sign > lid lag.
    c. lid lag > von Graefe's sign > lagophthalmos.
    d. von Graefe's sign > lagophthalmos > lid lag.

46. Before undertaking surgical correction of strabismus in Graves' ophthalmopathy, the angle of deviation should be stable for what period of time?
    a. 1 month.
    b. 3 months.
    c. 6 months.
    d. 1 year.

6

47. A 57-year-old woman presents with a blind painful left eye, which has secondarily developed perforation of the cornea. The patient underwent a surgical procedure for her condition (seen below). With regard to this patient, all of the following statements are correct, except
   a. The procedure is appropriate even in the setting of endophthalmitis.
   b. There is a future risk of developing granulomatous inflammation in the right eye.
   c. Posterior incisions in the sclera allow for placing a larger orbital implant.
   d. The cornea may be retained provided the epithelium and endothelium are removed.

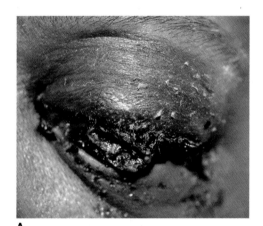

A

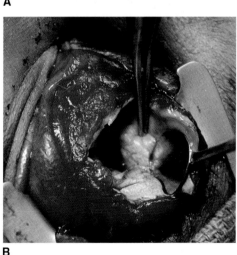

B

48. The most common postoperative complication of enucleation is
   a. socket contracture.
   b. enophthalmos.
   c. superior sulcus deformity.
   d. extrusion of implant.

49. A 68-year-old man presents with blind painful right eye, proptosis, and chemosis as photographed below. Which of the following treatments is most appropriate in the management of this patient?
   a. enucleation.
   b. retrobulbar alcohol injection.
   c. evisceration.
   d. diode laser cyclophotocoagulation.

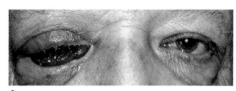

A

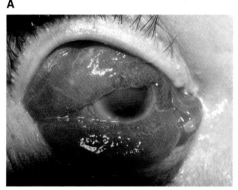

B

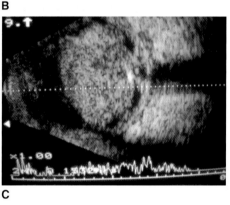

C

50. Which one of the following regarding a biopsy of orbital rhabdomyosarcoma is false?
   a. Metastatic workup includes lumbar puncture and bone marrow biopsy.
   b. The most malignant variant, alveolar rhabdomyosarcoma, occurs most frequently in the superior orbit.
   c. Electron microscopic studies may be used in facilitating the diagnosis, as cross-striations are more apparent on electron microscopy.
   d. The embryonal pattern is the most common pathologic variant, accounting for more than 80% of total cases.

51. A patient with known neurofibromatosis presents with pulsating proptosis of long duration. CT scan of the orbit will most likely reveal
    a. orbital neurofibroma.
    b. abnormality of the sphenoid bone.
    c. optic nerve glioma.
    d. carotid–cavernous fistula.

52. A 33-year-old patient with type I diabetes mellitus presents with a 2-week history of gradually progressive proptosis, redness, and irritation in the left eye. Visual acuities are 20/20 in the right eye and 20/100 in the left eye. There is an afferent pupillary defect on the left, along with 4 mm of proptosis and moderate conjunctival injection. Ductions are normal on the right and globally reduced on the left. CT scanning reveals left ethmoid and maxillary sinusitis with evidence of orbital involvement. The next step in the proper evaluation of this patient is
    a. complete blood count.
    b. oral temperature.
    c. blood glucose.
    d. careful ear, nose, and throat evaluation.

53. Which one of the following papillomatous lesions of the eyelid is considered premalignant?
    a. acanthosis nigricans.
    b. actinic keratosis.
    c. seborrheic keratosis.
    d. verruca vulgaris.

54. Which of following papillomatous lesions of the eyelid may be associated with underlying systemic malignancy?
    a. acanthosis nigricans.
    b. verruca vulgaris.
    c. ephelis.
    d. actinic keratosis.

55. What preoperative medication is most appropriate for reducing the chance of irreversible scarring in patients prior to undergoing laser skin resurfacing?
    a. valacyclovir.
    b. prednisone.
    c. diphenhydramine.
    d. mitomycin-C.

56. Laser skin resurfacing is contraindicated in patients taking which one of the following medications?
    a. isotretinoin.
    b. hydrochlorothiazide.
    c. docetaxel.
    d. sildenafil citrate.

57. Elevation of what structure to its previous anatomic position is often used to perform midface rejuvenation?
    a. preseptal orbicularis.
    b. suborbicularis oculi fat.
    c. retroorbicularis oculi fat.
    d. medial canthal tendon.

58. All of the following are true regarding sebaceous carcinoma, except:
    a. The primary focus may be either eyelid or caruncle.
    b. Shave biopsy techniques are adequate.
    c. The hallmarks of the histopathology of the condition include skip areas and pagetoid intraepithelial spread of malignancy.
    d. Recognition is often delayed due to misdiagnosis as benign eyelid inflammation.

59. All of the following are true regarding malignant melanoma of eyelid skin, except:
    a. Lentigo maligna melanoma and nodular melanoma are the most common forms affecting the eyelid.
    b. Nodular melanoma is the most rare eyelid melanoma and has the worst prognosis.
    c. The factor of greatest prognostic significance is depth of invasion.
    d. Like conjunctival melanosis, eyelid melanoma may be controlled with cryotherapy.

60. A 14-year-old patient presents with a left upper eyelid lesion as photographed at the top of the next page. Histopathology of the lesion showed shadow cells and areas of calcification surrounded by basophilic cells. All of the following are true of the patient's condition, except:
    a. Young adults are most often affected.
    b. The lesion is epithelial in origin.
    c. Surgical excision of the lesion is curative.
    d. The eyebrow is also a common site of involvement.

132

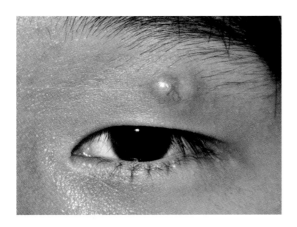

61. Typical manifestations of idiopathic orbital inflammation (pseudotumor) include all of the following, except
    a. dacryoadenitis.
    b. optic perineuritis.
    c. periscleritis.
    d. peripheral ulcerative keratitis.

62. Compared with adults, all of the following findings are more common in pediatric idiopathic orbital inflammation (orbital pseudotumor), except
    a. uveitis.
    b. optic disc edema.
    c. unilateral presentation.
    d. eosinophilia.

63. All of the following disorders may be associated with a clinical presentation indistinguishable from typical inflammatory orbital pseudotumor, except
    a. Wegener's granulomatosis.
    b. Churg-Strauss syndrome.
    c. sarcoidosis.
    d. polyarteritis nodosa.

64. All Le Fort fractures (I, II, and III) must extend posteriorly through what bone?
    a. pterygoid plates.
    b. maxillary bone.
    c. zygomaticomaxillary complex.
    d. naso-orbital-ethmoidal.

65. The optimal time for surgical repair of orbital floor fractures is generally considered to be
    a. within 24 hours of injury.
    b. 1 to 3 days following injury.
    c. 2 weeks following injury.
    d. 6 weeks following injury.

66. A 76-year-old patient is referred for left upper eyelid ptosis. Examination shows an incomitant strabismus and a lesion of the left lower eyelid, lateral canthus, and conjunctiva (see image below). The patient has a history of prior basal cell carcinoma of the left lower eyelid. A biopsy confirms recurrence of basal cell carcinoma. CT scan shows a mass extending deeply in the lateral orbit. What treatment is recommended?
    a. orbital exenteration.
    b. full-thickness pentagonal wedge resection.
    c. cryotherapy.
    d. radiation therapy.

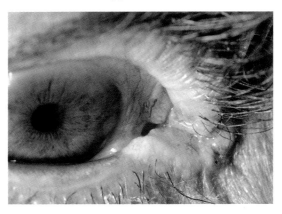

67. Consultation is requested for a patient who sustained massive facial trauma. Which of the following statements accurately characterizes the condition shown in the image below by the metal probe?
    a. After surgical repair, stents are left in place for 3 weeks.
    b. Direct suturing of the cut ends is required.
    c. Irrigation using methylene blue may facilitate intraoperative visualization.
    d. Repair of all such injuries is recommended.

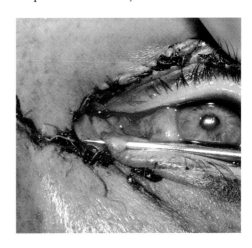

133

83. A patient sustained a severe motor vehicle accident, which included a tree branch penetrating the left medial orbit. The avulsed globe was found at the site of the accident. The entire length of superior oblique tendon is seen draped along the posterior and inferior aspects of the globe. The optic nerve starts at the 4.9 cm mark and attaches to the back of the eye at the 8.1 cm mark on the ruler. What is the name of the region of optic nerve at the cut (avulsed) end?
    a. intraocular.
    b. intraorbital.
    c. intracanalicular.
    d. intracranial.

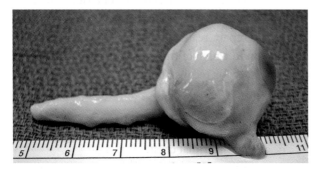

84. A patient photographed in the image A below reports the acute onset of left eye proptosis and painful diplopia after prolonged retching following an episode of alcohol binge drinking. CT scan shows a space-occupying mass (see image B at the top of the right column). The patient has decreased vision, a relative afferent papillary defect, elevated intraocular pressure, and optic disc hyperemia. What is the most appropriate management recommendation?
    a. aqueous suppressant medications.
    b. surgical drainage.
    c. observation.
    d. anterior chamber paracentesis.

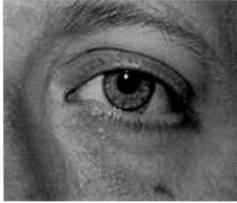

A

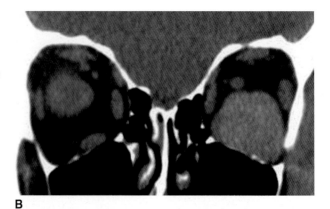

B

85. The systemic disorder most commonly associated with the blepharophimosis syndrome is
    a. diabetes mellitus.
    b. primary amenorrhea.
    c. hypospadias.
    d. coarctation of the aorta.

86. A 45-year-old woman presents with an encapsulated well-circumscribed retrobulbar mass of the left orbit demonstrated in the image below. All of the following are potential diagnoses, except
    a. neurilemoma.
    b. hemangiopericytoma.
    c. lymphangioma.
    d. fibrous histiocytoma.

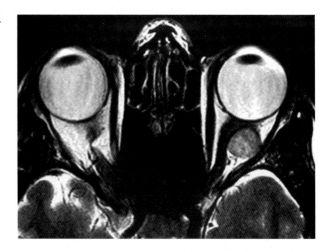

136

87. Which one of the following regarding dermoid and epidermoid cysts is false?
    a. They share a common pathophysiology.
    b. The key distinguishing feature between the two is the nature of the wall of the cystic cavity.
    c. In adults, nearly all of these lesions are anterior to the orbital septum.
    d. Superficial cysts present more often during childhood.

88. An image of a left orbit is shown below. What lettered location best represents the most common site of adherence for a dermoid cyst?
    a. location A.
    b. location B.
    c. location C.
    d. location D.

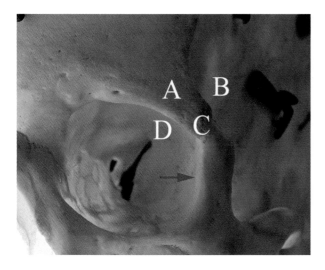

89. In question 88, a blue arrow is seen in the figure. The arrow points to a small palpable structure just inside the orbital rim. All of the following structures attach to the site indicated by the blue arrow, except
    a. superior transverse ligament of the orbit.
    b. aponeurosis of the levator palpebrae superioris muscle.
    c. suspensory ligament of the eyeball.
    d. lateral check ligament of the inferior oblique muscle.

90. A patient presents with slowly progressive proptosis of the right eye. Excisional biopsy confirms large cavernous spaces containing erythrocytes (images A,B, and C below). All of the following may be seen in this condition, except
    a. accelerated growth of the lesion in a pregnant patient.
    b. anterior displacement of the far point plane of the eye.
    c. more than one type of optic neuropathy.
    d. radiodense phleboliths present on CT scan imaging.

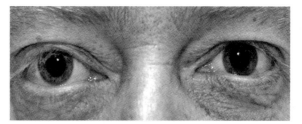

A

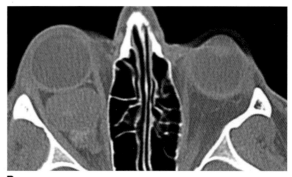

B

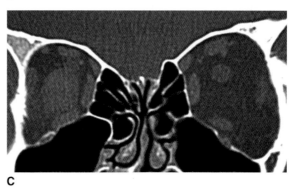

C

91. What is the expected reflectivity on A-scan ultrasonography of the capsule of the lesion in the previous question?
    a. none.
    b. low.
    c. medium.
    d. high.

6

92. In patients with eyelid ptosis, which of the following is the most important measure in determining the type of surgery to perform?
    a. margin reflex distance.
    b. eyelid excursion.
    c. response to phenylephrine testing.
    d. palpebral fissure.

93. If one makes an incision 15 mm above the eyelid margin through the full thickness of the central upper eyelid, what is the correct order of the anatomic structures encountered?
    a. skin, orbicularis oculi muscle, orbital septum, orbital fat, levator aponeurosis, Müller's muscle, conjunctiva.
    b. skin, orbital septum, orbicularis oculi muscle, orbital fat, levator aponeurosis, Müller's muscle, conjunctiva.
    c. skin, orbicularis oculi muscle, orbital septum, orbital fat, Müller's muscle, levator aponeurosis, conjunctiva.
    d. skin, orbicularis oculi muscle, orbital fat, orbital septum, levator aponeurosis, Müller's muscle, conjunctiva.

94. A 2-year-old child presents with bilateral proptosis. Which of the following is the least likely diagnosis?
    a. metastatic neuroblastoma.
    b. leukemia.
    c. capillary hemangioma.
    d. orbital pseudotumor.

95. The average distance from lacrimal punctum to nasolacrimal sac is
    a. 2 mm.
    b. 8 mm.
    c. 10 mm.
    d. 30 mm.

96. What is the organism that most commonly causes canaliculitis?
    a. *Nocardia asteroides*.
    b. *Staphylococcus*.
    c. *Candida albicans*.
    d. *Actinomyces israelii*.

97. All of the following medications are known to potentially cause canalicular obstruction, except
    a. phospholine iodine.
    b. 5-fluorouracil.
    c. doxorubicin.
    d. idoxuridine.

98. What type of epithelium are the lacrimal canaliculi lined by?
    a. stratified cuboidal.
    b. pseudostratified ciliated columnar.
    c. stratified squamous.
    d. bilayered cuboidal.

99. An infant with congenital nasolacrimal duct obstruction undergoes lacrimal probing. Starting from the punctum, what distance will the probe travel before reaching the inferior meatus?
    a. 12 mm.
    b. 20 mm.
    c. 24 mm.
    d. 30 mm.

100. In adults, the average distance from lacrimal punctum to inferior nasal meatus is
    a. 2 mm.
    b. 8 mm.
    c. 10 mm.
    d. 30 mm.

101. What is the most commonly performed clinical test in the evaluation of the adult patient with epiphora?
    a. Jones I test.
    b. Jones II test.
    c. lacrimal irrigation.
    d. dye disappearance test.

102. Which one of the following functional tests of lacrimal drainage is most likely to yield a false-positive result?
    a. lacrimal scintigraphy.
    b. secondary dye test (Jones II test).
    c. dye disappearance test.
    d. primary dye test (Jones I test).

103. Which one of the following functional tests of lacrimal drainage allows identification of a failure of the lacrimal pump mechanism?
   a. Schirmer's test.
   b. primary dye test (Jones I test).
   c. dye disappearance test.
   d. secondary dye test (Jones II test).

104. A 75-year-old patient is brought in from the nursing home for acute dacryocystitis. Which of the following is the most appropriate initial step in the treatment of this patient?
   a. dacryocystorhinostomy.
   b. broad-spectrum antibiotics.
   c. nasolacrimal duct probing.
   d. canalicular irrigation.

105. The most important predisposing factor for acute dacryocystitis is
   a. chronic blepharitis.
   b. acute bacterial conjunctivitis.
   c. dry eye.
   d. tear stasis of any etiology.

106. When performing an endoscopic dacryocystorhinostomy, all of the following bones are often removed, except
   a. nasal.
   b. maxilla.
   c. lacrimal.
   d. ethmoid.

107. Acute, lancinating pain in the medial canthal region with minimal noninflamed enlargement of the lacrimal sac is most suggestive of
   a. impacted dacryolith.
   b. acute dacryocystitis.
   c. chronic dacryocystitis.
   d. Wegener granulomatosis.

108. The most common site of organic obstruction in acquired nasolacrimal obstruction is
   a. intraosseous nasolacrimal duct.
   b. punctum.
   c. valve of Hasner.
   d. canaliculus.

109. All of the following may occur in a patient with a palsy of the seventh cranial nerve, except
   a. epiphora.
   b. keratitis.
   c. ectropion.
   d. ptosis.

110. An image of a right orbit is shown below. There are two numbered sites. Which of the following series correctly pairs the number with the correct bones of the orbit?
   a. (1) zygomatic bone, (2) greater wing of the sphenoid bone.
   b. (1) greater wing of the sphenoid bone, (2) lesser wing of the sphenoid bone.
   c. (1) zygomatic bone, (2) ethmoid bone.
   d. (1) maxillary bone, (2) greater wing of the sphenoid bone.

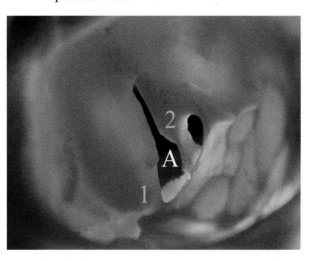

111. An image of a right orbit is shown in question 110. All of the following structures pass through the space depicted by the letter A, except
   a. sympathetic nerve fibers.
   b. superior ophthalmic vein.
   c. trochlear nerve.
   d. zygomatic nerve.

112. Which sinus system aerates first?
   a. maxillary.
   b. frontal.
   c. sphenoid.
   d. ethmoid.

113. The most common sinus lesion that invades the orbit is the
    a. osteoma.
    b. inverted papilloma.
    c. mucocele.
    d. squamous cell carcinoma.

114. The medial aspect of a left orbit is shown below. What bone is depicted by number (1) and what structure originates from the point shown by number (2)?
    a. (1) lacrimal bone, (2) medial canthal tendon.
    b. (1) lacrimal bone, (2) inferior oblique muscle.
    c. (1) maxillary bone, (2) inferior oblique muscle.
    d. (1) maxillary bone, (2) medial canthal tendon.

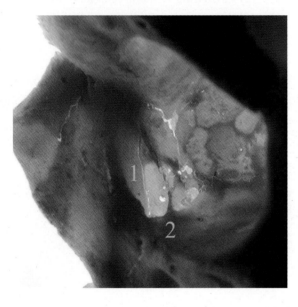

115. What tissue plane is the temporal branch of the facial nerve located in superior to the zygomatic arch?
    a. deep temporal fascia.
    b. loose areolar tissue.
    c. subcutaneous tissue.
    d. temporoparietal fascia.

116. The normal upper eyelid cross-sectional anatomy from the left orbit of a Caucasian cadaver is shown below. The presence of what lettered structure when clinically evaluating a patient with an eyelid laceration should raise the suspicion of a concomitant corneoscleral laceration?
    a. structure A.
    b. structure B.
    c. structure C.
    d. structure D.

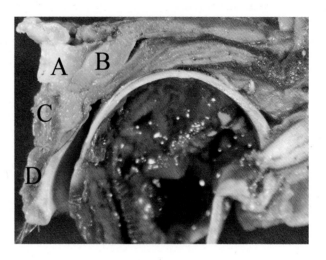

117. All of the following surgeries may be performed by making an incision at the site of the green asterisk in the image from question 116, except
    a. blepharoplasty.
    b. internal blepharoptosis repair.
    c. lateral orbitotomy.
    d. optic nerve sheath fenestration.

118. All of the following are true regarding the levator palpebrae superioris, except
    a. It runs from the posterior lacrimal crest medially to the lateral orbital tubercle laterally.
    b. Its superficial portion inserts into the orbicularis muscle and subcutaneous tissues.
    c. It originates in close proximity to the superior rectus origin, just above the annulus of Zinn.
    d. The muscular portion is shorter than the aponeurotic portion.

119. The structure that gives rise to the gray line of the eyelid margin is best represented by
    a. meibomian glands.
    b. tarsal border.
    c. mucocutaneous junction.
    d. orbicularis muscle.

120. The capsulopalpebral fascia is analogous to which upper eyelid structure?
    a. levator aponeurosis.
    b. orbital septum.
    c. superior transverse ligament.
    d. Müller's muscle.

121. The normal horizontal extent of the human palpebral fissure is approximately
    a. 20 mm.
    b. 25 mm.
    c. 30 mm.
    d. 35 mm.

122. The most likely outcome following inadvertent suturing of the orbital septum into subcutaneous tissues while repairing a partial-thickness eyelid laceration is
    a. ectropion.
    b. lid retraction in downgaze.
    c. entropion.
    d. blepharoptosis.

123. All of the following are characteristic of features of blepharochalasis, except
    a. lacrimal gland atrophy.
    b. excess eyelid skin.
    c. blepharoptosis.
    d. blepharophimosis.

124. What is the treatment of choice for a patient with an optic nerve sheath meningioma confined to the orbit and with progressive visual loss?
    a. observation.
    b. surgical excision.
    c. chemotherapy.
    d. radiation therapy.

125. An 86-year-old patient presents with left eye proptosis, diplopia, and a subconjunctival lesion photographed at the top of the right column. Which of the following is the most appropriate next step?
    a. biopsy.
    b. B-scan ultrasonography.
    c. corticosteroids.
    d. orbital imaging.

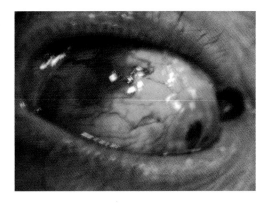

126. A 7-year-old boy presents with a 3-day history of progressive proptosis, injection, and pain of the left eye. He is systemically well with normal temperature. White blood cell count is normal, and emergent orbital CT scanning reveals superonasal orbital infiltration with bony erosion. The most likely diagnosis at this point is
    a. frontal sinus mucocele.
    b. rhabdomyosarcoma.
    c. bacterial orbital cellulitis.
    d. optic nerve glioma.

127. An image of a skull centered on the left orbit is shown below. What lettered location indicates a bone that is not part of the orbit?
    a. location A.
    b. location B.
    c. location C.
    d. location D.

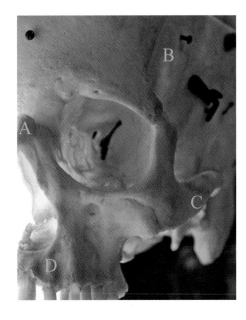

6

128. Which one of the following histiocytic disorders is most likely to involve orbital bone?
    a. sinus histiocytosis.
    b. Hand–Schüller–Christian disease.
    c. Letterer–Siwe disease.
    d. eosinophilic granuloma.

129. Which of the following is one of the most common mesenchymal tumor of the orbit?
    a. hemangiopericytoma.
    b. fibrous histiocytoma.
    c. osteogenic sarcoma.
    d. ossifying fibroma.

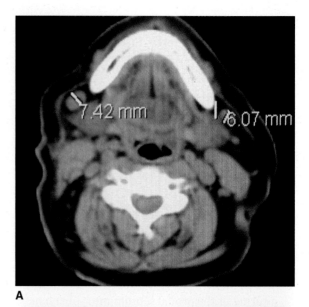

A

130. The most common site of a primary tumor metastatic to the orbit in men is
    a. lung.
    b. colon.
    c. prostate.
    d. melanoma.

131. All of the following conditions may present with epiphora secondary to impaired blink function (abnormal blink), except
    a. Sjögren's syndrome.
    b. Parkinson's disease.
    c. scleroderma.
    d. progressive supranuclear palsy.

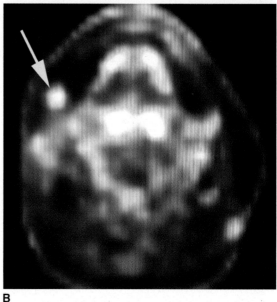

B

132. A patient with biopsy-proven sebaceous carcinoma of the eyelid presents with positive lymphadenopathy, as seen on PET-CT scans at the top of the right column. Based on both the most likely eyelid affected by sebaceous carcinoma and the involved node, which of the following is most likely to be the location of this patient's eyelid neoplasm?
    a. medial, lower eyelid.
    b. lateral, lower eyelid.
    c. medial, upper eyelid.
    d. lateral, upper eyelid.

133. Components in the evaluation of corneal protective mechanisms prior to ptosis surgery include all of the following, except
    a. examination for lagophthalmos.
    b. Jones (primary dye) testing.
    c. assessment of Bell's phenomenon.
    d. evaluation of corneal sensation.

134. The primary abnormality seen in simple congenital ptosis is in the
    a. levator muscle.
    b. levator aponeurosis.
    c. levator innervation.
    d. Müller's muscle.

135. The primary abnormality seen in ptosis after cataract surgery is in the
   a. levator aponeurosis.
   b. Müller's muscle.
   c. levator innervation.
   d. levator muscle.

136. The procedure of choice in a patient with ptosis following cataract surgery (good levator function and a high or effaced upper eyelid crease) would be
   a. levator muscle resection.
   b. unilateral frontalis suspension.
   c. Müller's muscle resection.
   d. reinsertion of levator aponeurosis.

137. A patient is referred for surgical repair of the bilateral eyelid condition shown in the image below. On examination, he has papillary conjunctivitis and an upper eyelid margin reflex distance (MRD1) of 1 mm bilaterally. What effect will full thickness wedge resection (FTWR) to tighten the eyelids horizontally most likely have on the height of the upper eyelids?
   a. A FTWR will slightly raise the eyelid.
   b. A FTWR is not expected to affect the eyelid position.
   c. A FTWR will slightly lower the eyelid.
   d. A FTWR will cause eyelid retraction.

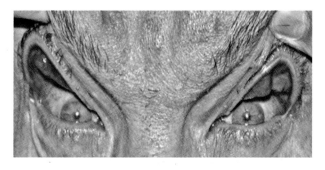

138. Which of the following is characteristic of the histopathology of the eyelid condition shown in question 137?
   a. decrease in tarsal elastin fibers.
   b. decrease in conjunctival inflammation.
   c. decrease in tarsal collagen type I.
   d. decrease in tarsal collagen type III.

139. Which of the following extraocular muscles is least likely to be injured during upper or lower blepharoplasty?
   a. inferior oblique.
   b. inferior rectus.
   c. superior oblique.
   d. superior rectus.

140. The most significant complication of blepharoplasty is
   a. orbital hemorrhage.
   b. diplopia.
   c. overcorrection.
   d. cellulitis.

141. The most common cause of indirect traumatic optic neuropathy is blunt trauma to which bone?
   a. maxillary.
   b. zygomatic.
   c. frontal.
   d. temporal.

142. What percentage of tear loss is evaporative in nature in young and elderly patients, respectively?
   a. 5% and 10%.
   b. 10% and 20%.
   c. 15% and 30%.
   d. 20% and 40%.

143. Which of the following is least likely to be associated with a zygomaticomaxillary complex (ZMC) fracture?
   a. inferior rectus entrapment.
   b. trismus.
   c. globe ptosis.
   d. lateral canthal dystopia.

144. Besides pharmacologic testing with edrophonium chloride (Tensilon), which of the following is another clinical test specifically used in diagnosing myasthenia gravis (MG)?
   a. exercise stress test.
   b. ice pack test.
   c. thyroid-stimulating hormone (TSH) receptor antibody test.
   d. three-step test.

6

143

145. An 11-year-old patient in the figures below presents gradually increasing proptosis of the right eye. Based on patient's most likely diagnosis, which one of the following clinical features would be considered inconsistent with the diagnosis?
    a. unilaterality.
    b. insidious onset.
    c. afferent pupillary defect.
    d. pain.

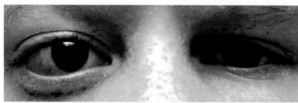

A

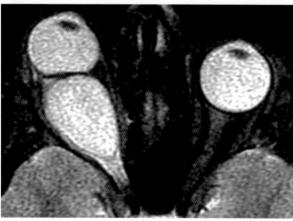

B

146. The systemic evaluation of a patient with biopsy-proven orbital lymphoma generally includes all of the following except
    a. lumbar puncture.
    b. bone scan.
    c. serum immunoelectrophoresis.
    d. bone marrow biopsy.

147. Which of the following answers would be the best treatment option for a localized orbital lymphoproliferative lesion?
    a. radiation and systemic corticosteroids.
    b. radiation therapy alone.
    c. surgical excision combined with chemotherapy.
    d. surgical excision combined with radiation.

148. A 5-month-old baby is seen in consultation for the condition shown below. All of the following characteristic of this condition, except
    a. autosomal dominant.
    b. lower eyelid entropion.
    c. lop ears.
    d. hypoplasia of the superior orbital rims.

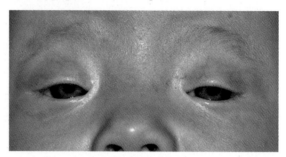

149. A patient undergoes placement of hard palate graft for lower eyelid retraction. Which of the following best characterizes the epithelium of the graft?
    a. retention of native epithelium.
    b. metaplasia into nonkeratinized epithelium.
    c. survival of submucosal glands.
    d. conjunctivalization of epithelium.

150. A 73-year-old patient in the photograph below is referred in consultation for chronic left eye irritation. He has a snap back test of greater than 6 mm and normal palpebral and forniceal conjunctiva. Based on the patient's diagnosis, all of the following are true statements regarding the patient's diagnosis, except
    a. no inferior movement of lower eyelid during downgaze.
    b. deeper than usual inferior fornix.
    c. presence of a white subconjunctival line below the inferior tarsal border.
    d. lower than normal position of lower eyelid.

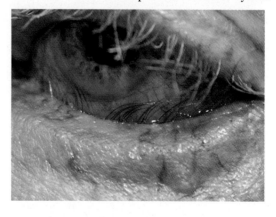

Answers

1. **c.** A superficially placed gold weight implant (GWI) is shown in the figure. The concern is that the implant may become exposed. The GWI is commonly placed in a pretarsal location underneath the orbicularis oculi muscle, rather than directly underneath the surface of the skin.

2. **c.** The periocular concerns of patients with facial nerve palsy include lagophthalmos, paralytic ectropion, and eyebrow ptosis, which are addressed surgically by choices a, b, and d, respectively. Blepharoplasty to correct dermatochalasis is unrelated to the patient's condition.

3. **b.** Choices a and d describe potential serious side effects. Other major side effects of edrophonium include bradycardia, bronchospasm, and cholinergic crisis. Besides choice c, a number of minor side effects may occur such as nausea, diaphoresis, salivation, abdominal cramping, and lacrimation.

4. **c.** A CT scan of the chest is appropriate to rule out thymoma, which occurs in about 10% of patients with MG. Conversely, about a third of patients with a thymoma have MG.

5. **a.** The lesion shown is classic-appearing example of a keratoacanthoma (KA). KA characteristically erupts rapidly and is considered a subtype of squamous cell carcinoma. The central crater is keratin filled. Of note, KA associated with sebaceous neoplasms may occur as part of the Muir-Torre syndrome (visceral malignancy).

6. **a.** Marcus Gunn jaw-winking ptosis results from synkinesis of the third and fifth (motor division) cranial nerves.

7. **b.** Eyelid synkinesis is associated with choices a, c, and d. While not considered synkinesis, a brief eyelid twitch, lasting seconds, may occur in a patient with ocular myasthenia gravis. The twitch, known as Cogan lid-twitch, may be seen when the patient looks from down to upgaze.

8. **c.** The patient has an age, history, and external examination consistent with involutional ptosis. The patient shown also has dermatochalasis. Involutional ptosis is characterized by normal levator function and a high eyelid crease. In contrast to pediatric ptosis, which exhibits lid lag, involutional ptosis worsens in the reading (downgaze) position. The supratarsal tissues are thinned. Dehiscence of the levator aponeurosis is the most commonly accepted mechanism for ptosis following cataract and other eye surgeries.

9. **d.** The patient has rhabdomyosarcoma. Incisional biopsy is necessary for making the diagnosis. If the tumor can be safely removed at the time of surgery, then excisional biopsy is more appropriate. Observation does not have a role in this patient's care. Chemotherapy is used to treat the condition once the diagnosis has been made. Bone marrow biopsy may be coordinated to coincide with biopsy of the orbital mass.

10. **b.** The gross examination shown is of an exenteration specimen of a patient with sebaceous carcinoma. The appropriate management of primary orbital rhabdomyosarcoma involves radiation therapy and systemic chemotherapy. Although historically, rhabdomyosarcoma was treated with exenteration, currently, such surgery is used only in recurrent cases.

11. **d.** Choices a–c are related to adenoid cystic carcinoma. Both benign mixed tumor (pleomorphic adenoma) and adenoid cystic carcinoma tend to occur in middle-aged patients.

12. **a.** Bony remodeling (fossa formation) occurs in benign mixed tumor due to its gradual growth pattern. Bony erosion is seen with infiltrative lesion such as adenoid cystic carcinoma. Lymphoid tumors tend to conform to the shape of the surrounding structures.

6

13. **a.** The peripheral arterial arcade lies just above the superior tarsal border between the levator aponeurosis and Müller's muscle. It is a distinct structure from the marginal arcade, which lies on the tarsal surface of each eyelid margin.

14. **c.** Lacrimal sac distention above the medial canthal tendon raises the suspicion of a lacrimal malignancy in adults and an encephalocoele in newborn patients, respectively.

15. **b.** The nasolacrimal drains inferiorly and runs slightly lateral and posterior.

16. **c.** The patient has a cicatricial ectropion. Choices a, b, and d are appropriate aspects of the surgical management of the condition. Eyelid retractor repair is an important component in the repair of involutional entropion and occasionally involutional ectropion.

17. **c.** The proptosis of optic nerve sheath meningioma is usually axial. Lacrimal gland malignancies may produce proptosis, which is typically down and medial. Maxillary sinus tumors typically push the eye superiorly.

18. **a.** The history of proptosis due to benign mixed tumor of the lacrimal gland (pleomorphic adenoma) is characteristically greater than 6 to 12 months.

19. **d.** The patient's raised pearly lesion with overlying telangiectatic vessels and madarosis is typical of nodular basal cell carcinoma. Once the diagnosis is confirmed by incisional biopsy, a more invasive full-thickness wedge resection (excisional biopsy) may be undertaken.

20. **d.** Choices a–c are true of botulinum toxin type B. It is type A that has a longer duration of action.

21. **c.** Hemifacial spasm is rarely bilateral and is usually due to vascular compression of the seventh cranial nerve at the brainstem and can result in synchronous contractions of the entire side of the face. Along with partial complex seizures and myoclonic epilepsy, essential blepharospasm is effaced by sleep.

22. **b.** The long-term use of hard contact lenses has been associated with acquired aponeurotic ptosis due to repetitive traction. Involutional attenuation is an age-related condition also associated with dehiscence of the levator aponeurosis. Levator muscle dysgenesis is seen in congenital ptosis. Myogenic ptosis occurs in muscular diseases such as myasthenia gravis, muscular dystrophy, oculopharyngial dystrophy, and chronic progressive external ophthalmoplegia.

23. **d.** Orbital cellulitis is the most common cause of unilateral proptosis in children. Thyroid eye disease is the most common cause of both unilateral and bilateral proptosis in adults.

24. **d.** A bluish bulge *above* the medial canthal tendon is typically a meningocele, whereas one *below* is typically a dacryocele.

25. **c.** The patient has a direct (high-flow) carotid cavernous (CC) sinus fistula. Indirect (low-flow) dural cavernous fistulas tend to occur in elderly women, whereas the direct dural cavernous fistulas occur after a basal skull fracture. Arteriography is used to differentiate between the two types of fistula. A cranial bruit is characteristic of a direct CC fistula. Extraocular muscle enlargement may occur due to orbital congestion.

26. **b.** This is a classic presentation of a cavernous sinus wall–dural shunt, featuring lower arterial flow and an insidious onset.

27. **d.** The orbits of patients with craniosynostoses are usually shallow and small, with resultant proptosis and exposure. V-pattern exotropia is also common.

28. **b.** Choices a, c, and d are risk factors for orbital cellulitis. Recent skin trauma is the most common risk factor for preseptal cellulitis.

29. **a.** Breast cancer is the most common primary source of metastases to the orbit in women. Hormone therapy is used in estrogen-receptor–positive tumors. Extraocular involvement is more common than bony involvement. Although the scirrhous subtype can present with enophthalmos, the majority of patients with metastatic breast cancer present with proptosis. Clinically, the patient in this case had 7 mm of proptosis in the left eye, which is consistent with the radiographic appearance of the space occupying mass lesion.

30. **c.** The patient has complete left upper eyelid ptosis and compensatory right upper eyelid retraction (Hering's law).

31. **b.** The patient has a capillary hemangioma, which is causing mechanical ptosis. Although the lesion may involute over time, deprivation amblyopia is an urgent concern in the management of this patient and thus early treatment is warranted.

32. **a.** Choices b–d have been used in the treatment of capillary hemangioma. Intralesional steroid injection is often the first line approach. However, the use of propranolol is an area of active evolution in the treatment of patients with capillary hemangioma.

33. **c.** Kasabach-Merritt syndrome is a platelet sequestration disorder associated with multiple large capillary hemangiomas, which results in thrombocytopenia.

34. **a.** Cavernous sinus thrombosis is one of the most dreaded complications of orbital cellulitis, with a significant increase in systemic morbidity and mortality.

35. **a.** Telecanthus is defined as an abnormally large distance between medial canthi, regardless of intraorbital distance. Telecanthus and rounding of the medial canthus are characteristic findings in direct naso-orbital-ethmoid fractures.

36. **c.** Orbital floor fractures usually produce vertical limitations of gaze. Global motility deficits generally indicate blunt trauma with muscle and/or nerve contusion.

37. **d.** The images show a fracture of the right orbital roof (the most common orbital fracture in young children). The lack of a pneumatized frontal sinus predisposes the early childhood age group to roof fractures. Choice c is incorrect in that the injury can occur in a fall from a height of less than 10 ft. Choice d is characteristic clinical finding associated with roof fractures. Treatment is indicated only for significantly displaced roof fractures; a multidisciplinary approach works best for the minority of patients that require surgery.

38. **d.** Choices a–c, as well as scirrhous breast carcinoma, are associated with enophthalmos. In contrast, malar hypoplasia may create an appearance of proptosis (relative exophthalmos).

39. **d.** The nevus flammeus (port-wine stain) is a cavernous hemangioma of the dermis. It can be seen in Sturge-Weber syndrome, Klippel-Trénaunay-Weber syndrome, and as an idiopathic finding. Some pathology references also refer to the lesion as a dermal telangiectasia.

40. **a.** Although not usually present at birth, the majority of capillary hemangiomas become apparent within the first several weeks of life.

41. **b.** Capillary hemangiomas generally start to involute spontaneously by 12 months of age. 40% of tumors completely regress by age 4. 80% of tumors completely regress by age 8.

42. **b.** Capillary hemangiomata will blanch with pressure, whereas the nevus flammeus does not. There is considerable overlap between the other features listed.

43. **c.** Choice correctly identifies the approximate percentages of the different patients with the thyroid eye disease.

6

147

44. c. The enlargement generally features smooth contours. Although sometimes only a single muscle is enlarged, this should be considered an atypical finding.

45. d. Eyelid retraction is the most commonly occurring eyelid finding in patients with Graves' ophthalmopathy (seen in about 38% of patients). Von Graefe's sign, lagophthalmos, and lid lag occur in about 36%, 16%, and 8% of patients with Graves' ophthalmopathy, respectively.

46. c. Waiting for a period of 6 months allows adequate time for stability of the condition to be established, allowing for a more predictable outcome.

47. d. Preoperative and intraoperative images of a patient who underwent evisceration surgery are shown. The cornea should be removed in cases of active corneal disease. Choices a–c are correct.

48. c. A superior sulcus deformity results from inadequate volume replacement when the eye is removed from the orbit.

49. a. The patient has choroidal melanoma. The intraocular mass (with characteristic low internal reflectivity) is seen on the ultrasound examination. Removal of the eye is the most appropriate treatment. Evisceration should never be performed in the presence of an intraocular mass.

50. b. Alveolar rhabdomyosarcoma has a predilection for the inferior orbit. The embryonal variant is more common superonasally. Metastatic workup includes lumbar puncture and bone marrow biopsy, best done under anesthesia.

51. b. Dysplasia or aplasia of the sphenoid bone creates large posterior orbital defects. This leads to pulsating exophthalmos, as brain tissue herniates outward.

52. d. Orbital phycomycosis generally results from invasion by necrotizing fungal sinusitis. Black eschar in the nasal cavity is virtually diagnostic, but is a late finding. (Its absence does not exclude the diagnosis.)

53. b. Acanthosis nigricans is associated with internal malignancy but not transformation. Actinic keratosis is the most common premalignant skin lesion. It is related to ultraviolet (UV) exposure and may develop into squamous cell carcinoma. Although actinic keratoses resolve spontaneously within a year in up to 25% of cases, patients with multiple actinic keratoses have a 12% to 16% risk of developing squamous cell carcinoma.

54. a. Suddenly appearing multiple seborrheic keratoses may in fact be evolving acanthosis nigricans. This is known as the Leser-Trélat sign and is usually associated with a GI malignancy.

55. a. Anti-herpetic medication is given to patients. Oral antibiotic medication is also often prescribed preoperatively.

56. a. Use of isotretinoin (Accutane) within the preceding 12 months is a contraindication for laser skin resurfacing due to impaired ability of reepithelialization.

57. b. Suborbicularis oculi fat (SOOF) elevation provides a youthful midface appearance. It is usually accessed through a transconjunctival or subciliary approach.

58. b. There may be multicentric foci of tumor with skip areas. Negative margins do not necessarily imply complete excision of the tumor. Wide surgical margins should be used, with map biopsies taken over the area surrounding the lesion.

59. d. Cryotherapy selectively destroys melanocytes but is insufficient for cutaneous melanoma and should be considered a palliative treatment.

60. b. A patient with a pilomatricoma of the central, left upper eyelid is shown. The lesion has a characteristic histopathologic appearance (includes shadow cells), which is described in the question stem. It is classified as a benign tumor of hair follicle (i.e., skin adnexal, rather than epithelial) origin. Clinically, the lesion can be mistaken for a cyst.

61. **d.** Changes in corneal sensation may occur, but frank ulceration—especially peripherally—is unusual.

62. **c.** Bilateral presentation of orbital pseudotumor is more common in children (occurs in about one-third of cases). Choices a, b, and d are true.

63. **c.** Sarcoidosis is generally not associated with pain and usually spares orbital soft tissues.

64. **a.** All Le Fort fractures by definition must involve the pterygoid plates. The Le Fort I fracture is the only one of the three that does not involve the orbit. In actuality, mixed presentations of the three types frequently occur.

65. **c.** Two weeks provides a chance for orbital swelling and "contusion diplopia" to resolve and yet is early enough to avoid problems with scarring of a significant floor fracture.

66. **a.** The patient has basal cell carcinoma invasive to the orbit. Exenteration is an appropriate treatment strategy, as long as the tumor has not invaded too deeply that complete resection is not possible.

67. **d.** The patient has a canalicular laceration. Canalicular involvement should be suspected in any eyelid laceration medial to the corneal limbus. Direct suturing of the ends in not required; however, stenting is necessary. Canalicular stents are ideally left in place for 3 to 6 months (not weeks). While irrigation with fluorescein can be helpful to localize the cut ends of the canaliculus, methylene blue is not recommended as it stains the whole surgical field.

68. **a.** The trochlea is the only cartilaginous structure in the normal orbit.

69. **b.** Rituximab is a monoclonal antibody that targets the B cell CD20 receptor.

70. **c.** About half of newborns are born with an imperforate valve of Hasner. Most (>90%) congenital nasolacrimal duct obstructions resolve within the first 12 months of life.

71. **c.** The sphenopalatine ganglion receives parasympathetic fibers from the greater superficial petrosal nerve (a division of CN VII).

72. **d.** Tear production commences by the first 6 weeks of life.

73. **c.** Benign mixed tumor (pleomorphic adenoma) is the most common lacrimal gland neoplasm.

74. **a.** Adenoid cystic carcinoma is the most common *malignant* neoplasm of the lacrimal gland.

75. **d.** The levator aponeurosis divides the lacrimal gland into palpebral and orbital lobes.

76. **a.** The most likely diagnosis is that of benign mixed cell tumor. The male–female ratio is 3:2. The tumor should be approached through a lateral orbitotomy with careful excision to avoid rupture of the tumor's pseudocapsule. Incisional or incomplete biopsy techniques can lead to infiltrative tumor recurrence and, occasionally, malignant transformation.

77. **a.** An encephalocele is not associated with reflex hypersecretion.

78. **c.** A dermoid cyst is an example of a choristoma. The lesion is lined by keratinizing epithelium. The condition most commonly occurs at the lateral brow at the frontozygomatic suture. The superonasal location (e.g., the frontolacrimal and frontoethmoidal sutures) is the next most common location. An eyelid crease incision is frequently used to provide surgical access (including in the patient shown).

6

149

79. b. When ocular or optic disc perfusion is severely compromised by an orbital compartment syndrome, immediate canthotomy with cantholysis should be performed to decompress the orbit.

80. a. In cases where the ocular examination suggests optic nerve trauma (afferent pupillary defect, poor vision), neuroimaging is indicated to rule out direct optic nerve injury (e.g., optic canal fracture).

81. d. Reattachment of the posterior crus of the medial canthal tendon to the posterior lacrimal crest is necessary for reconstruction of the normal eyelid contour at the medial canthus. In the setting of a fracture, either transnasal wiring or Y-shaped miniplate fixation is required.

82. c. Traumatic ptosis is repaired after 6 months of observation. Ptosis repair prior to the possible spontaneous return of function may lead to lagophthalmos.

83. c. The intraorbital portion of the optic nerve measures about 28 to 30 mm in length. The avulsed globe shown in the figure has a 32 mm segment of optic nerve attached. Thus the avulsion has occurred at the intracanalicular portion (note in the figure the last 2 mm appear slightly different).

84. b. The patient has an orbital hemorrhage associated with the inferior rectus muscle. The condition may occur spontaneously and complete resolve without intervention. In cases without optic neuropathy, observation is advised. The patient presented has decreased vision and surgical drainage is recommended.

85. b. Primary amenorrhea is the most common condition associated with blepharophimosis.

86. c. A patient has a cavernous hemangioma, which is an encapsulated tumor. Choices a, b, and d are also encapsulated tumors. Lymphangioma, however, is not encapsulated.

87. c. Both types are ectopic epithelial rests created by aberrant "pinching off" *in utero*. The variety that is silent until adulthood is generally intraorbital (retroseptal).

88. c. Dermoid cysts are often adherent to suture lines; the frontozygomatic suture (marked location C) is the most common location. Anterior cysts also occur along the frontolacrimal and frontoethmoidal sutures.

89. d. The arrow marks the lateral orbital tubercle of Whitnall, which is a palpable structure about 11 mm below the frontozygomatic suture. In addition to Choices a–c, the lateral canthal tendon and the check ligament of the lateral rectus muscle also attach to Whitnall's tubercle. Other attached structures include the deep pretarsal orbicularis insertion and an expansion of the superior rectus muscle sheath. During horizontal eyelid tightening surgery (e.g., lateral tarsal strip) the lateral eyelid is reattached to the tubercle.

90. b. The patient has a cavernous hemangioma (CH). The growth of CH may accelerate during pregnancy. CH may exert pressure on the globe (raising intraocular pressure) and optic nerve, leading to glaucomatous and compressive optic neuropathies, respectively. Pressure on the globe can cause hyperopic shift (posterior displacement of the far point of the eye). CT scan may demonstrate radiodense phleboliths in older lesions.

91. d. As described, the lesion is a CH, which generally have high (especially the capsule) reflectively on A-scan.

92. b. The levator function (also known as eyelid excursion) is the critical measurement in guiding the type of ptosis surgery to perform.

93. a. Choice a indicates the correct order of the anatomic structures encountered.

94. c. Choices a, b, and d can commonly present bilaterally.

95. c. The distance is 2 mm down (ampulla), then 8 mm across (canaliculus).

96. d. *Actinomyces israelii* is most common bacterial cause of canaliculitis.

97. c. Docetaxel (Taxotere) is a chemotherapeutic agent used in the treatment of breast, ovarian, and nonsmall cell lung cancer. The drug is secreted in the tear film and can cause canalicular stenosis. Doxorubicin (Adriamycin) is also a chemotherapeutic agent that is known for cardiac side effects but does not lead to canalicular stenosis. Choices a, b, and d may cause canalicular stenosis.

98. c. The canaliculi are lined by stratified squamous epithelium.

99. b. The total length of the infant nasolacrimal system measures about 20 mm.

100. d. Besides the 10 mm distance from lacrimal punctum to sac, the length of the lacrimal sac and nasolacrimal duct adds another 20 to 25 mm. Thus in adults, the total length is 30 mm from lacrimal punctum to inferior meatus.

101. c. The Jones tests are not often performed in the clinical setting. Lacrimal irrigation is most commonly performed in the evaluation of epiphora.

102. d. The Jones I test consists of placing 2% fluorescein in the conjunctival fornices and attempting to recover fluorescein with a swab at the inferior meatus. Unfortunately, one-third of normal patients will have abnormal results with this test.

103. d. The Jones II test is performed after a dye disappearance test or after Jones I indicates blockage. The fornix is irrigated, and the lacrimal sac cannulated and irrigated. If dye is recovered in the inferior meatus, then incomplete blockage of the nasolacrimal duct, patent upper system, and functioning lacrimal pump is indicated. However, if only clear fluid is recovered, then a nonfunctioning lacrimal pump or blocked upper system is indicated.

104. b. The initial management of a patient with acute dacryocystitis includes broad-spectrum antibiotics. Dacryocystorhinostomy is performed once the initial inflammation subsides. Probing does not have a role in the management of adult nasolacrimal disorders. Canalicular irrigation is a treatment for canaliculitis.

105. d. Strictures, narrow or long ducts, and nasal and sinus inflammatory disease may cause tear stasis and lead to acute dacryocystitis.

106. a. The lacrimal and maxillary bones are invariably removed. In some cases, removal of anterior ethmoid air cells is performed to provide access to the lacrimal sac fossa. The nasal bone is not removed.

107. c. This is the ocular equivalent of a kidney stone.

108. a. In congenital obstruction, the blockage is at the valve of Hasner. In acquired cases, the blockage is within the intraosseous nasolacrimal duct. Involutional stenosis is one of the most common causes of acquired nasolacrimal duct obstruction.

109. d. Choices a–c occur with facial nerve palsy. Such patients have impaired eye closure (lagophthalmos), not eyelid ptosis.

110. b. The two wings of the sphenoid bone are marked. The two parts: (1) greater wing and (2) lesser wing are correctly labeled in choice b. The sphenoid bone makes up part of the orbital roof and lateral and medial walls of the orbit.

111. d. The marked space (A) is the superior orbital fissure. Choices a–c pass through the superior orbital fissure.

6

112. **a.** The maxillary sinus aerates first.

113. **c.** The most common sinus lesion to invade the orbit is mucocele. The most common neoplasm to invade the orbit is squamous cell carcinoma.

114. **c.** The lacrimal sac fossa, including the suture line separating the lacrimal and maxillary bones, is shown. The thinner lacrimal bone is seen to the right of the 1. The anterior process of the maxilla is marked (1). Lateral to the fossa, just inside the inferior orbital rim, is the origin (2) of the inferior oblique muscle. The medial canthal tendon attaches to the anterior and posterior crests of the lacrimal sac fossa.

115. **d.** The temporal branch of the facial nerve runs superficially (in the temporoparietal fascia) superior to the zygomatic arch.

116. **b.** The labeled structures are as follows: (A) brow fat, (B) preaponeurotic fat, (C) preseptal orbicularis muscle, and (D) pretarsal orbicularis muscle. A complete eye examination is important in all ocular and periocular trauma. Moreover, an eyelid laceration with visible adipose tissue present, specifically fat from the orbit, should raise concern for the possibility of injury to the globe.

117. **b.** The eyelid crease is marked by the asterisk. The crease occurs at the superior tarsal border in Caucasians. Choices a, c, and d may all be performed through an eyelid crease incision. Choice b is performed through the posterior approach by everting the eyelid.

118. **d.** The muscular portion is longer than the aponeurotic portion.

119. **d.** The gray line is an isolated bundle of pretarsal orbicularis muscle also known as the muscle of Riolan.

120. **a.** The capsulopalpebral fascia is analogous to the levator aponeurosis.

121. **c.** The normal adult palpebral fissure is 27 to 30 mm horizontally and 8 to 11 mm vertically.

122. **b.** The patient will have a deficiency of the middle lamella. Incorporation of the orbital septum will lead to lid retraction in downgaze.

123. **a.** The term blepharochalasis is sometimes confused with dermatochalasis. Blepharochalasis, a rare disorder, is considered a familial type of angioneurotic edema. The condition, characterized by repeated bouts of painless eyelid edema, often presents in children and adolescents. Patients may have prolapse (not atrophy) of the lacrimal gland. Other features include lower eyelid retraction, pseudoepicanthal folds, proptosis, blepharoptosis, blepharophimosis, and atrophic wrinkled excess eyelid skin.

124. **d.** The tumor may be observed unless there is loss of vision, in which case radiation therapy is advisable.

125. **d.** A salmon patch subconjunctival lesion is shown. The presence of proptosis and diplopia warrant imaging for an orbital mass, which was present in this patient with orbital lymphoma.

126. **b.** Orbital cellulitis does not usually cause bony erosion. In addition, the white blood cell count and temperature would be expected to be elevated (unless the child were immunocompromised). Mucocele and glioma are not typically so inflammatory. Rhabdomyosarcoma responds well to treatment and should be promptly diagnosed.

127. **a.** The labeled bones are as follows: (A) nasal, (B) frontal, (C) zygomatic, and (D) maxillary. The nasal bone is not part of the orbit. The adjacent frontal process of the maxilla lies just to the right of the nasal bone in the figure.

128. **d.** Eosinophilic granuloma frequently involves the orbital bones. The classic triad of Hand-Schüller-Christian disease consists of proptosis,

lytic skull lesions, and diabetes insipidus. Orbital involvement is rare in Letterer-Siwe disease. Prior characterization of histiocytic disorders using these terms is being replaced by the terms diffuse soft tissue histiocytosis and unifocal/multifocal eosinophilic granuloma of bone.

129. **b.** Most fibrous histiocytoma are benign (more than 90%), and have a storiform, or matlike, pattern on histopathology. The lesion is usually very firm and can displace other orbital structures.

130. **a.** An orbital metastasis is more likely to be the mode of presentation for bronchogenic carcinoma than for a breast primary.

131. **a.** A normal blink is necessary for the pump function of the lacrimal drainage system to work. Choices b–d are conditions with impaired blink function. Sjögren's syndrome causes a dry eye state.

132. **c.** The PET-CT scans show a positive submandibular node. The medial eyelid lymphatics drain to the submandibular nodes. In contrast, the lateral eyelid lymphatics drain to the preauricular nodes. Sebaceous carcinoma most commonly involves the upper eyelid. The patient shown had a sebaceous carcinoma of the medial right upper eyelid with regional spread to the submandibular nodes.

133. **b.** Jones testing will give information regarding patency of the lacrimal drainage system. Patients with positive Jones tests will have difficulties with epiphora, which can usually be managed independently.

134. **a.** Congenital myogenic ptosis results from a maldevelopment of the levator muscle.

135. **a.** Aponeurotic dehiscence has been blamed on anesthetic injections, lid specula, and bridle sutures. The exact cause is not clear.

136. **d.** Reinsertion of the levator aponeurosis would best correct the underlying anatomic defect.

137. **a.** The patient has floppy eyelid syndrome. Unlike in patients without eyelid laxity, patients with eyelid laxity tend to experience a slight elevation in the eyelid height after FTWR.

138. **a.** There is a decrease in tarsal elastin fibers.

139. **d.** The inferior rectus and inferior oblique are at risk during lower blepharoplasty. The superior oblique is at risk during upper blepharoplasty during excision of nasal fat.

140. **a.** Injury to orbital fat pads, vessels, or orbicularis may result in retrobulbar hemorrhage that dissects into the posterior orbit and compresses the optic nerve.

141. **c.** Blunt trauma to the frontal bone is the usual mechanism by which indirect traumatic optic neuropathy occurs.

142. **b.** Children have less evaporative tear loss than older individuals, 10% and 20%, respectively.

143. **a.** A ZMC fracture may involve the orbital floor; however, inferior rectus muscle entrapment is not common. Choices b–d may commonly occur.

144. **b.** The ice pack test is used in diagnosing MG. Testing for MG after exercise may help in confirming a positive result; however, this is not the same as the exercise stress testing, which is used as a method of screening for cardiac health. The three-step test is used for vertical strabismus. Due to the relatively nonspecific patterns of extraocular motility dysfunction in MG, the test has no role in the confirming a diagnosis of MG. The acetylcholine-receptor antibody test is related to MG, in that elevated serum values are seen in about 50% to 70% of patients with ocular MG and in 90% of those with systemic MG. Although about 5% of patients with MG also have thyroid eye disease, the TSH-receptor antibody test is not used to diagnose MG.

6

145. d. The patient has an optic nerve glioma. Choices a–c are considered typical. Pain would be unusual.

146. a. The central nervous system (CNS) is not routinely surveyed in patients with orbital lymphoma. This is in distinction to patients with intraocular lymphoma. When CNS involvement is suspected, CT or MRI is the starting point.

147. b. Surgical excision is not recommended, and neither are systemic corticosteroids. Radiation is the treatment of choice for these lesions.

148. b. The patient has blepharophimosis syndrome, an autosomal dominant disorder. The classic triad of epicanthus inversus, telecanthus, and ptosis are all seen in the photograph. Also seen is the characteristic poorly developed nasal bridge. The superior orbital rims are hypoplastic. This patient also had lop ears (cropped from the photograph). Patients with the syndrome may develop lateral lower eyelid ectropion due to anterior lamellar deficiency. Hypertelorism may also occur. Surgical correction must be individualized and may include ptosis repair (frontalis sling if poor levator function), Y-V plasty (or transnasal wiring), ectropion repair, and buildup of the hypoplastic orbital rims.

149. a. Full-thickness mucosal grafts have been shown to maintain their original epithelium after transplantation onto the ocular surface; however, submucosal glands typically do not survive.

150. d. The patient has involutional entropion. Choices a–c are true. In addition, the lower eyelid position is usually higher than normal due to the disinsertion of the lower eyelid retractors. Other features include overriding of the orbicularis oculi muscle, horizontal eyelid laxity, and (more recently) relative enophthalmos.

CHAPTER 7

Intraocular Inflammation and Uveitis

▌ Questions

1. Adaptive immunity
   a. works in an antigen-independent manner.
   b. is preprogrammed by evolution.
   c. is based on environmental stimulus.
   d. uses only nonspecific macrophages and PMNs to destroy offending agents.

2. Which of the following lymphocytes has cytotoxic activity without a specific antigen receptor and is not antigen specific?
   a. T lymphocytes.
   b. B lymphocytes.
   c. natural killer (NK) cells.
   d. macrophages.

3. Which of the following is exclusively part of the adaptive immunity system?
   a. antigen memory.
   b. use of macrophages/neutrophils to combat offending agents.
   c. inflammatory response.
   d. leukocyte receptor activation.

4. Which of the following cells are used by only the adaptive immunity system?
   a. monocytes.
   b. lymphocytes.
   c. neutrophils.
   d. eosinophils.

5. The first cell that an antigen typically comes in contact with during the cascade of the immune response is the
   a. NK cell.
   b. T lymphocyte.
   c. B lymphocyte.
   d. macrophage.

6. A 70-year-old man infected with virus A. He has never been exposed to this virus in the past. What subtype of immunoglobulin will be made in response to the initial exposure to the virus?
   a. IgA.
   b. IgD.
   c. IgM.
   d. IgG.

7. Which type of immunoglobulin will the man in question 6 form against virus A other than IgM?
   a. IgA.
   b. IgD.
   c. IgE.
   d. IgG.

8. Class I MHC
   a. are present on almost all nucleated cells.
   b. refer to HLA-DR, HLA-DP, and HLA-DQ.
   c. work with CD4 helper T cells.
   d. are best at processing endocytosed antigens.

9. What is the most abundant antibody subtype present in the tear film?
   a. IgE.
   b. IgM.
   c. IgA.
   d. IgG.

10. The major histocompatibility antigen complex in humans (human leukocyte antigen [HLA] system) is coded for by genes located on chromosome
    a. 6.
    b. 11.
    c. 13.
    d. 18.

11. What component of the conjunctiva is the most important for immune regulation?
    a. epithelium.
    b. substantia propria.
    c. lymphoid tissue.
    d. goblet cells.

12. Presumed ocular histoplasmosis syndrome is associated with which HLA marker?
    a. A29.
    b. B5.
    c. B7.
    d. B8.

13. Sympathetic ophthalmia (S.O.) and Vogt-Koyanagi-Harada (VKH) syndrome are associated with which HLA marker?
    a. B5.
    b. B44.
    c. B51.
    d. DR4.

14. Which immunoglobulin class has the highest individual molecular weight?
    a. IgA.
    b. IgD.
    c. IgE.
    d. IgM.

15. Which immunoglobulin molecule has the longest serum half-life?
    a. IgA.
    b. IgM.

c. IgE.
d. IgG.

16. Which is the most abundant immunoglobulin class to cross the human placenta?
    a. IgA.
    b. IgD.
    c. IgE.
    d. IgG.

17. What is the most common type of uveitis?
    a. anterior.
    b. intermediate.
    c. posterior.
    d. panuveitis.

18. Anaphylactoid reactions are grouped into what type of hypersensitivity reactions?
    a. type I.
    b. type II.
    c. type III.
    d. type IV.

19. What type of hypersensitivity is associated with immune-complex reactions?
    a. type II.
    b. type III.
    c. type IV.
    d. type V.

20. Which immunoglobulin class is probably the oldest phylogenetically?
    a. IgA.
    b. IgD.
    c. IgM.
    d. IgG.

21. What type of cells have a particular affinity for IgE immunoglobulins?
    a. eosinophils.
    b. mast cells.
    c. basophils.
    d. macrophages.

22. Which of the following medications is an alkylating agent?
    a. cyclophosphamide.
    b. methotrexate.
    c. azathioprine.
    d. mycophenolate mofetil.

23. Which complement component is present in the highest serum concentrations?
    a. C1q.
    b. C3.
    c. C4.
    d. C5.

24. What complement component is part of the membrane attack complex?
    a. C3a.
    b. C4a.
    c. C5a.
    d. C6.

25. Which of the following substances is NOT produced by the cyclooxygenase pathway?
    a. prostacyclins.
    b. thromboxane.
    c. leukotrienes.
    d. prostaglandins.

26. What complement component begins the complement pathway?
    a. C3a
    b. C3b.
    c. C4a.
    d. C5a.

27. A 50-year-old man presents with decreased vision. His medical history is positive for end-stage AIDS and current IV drug use. His fundus photo is present below. What is the diagnosis?
    a. *Candida* endogenous endophthalmitis.
    b. CMV retinitis.
    c. ocular lymphoma.
    d. HIV retinopathy.

28. The Arthus reaction is what type of hypersensitivity?
    a. I.
    b. II.
    c. III.
    d. IV.

29. Immune recovery uveitis (IRU)
    a. occurs in patients with HZV and HSV retinitis.
    b. occurs only in CMV-infected eyes.
    c. does not cause macular edema.
    d. does not cause epiretinal membrane formation.

30. Graves' disease is a manifestation of what type of hypersensitivity?
    a. type I.
    b. type II.
    c. type IV.
    d. type V.

31. Which immunoglobulin has NOT been detected in tear samples?
    a. IgA.
    b. IgD.
    c. IgE.
    d. IgG.

32. Wessely rings represent what type hypersensitivity?
    a. type I.
    b. type II.
    c. type III.
    d. type IV.

7

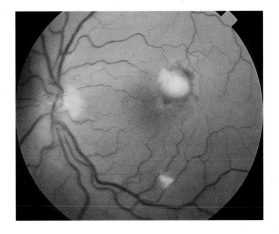

157

Questions 33–36. Refer to vignette below.
A 34-year-old man presents with a 1-week history of right eye pain and light sensitivity. The left eye is without symptoms. There are 2+ cells and 2+ flare in the anterior chamber. There is no posterior inflammation present. Upon further questioning, he has had lower back stiffness and pain upon awakening for several years. The back pain improves during the day. He has no other general medical symptoms. His social history is negative for promiscuous sexual history.

33. What is the most likely diagnosis?
   a. syphilis.
   b. Reiter's syndrome.
   c. ankylosing spondylitis.
   d. toxoplasmosis.

34. What radiographic test would be appropriate and most cost effective in this scenario?
   a. CT scan of head.
   b. MRI of spinal column.
   c. sacroiliac x-ray films.
   d. CT scan of thoracic spine.

35. What percentage of patients with this pathology possess the HLA-B27 gene?
   a. 10%.
   b. 25%.
   c. 50%.
   d. over 75%.

36. Not including the eye and lumbosacral spine, what other area may rarely be inflamed?
   a. heart.
   b. brain.
   c. kidneys.
   d. aorta.

37. Which of the following is INCORRECT regarding Dalen-Fuchs nodules?
   a. They consist of RPE and epitheloid cells.
   b. They are present in sympathetic ophthalmia.
   c. They are present in Vogt-Koyanagi-Harada syndrome.
   d. They are present in Behcet's disease.

38. The most common cause of anterior uveitis in the adult population is
   a. herpes simplex keratouveitis.
   b. idiopathic.
   c. HLA-B27 iridocyclitis.
   d. herpes zoster.

39. The most common cause of posterior uveitis in the adult population is
   a. toxocariasis.
   b. sarcoidosis.
   c. toxoplasmosis.
   d. idiopathic posterior uveitis.

40. Patient presents with unilateral anterior segment uveitis. On slit-lamp exam, the corneal endothelium is diffusely covered with stellate KPs. There are 1+ cells in the anterior chamber. The iris has atrophy. There are no iris nodules or posterior synechiae. What is the most likely diagnosis pictured below?
   a. syphilitic uveitis.
   b. HLA-B27 uveitis.
   c. Fuchs' iridocyclitis.
   d. sarcoidosis.

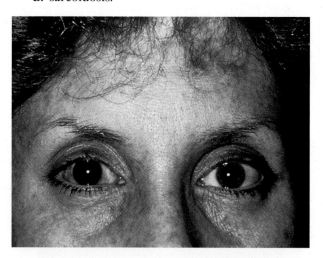

41. Which of the following is true regarding the condition seen above?
   a. Hyphema may be seen after cataract surgery.
   b. There is no association with glaucoma or cataract.
   c. The majority of cases need aggressive steroid treatment.
   d. Patient's usually have severe discomfort when the condition is active.

42. Which condition below has inflammation that primarily affects the venules?
    a. Eales' disease.
    b. systemic lupus erythematosus.
    c. acute retinal necrosis.
    d. polyarteritis nodosa.

43. Which of the following is true regarding Reiter's Syndrome?
    a. There are only three major diagnostic criteria.
    b. The syndrome can be triggered by dysentery.
    c. Iritis is the most common finding in Reiter's syndrome.
    d. The syndrome has no dermatologic manifestations.

44. Which of the following conditions are NOT associated with iris nodules and skin findings?
    a. sarcoidosis.
    b. juvenile xanthogranuloma.
    c. neurofibromatosis.
    d. pseudoxanthoma elasticum.

45. The most common cause of decreased vision in intermediate uveitis is
    a. disc edema.
    b. posterior subcapsular cataract.
    c. vitritis.
    d. cystoid macular edema.

46. The prevalence of HLA-B27 in the general population is
    a. 1%–8%.
    b. 10%–25%.
    c. 25%–50%.
    d. 50%–75%.

47. Which of the following antiretroviral agents has been shown to increase the CD8+ lymphocyte count in HIV-positive patients?
    a. zidovudine (ZDV, AZT).
    b. ritonavir.
    c. didanosine (ddI).
    d. zalcitabine (ddC).

48. What is false regarding Fuchs' uveitis syndrome?
    a. Glaucoma is common in this condition.
    b. Synechiae are commonly observed in this condition.
    c. Cataract is common in this condition.
    d. Vitreous and retinal findings may be present.

49. What is the probability, given HLA-B27 genotype, of sacroiliac disease?
    a. <5%.
    b. 10%.
    c. 25%.
    d. 50%.

50. The most important component of long-term therapy in a young man who is HLA-B27 positive is
    a. cardiac ultrasound.
    b. annual tonometry.
    c. systemic (oral) nonsteroidal antiinflammatory therapy.
    d. physical therapy.

51. Which one of the following concerning Reiter's syndrome is false?
    a. 90% of cases are in men.
    b. It may follow a bout of either urethritis.
    c. Skin lesions are present at times.
    d. The most common ocular finding is an acute nongranulomatous anterior uveitis.

52. Which of the following is true regarding acute iritis?
    a. It is more frequently present in Crohn's disease compared to ulcerative colitis.
    b. It is usually present in psoriatic patients *without* arthritis.
    c. It can occur with nephritis.
    d. Signifies only inflammation and NOT infection.

53. The patient below is a 4-year-old girl. What is the most likely diagnosis?
    a. sarcoidosis.
    b. syphilis.
    c. toxocara.
    d. juvenile rheumatoid arthritis.

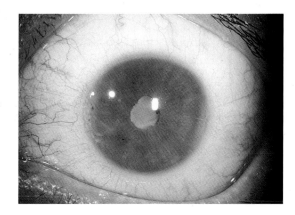

7

159

54. Which of the following lab values are most consistent with the clinical scenario presented in question 53?
    a. ANA+, RF+.
    b. ANA+, RF−.
    c. ANA−, RF+.
    d. ANA−, RF−.

55. Which of the following is NOT a risk factor for developing iridocyclitis in JRA?
    a. associated type I diabetes.
    b. pauciarticular arthritis.
    c. female gender.
    d. ANA positivity.

56. Which of the following is usually false with regard to JRA?
    a. Still's disease has a low rate of uveitis.
    b. The involved eye is red and inflamed.
    c. Methotrexate is a possible treatment option.
    d. Cataract formation is a major issue in management of these children.

57. Which one of the following concerning Behçet's disease is false?
    a. The disease is more common among Japanese than Americans.
    b. The classic acute uveitis of Behçet's disease is typically associated with a hypopyon.
    c. Anterior uveitis is more common in Behçet's disease in men than posterior uveitis.
    d. Characteristic aphthous ulcers develop on mucous membranes, including the mouth and genital tract.

58. Which of the following is true regarding Behçet's disease?
    a. The course of the ocular disease generally is self-limited.
    b. There is no cardiovascular association in Behçet's disease.
    c. A shifting hypopyon may be present in the anterior chamber.
    d. Steroids are generally the only long-term therapy.

59. The patient at the top of the right column presents to the clinic. What is the diagnosis?
    a. episcleritis.
    b. oculodermal melanocytosis.

c. conjunctival melanoma.
d. scleromalacia perforans.

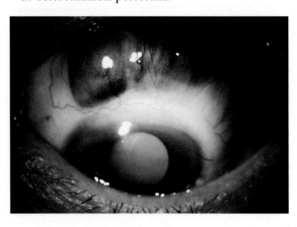

60. Which one of the following concerning Kawasaki's disease is false?
    a. The vast majority of affected patients are children under the age of 10 years.
    b. The hallmark of the eye findings is a bilateral conjunctival congestion that spares the limbus.
    c. The hallmark of the dermatologic findings is a shedding rash affecting the extremities.
    d. Corticosteroids are agents of choice to treat the underlying disease.

For Questions 61–64, refer to the below given photograph.

A 10-year-old boy presents with the complaint of new floaters in both eyes. He has stated his vision is blurry at school. He has previous had no refractive error. Upon workup, he has no systemic illness. On exam there are white clumps of debris seen inferiorly at the vitreous base in both eyes.

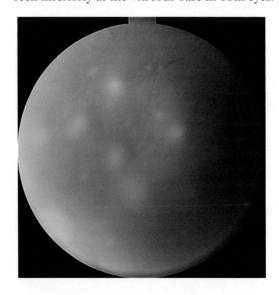

For Questions 61–64, refer to vignette and clinical photograph on page 160 (bottom of the right column).

61. Which of the following is true regarding the clinical scenario?
    a. It is the most common form of intermediate uveitis.
    b. There is usually a definable cause.
    c. It is present in young people only.
    d. There are no HLA associations.

62. What is a major cause of vision loss in patients with this process?
    a. venous sheathing.
    b. chronic cystoid macular edema.
    c. retinal venous sheathing.
    d. anterior chamber cells.

63. What medical condition is associated with this process?
    a. syphilis.
    b. sarcoidosis.
    c. toxocariasis.
    d. multiple sclerosis.

64. First line therapy for this process is usually which of the following?
    a. laser ablation.
    b. methotrexate.
    c. corticosteroids.
    d. cryotherapy.

65. Which of the following generally does NOT occur in patients with lupus?
    a. choroidal neovascularization.
    b. choroidal infarction.
    c. nerve fiber layer infarct.
    d. retinitis.

66. In reference to Wegner's granulomatosis, which of the following is false?
    a. Skin involvement can occur.
    b. P-ANCA is a diagnostic test for this disease.
    c. Glomerunephritis is a serious issue in these patients.
    d. Uveitis may be anterior, intermediate, or posterior in this disease.

67. The patient presents with blurred vision, photophobia, and the below findings. What is the most likely diagnosis?
    a. herpes.
    b. Behçet's disease
    c. sarcoidosis.
    d. reactive arthritis.

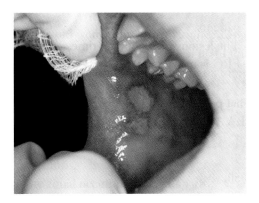

For Questions 68–71, refer to vignette and clinical the below given photograph.

A 69-year-old woman presents with decreased vision in both eyes. She states she has noted more floaters lately in both eyes. She is also having difficulty driving at night.

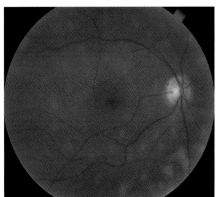

A

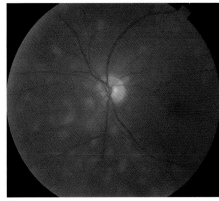

B

85. The type of bacteria most commonly isolated in bleb-associated endophthalmitis is
    a. *Staphylococcus*.
    b. *Neisseria*.
    c. *Propionibacterium*.
    d. *Streptococcus*.

86. Which of the following is false in regards to endophthalmitis?
    a. The Endophthalmitis Vitrectomy Study gives guidance for management of postoperative infectious endophthalmitis.
    b. Endophthalmitis does not occur after extra-ocular surgery such as pterygium excision.
    c. Endophthalmitis may come from an endogenous source.
    d. Other uveitic conditions may masquerade as endophthalmitis.

87. What organism is classically implicated in the pathogenesis of chronic postoperative endophthalmitis?
    a. *Pseudomonas*.
    b. *Neisseria*
    c. *Propionibacterium acnes*.
    d. *Serratia* species.

88. Which endophthalmitis has the worst prognosis?
    a. acute postoperative endophthalmitis.
    b. chronic postoperative endophthalmitis.
    c. posttraumatic endophthalmitis.
    d. bleb-associated endophthalmitis.

89. The organism responsible for approximately 25% of posttraumatic endophthalmitis is
    a. *Staphylococcus aureus*.
    b. *Streptococcus pneumoniae*.
    c. *Aspergillus*.
    d. *Bacillus cereus*.

90. The organism with the poorest prognosis in post-traumatic endophthalmitis is
    a. *Staphylococcus aureus*.
    b. *Streptococcus pneumoniae*.
    c. *Aspergillus*.
    d. *Bacillus cereus*.

91. The picture below is a 60-year-old woman who complains of photopsias and blurred vision in both eyes. The left eye has similar changes. What is the diagnosis?
    a. choroideremia.
    b. acute zonal occult outer retinopathy (AZOOR).
    c. multifocal choroiditis (MFC).
    d. multiple evanescent white dot syndrome (MEWDS).

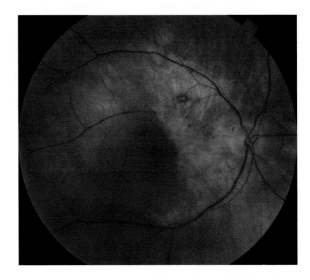

92. Which one of the following concerning fungal endophthalmitis is false?
    a. *Candida* is the most common etiology.
    b. The classic vitritis follows an earlier retinochoroiditis.
    c. The majority of patients with endogenous *Candida* endophthalmitis will have positive blood cultures.
    d. Approximately 10% of patients with candidemia will eventually develop endophthalmitis.

93. Which of the following is false regarding sympathetic ophthalmia?
    a. It is associated with previous ocular surgery or trauma.
    b. It characteristically affects the choriocapillaris.
    c. It is associated with retinal detachments.
    d. It is a diffuse ocular process.

94. Which of the following is false concerning Vogt-Koyanagi-Harada (VKH) disease?
    a. Skin findings precede ocular disease.
    b. Auditory symptoms may be present.
    c. Retinal detachments may cause vision loss.
    d. There is thickened choroidal signal on B-scan ultrasound.

95. Which one of the following concerning toxoplasmosis is true?
    a. The manifestations are strictly posterior in nature.
    b. The retinal vessels are spared in ocular toxoplasmosis.
    c. ELISA testing for antitoxoplasma antibodies is important in the diagnosis of atypical lesions.
    d. The definitive hosts of *Toxoplasma gondii* is a species of small rodent.

96. Potential adverse affects of the pharmacologic management of toxoplasmosis include all of the following except
    a. pseudomembranous colitis.
    b. Stevens-Johnson syndrome.
    c. aggravation of diabetes mellitus.
    d. microcytic anemia.

97. Which one of the following regarding onchocerciasis is false?
    a. *Onchocerca volvulus* is transmitted by the bite of the Simulium black fly.
    b. Skin findings are rare in this condition.
    c. Microfilariae may be seen swimming in the anterior chamber and may induce a severe anterior uveitis with glaucoma and cataract.
    d. Chorioretinal and optic atrophy are common in advanced disease.

98. What is the most likely diagnosis in the patient pictured at the top of the right column?
    a. syphilis.
    b. herpetic disease.
    c. scleritis.
    d. sarcoidosis.

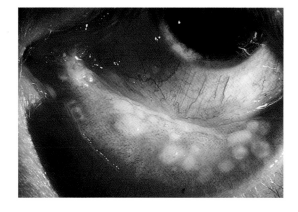

99. The picture below is from a 50-year-old man with AIDS. He is not on antiretroviral therapy. He presents with decreased vision and photopsias in the left eye. What is the most likely diagnosis given this clinical scenario?
    a. sarcoidosis.
    b. Lyme disease.
    c. cytomegalovirus infection.
    d. Behçet's disease.

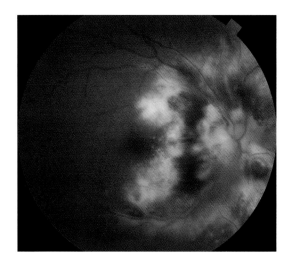

100. Which one of the following concerning cytomegalovirus (CMV) infection is false?
    a. The congenital form may be heralded by fever, pneumonia, or hepatosplenomegaly.
    b. The eye findings in congenital disease include cataract and peripheral retinal lesions, both atrophic and hyperpigmented.
    c. Retinal detachment is uncommon in CMV retinitis.
    d. Posterior segment involvement generally starts as a retinitis and secondarily involves the choroid.

7

165

101. Which of the following choices is NOT a thera-peutic option for the above patient?
   a. oral valganciclovir.
   b. IV acyclovir
   c. IV ganciclovir
   d. intravitreal foscarnet.

102. Which of the following is not a risk factor for *Candida* endophthalmitis?
   a. recent total parenteral nutrition.
   b. intravenous drug abuse.
   c. organ transplantation.
   d. AIDS.

103. Which one of the following concerning acute retinal necrosis (ARN) is false?
   a. Anterior segment inflammation is variable.
   b. Posterior segment inflammation is generally heavy.
   c. Retinal detachments associated with ARN may benefit from the use of tamponade with silicone oil.
   d. Like other viral retinitides, affected patients are usually immunosuppressed.

104. The differential diagnosis for a patient with chronic vitreous cells does not include which of the following?
   a. retinitis pigmentosa.
   b. ocular histoplasmosis syndrome.
   c. retinal detachment.
   d. intraocular foreign body.

105. *Nocardia asteroids*
   a. usually has only a localized abscess.
   b. may present with pneumonia.
   c. commonly affects the eye.
   d. only causes a mild inflammatory response.

106. Which of the following concerning ocular toxocariasis is false?
   a. The definitive host for the parasite is the dog or cat.
   b. Ingested ova initially take up residence in the liver and lung.
   c. Manifestations may include chronic endophthalmitis, localized macular granuloma, or localized peripheral granuloma.
   d. Inflammation is usually bilateral.

107. Which of the following concerning the presumed ocular histoplasmosis syndrome (POHS) is true?
   a. The maculopathy generally precedes the formation of peripheral punched out lesions, or "histo spots."
   b. The vitritis associated with the condition may decrease vision.
   c. Fundus lesions in their acute phase represent a retinitis with a secondary choroidal reaction.
   d. A patient with a macular histo spot has about a one-in-four chance of active maculopathy over the next 3 years.

108. A 23-year-old healthy young man with no medical problems presents with scotomas in both eyes. His vision is 20/25 in both eyes. He states he had a chest cold last week (images below). What is most likely the diagnosis?
   a. sarcoidosis.
   b. pars planitis.
   c. acute multifocal posterior placoid epitheli-opathy (APMPPE).
   d. *Pneumocystis carinii.*

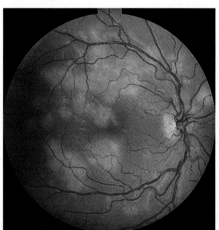

A

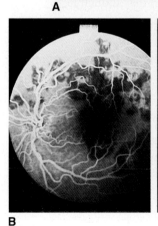
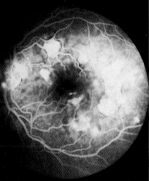

B

109. Berlin's nodules are located in which area of the eye?
    a. pupillary border.
    b. mid-iris.
    c. conjunctiva.
    d. angle.

110. Periocular steroid injection should be avoided in which of the following conditions?
    a. pars planitis associated with sarcoidosis and cystoid macular edema.
    b. necrotizing scleritis associated with rheumatoid arthritis.
    c. cystoid macular edema following cataract surgery.
    d. punctate inner choroidopathy.

111. Which of the following is false regarding diffuse unilateral subacute neuroretinitis (DUSN).
    a. The causative worms are thought to be Ancylostoma canium and Baylisascaris procyonis.
    b. Anti-helminthic medications are the only treatment options.
    c. Reinfection may occur.
    d. It is generally a unilateral condition.

112. What is false regarding the condition below?
    a. It may occur in eyes that have undergone vitrectomy.
    b. It may be seen in children.
    c. It is not related to chronic inflammation.
    d. Phthisical eyes may be associated with this condition.

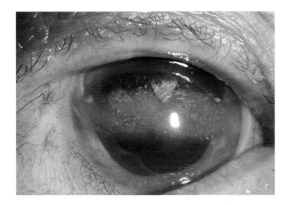

113. What is the most common retinopathy seen in patients with HIV/AIDS?
    a. toxoplasmosis.
    b. cytomegalovirus retinitis.

    c. *Pneumocystis carinii* retinitis.
    d. HIV retinopathy.

114. The most common intraocular opportunistic infection associated with HIV infection is
    a. toxoplasmosis.
    b. acute retinal necrosis secondary to herpes simplex virus.
    c. pneumocystis choroiditis.
    d. CMV retinitis.

115. Which of the following is believed to be a significant risk factor for the development of pneumocystis choroiditis?
    a. active *Pneumocystis carinii* pneumonia (PCP).
    b. treatment of *Pneumocystis carinii* pneumonia with aerosolized pentamidine.
    c. severe cachexia.
    d. absolute lymphocyte count below 500 cells/mm^3.

116. Kaposi's sarcoma may present in what ocular structure?
    a. retina.
    b. choroid.
    c. conjunctiva.
    d. orbit.

117. In the patient photographed below, which of the following is the most likely diagnosis?
    a. syphilitic uveitis.
    b. herpes uveitis.
    c. sarcoidosis.
    d. toxoplasmosis.

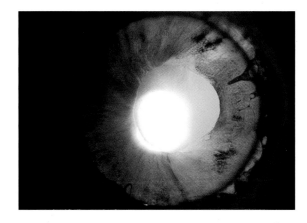

7

167

118. The patient pictured below is a 26-year-old female with blurred central vision in the left eye. Her refractive error is −4.00 OU in both eyes. She has no other medical problems. What is the most likely diagnosis?
    a. MEWDS.
    b. Birdshot chorioretinopathy.
    c. PIC.
    d. Krill's disease.

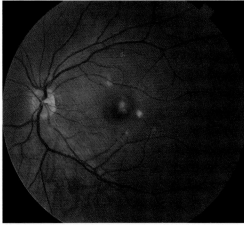

A

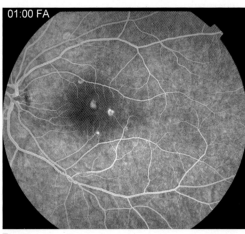

B

119. What percentage of patients with documented candidemia will develop Candida chorioretinitis?
    a. 0%.
    b. 5%.
    c. 10%
    d. 20%

120. Which of the following is true regarding intermediate uveitis and multiple sclerosis?
    a. The incidence of uveitis in MS is approximately 1%.
    b. Anterior uveitis is most commonly found in association with MS.
    c. Macular edema is more common in association with MS.
    d. HLA-DR51 is associated with MS and uveitis.

121. Clinical features distinguishing the progressive outer retinal necrosis (PORN) syndrome from the acute retinal necrosis (ARN) syndrome include each of the following, except
    a. relative lack of vitreous inflammation.
    b. relative lack of vasculitis.
    c. relative early involvement of the macula.
    d. better visual outcome.

122. One potential complication of cryotherapy for pars planitis is
    a. exacerbation of vitritis.
    b. exacerbation of posterior subcapsular cataract.
    c. exacerbation of CME.
    d. rhegmatogenous retinal detachment.

123. Each of the following regarding sympathetic ophthalmia is true, except
    a. The incidence following penetrating trauma is approximately 0.1%.
    b. The incidence following elective intraocular surgery is approximately 0.01%.
    c. An exciting eye with better visual potential than the sympathizing eye should not be removed.
    d. Initial treatment usually includes systemic cytotoxic agents.

124. What area of the eye has the highest blood flow?
    a. retina.
    b. choroid.
    c. cornea.
    d. iris.

125. What percentage of patients with primary CNS lymphoma (PCNSL) have ocular involvement?
     a. 5%.
     b. 10%.
     c. 25%.
     d. 50%.

126. What is the histology of most primary CNS lymphoma?
     a. Hodgkin T-lymphocyte lymphoma.
     b. Hodgkin B-lymphocyte lymphoma.
     c. non-Hodgkin B-lymphocyte lymphoma.
     d. non-Hodgkin T-lymphocyte lymphoma.

127. Which of the following is true regarding primary CNS lymphoma?
     a. Steroids may initially reduce ocular inflammation.
     b. All cases are derived from B lymphocytes.
     c. Vitreous biopsy is compulsory for diagnosis.
     d. Surgery is the main treatment option.

128. In men, choroidal metastases most commonly derive from a primary _____ tumor.
     a. lung.
     b. testicular.
     c. colon.
     d. prostate.

129. In women, choroidal metastases most commonly derive from a primary _____ tumor.
     a. lung.
     b. breast.
     c. colon.
     d. cervical.

130. Retinal metastases are most commonly from a primary _____.
     a. breast tumor.
     b. lung tumor.
     c. gastrointestinal tumor.
     d. cutaneous melanoma.

7

Answers

1. **c.** Innate immunity is preprogrammed by evolution to respond to offending agents. It has preprogrammed responses due to having preexisting receptors for particular stimuli. Adaptive immunity, on the other hand, is based on a specific environmental stimulus.

2. **c.** Natural killer (NK) cells are a distinct class of lymphocytes that have the ability to lyse a wide variety of cell types. It is felt that they represent the front-line defense against infections and neoplasia. NK cells may be involved in ocular protection against CMV retinitis or herpes simplex ocular infections.

3. **a.** "Memory" is exclusive to the adaptive system. On repeated exposure of an offending stimulus, the immune response is more aggressive. This is not true of innate immunity. This is based on memory B and T lymphocytes. The other choices are used by both innate and adaptive immunity.

4. **b.** The lymphocytes, both B and T, are used only by the adaptive immunity system. Macrophages, monocytes, neutrophils, eosinophils are common to both innate and adaptive immunity as nonspecific effector cells.

5. **d.** Macrophages can initiate the immune cascade by phagocytosing antigen and presenting it to T cells. Macrophages are also known as antigen-presenting cells.

6. **c.** IgM peaks earlier and disappears earlier than IgG during the primary immune response.

7. **d.** IgG is the major antibody formed following exposure to an antigen that has previously been encountered.

8. **a.** Class I MHC molecules, HLA-A, -B, -C, are used in CD8 regulatory T lymphocytes. They are present on almost all nucleated cells. Class II MHC, HLA-DR, HLA-DP, HLA-DQ, are used in CD4 helper T lymphocytes. Class II dependent APCs are best at dealing with endocytosed antigens from the environment.

9. **c.** IgA is the most abundant antibody in the tear film. IgA is present in mucosal secretions of the body.

10. **a.** The HLA complex governs immune response and surveillance.

11. **c.** Mucosa associated lymphoid tissue, or MALT, is the most important immune regulatory component of the conjunctiva. Similar types of lymphoid tissue are found in the gut, genitourinary tract, and respiratory tract.

12. **c.** B7 is associated with POHS.

13. **d.** DR 4 is associated with S.O. and VKH. Other HLA associations are listed below.

   A29—Birdshot chorioretinitis
   B7 and DR2—POHS and MS
   B8—Sarcoidosis, intermediate uveitis
   B27—Idiopathic iritis, psoriatic arthritis, inflammatory bowel disease, ankylosing spondylitis, Reiter's syndrome
   B44—Retinal vasculitis
   B51—Behçet's disease (in Asians only)
   DR4—JRA, VKH, sympathetic ophthalmia.

14. **d.** IgM is made of five units, each unit the size of one IgG.

15. **d.** IgG has the longest half-life, 21 to 23 days. IgA is second at about 6 days, followed by IgM (5 days), IgD (3 days), and IgE (2 days).

16. **d.** IgG transfer occurs both passively and by active transport to the placenta. (Minimal amounts of IgA also may cross by passive diffusion.)

17. a. Anterior uveitis is the most common type of uveitis.

18. a. Type I hypersensitivity reactions are anaphylactoid.

19. b. Type III. The types of hypersensitivity are listed below:

Type I: Anaphylactoid
Type II: Cytotoxic antibodies
Type III: Immune complex
Type IV: Cell-mediated
Type V: Stimulatory

20. c. IgM or IgM-like immunoglobulins tend to be the only type present in organisms with the most "rudimentary" immune systems.

21. b. Mast cells and IgE promote allergic reactions.

22. a. Cyclophosphamide and chlorambucil are alkylating agents. Methotrexate, azathioprine, and mycophenolate mofetil are antimetabolites.

23. b. C3 is present in serum at a concentration of approximately 1 mg/mL.

24. d. The membrane attack complex, or MAC, consists of C6–C9 complement components.

25. c. Leukotrienes are formed by the lipoxygenase pathway. Cyclooxygenase inhibitors (nonsteroidal agents) block production of all three end products.

26. b. C3b begins the complement pathway.

27. a. This is a classic picture of Candida endogenous endophthalmitis. Lesions begin in the choroid, progress anteriorly through the retina and break through into the vitreous cavity. Intravitreal and systemic therapy may be needed for treatment. Surgery may also be an option. The patient's history is strongly suggestive of Candida. The patient also needs an infectious disease/endocarditis work up.

28. c. The Arthus reaction (type III) results from formation of antigen–antibody complexes in tissue.

29. b. Immune recovery uveitis occurs in patients infected with HIV/AIDS and CMV. As the immune system improves, patients can suffer from anterior/intermediate uveitis and also develop CME. Epiretinal membranes may also be seen in this condition. It occurs only in eyes infected with CMV. In one study, IRU was associated with previous CMV retinal surface area infection of 25%. Intravitreal injections of steroids are avoided in this condition.

30. d. Graves' disease and myasthenia gravis are excellent examples of type V hypersensitivity. In these conditions, antibodies react with specific cell surface receptors and either stimulate or depress cellular function.

31. b. All major immunoglobulins classes except IgD have been detected in human tears. IgA (secretory immunoglobulin) is the primary immunoglobulin in tears.

32. c. Wessely rings, also known as immune rings, are ring infiltrates of the corneal stroma, parallel to the limbus. Some corneal rings are probably formed as antigen from a corneal infiltrate encounters antibody from peripheral corneal blood vessels. The infiltrate generally contains complement factors and PMNs.

33. c. Anklyosing spondylitis presents with acute iritis. The back pain and stiffness is usually worse after inactivity and improves with activity.

34. c. Sacroiliac x-ray films may display sclerosis and narrowing of the joint space. Sacroiliitis may also be present.

35. d. Up to 90% of patients with ankylosing spondylitis are positive for HLA-B27. HLA-B27 is also associated with several other diseases, although the chance that an HLA-B27 positive

7

individual will have a seronegative spondyloarthropathy or eye disease is approximately 25%. Fifty percent of patients with acute iritis may be HLA-B27 positive.

36. **d.** Aortitis occurs in 5% of cases. Aortic valve insufficiency may also be present.

37. **d.** Dalen-Fuchs nodules are focal accumulations of epithelioid-like cells between Bruch's membrane and the retinal pigment epithelium (RPE). They may include depigmented RPE cells. They are classically associated with sympathetic ophthalmia and VKH syndrome. They also may be found in tuberculous choroiditis and sarcoidosis.

38. **b.** Idiopathic iridocyclitis is the most common cause of anterior uveitis, making up at least 10% of all uveitis cases. HLA-B27 iridocyclitis is the second most common cause, and juvenile rheumatoid arthritis and herpes (simplex or zoster) follow in incidence.

39. **c.** Toxoplasmosis is the most common cause of posterior uveitis, accounting for up to 7% of total uveitis cases. Other causes of posterior uveitis include retinal vasculitis, necrotizing herpetic retinopathy, and idiopathic causes.

40. **c.** The differential diagnosis of diffusely distributed keratic precipitates includes Fuchs' heterochromic iridocyclitis, and rarely sarcoidosis, syphilis, and toxoplasmosis. The diffuse distribution, along with a gelatinous, stellate appearance, makes the KPs of Fuchs' iridocyclitis distinctive.

41. **a.** Postoperative hyphema can be seen due to rupture of delicate vessels that cross the angle. Cataract and glaucoma are frequently present. For unknown reasons, synechiae are unusual in Fuchs' heterochromic iridocyclitis. Some experts question the "inflammatory" nature of this disorder. Visual prognosis is usually good after cataract extraction. The majority of cases have minimal symptoms and do not require therapy.

42. **a.** Eales' disease, birdshot retinochoroidopathy, multiple sclerosis, sarcoidosis have inflammation that is centered on the venules. The other answers listed all primarily have vasculitis that is confined to the arterioles.

43. **b.** Reiter's syndrome is another HLA-B27 associated disease. The classic findings include urethritis, polyarthritis, and conjunctivitis. Iritis is seen but less commonly. It usually affects young males. It may be triggered by diarrhea or dysentery episodes, and has been associated with Chlamydia, Shigella, Salmonella, Yersina, and Ureaplasma urealyticum. Keratoderma blennorrhagicum and circinate balanitis can also be seen in this syndrome. Other associations include Achilles tendonitis, nail pitting, oral ulcers, plantar fasciitis.

44. **d.** Granulomas as well as Koeppe and Busacca nodules may appear as iris nodules in ocular sarcoidosis. Juvenile xanthogranuloma features yellow iris nodules, appearing during childhood and associated with spontaneous hyphema. Juvenile xanthogranuloma most frequently involves the skin. Raised orange lesions are typical. In neurofibromatosis, Lisch nodules, actually clusters of nevus cells, are definitive. Cutaneous neurofibromas, café-au-lait spots, and Lisch nodules are all important diagnostic criteria. Pseudoxanthoma elasticum is associated with "chicken skin" of the head and neck, but no iris nodules.

45. **d.** Intermediate uveitis accounts for 15% of all uveitis cases, and is associated with several systemic disorders including sarcoidosis, MS, Lyme disease, TB, and syphilis. Idiopathic intermediate uveitis, or pars planitis, accounts for more than 80% of cases. 80% of pars planitis cases are bilateral. Macular edema, followed by cataract, is the most consistent cause of decreased vision in pars planitis. Cystoid macular edema may complicate anterior or posterior uveitis, but much less frequently.

46. **a.** The HLA antigens are determined by a series of four gene loci located on chromosome 6. HLA-B27 is present in 1.4% to 8.0% of the general population.

47. b. Ritonavir is a protease inhibitor that can increase CD8+ lymphocyte counts.

48. b. In Fuchs' uveitis syndrome, or Fuchs' heterochromic iridocyclitis, cataract and glaucoma occur commonly. Synechiae are rarely seen. Macular edema, retinal scarring, and retinal vascular inflammation have been reported in this condition.

49. c. Up to 25% of individuals with HLA-B27 develop sacroiliac disease. Symptoms of sacroiliac disease may be subtle. Personal or family history of back problems in patients with iritis should prompt the physician to obtain sacroiliac radiographs.

50. d. Asymptomatic sacroiliac disease can be seen in patients with HLA-B27 spondylitis, particularly in young men. Because irreversible damage may occur before the onset of significant symptoms and simple physical therapy is effective in limiting disability, physical therapy, consisting of back flexibility and stretching exercises, is recommended in young men who are found to be HLA-B27 positive.

51. d. The most common eye finding in Reiter's syndrome is a nonspecific conjunctivitis. Nongranulomatous iritis, which can be bilateral and chronic, is less common. Keratoderma blennorrhagicum and circinate balanitis are also diagnostic criteria for the disease.

52. c. Although it is associated with both forms of inflammatory bowel disease, iritis occurs more commonly in patients with ulcerative colitis. Less than 15% of patients with ulcerative colitis and <5% of patients with Crohn's disease develop acute anterior uveitis. Acute anterior uveitis is associated with psoriatic arthritis, but usually not with psoriasis without arthritis. Tubulointerstitial nephritis uveitis (TINU) occurs in women from adolescence to early 30s. Infectious sources must always be kept in mind in a uveitic condition.

53. d. Juvenile rheumatoid arthritis (JRA) is the most common systemic disease with iridocyclitc association in children.

54. b. ANA+, RF− are risk factors for development of chronic iridocyclitis.

55. a. Diabetes is not a risk factor. The other listed answers are risk factors for development of iridocyclitis.

56. b. On external examination, these eyes are usually white. The disease progresses in an insidious nature. This is why there can be hidden damage done to the eye. This disease is divided into systemic (Still's disease), polyarticular onset, and pauciarticular onset. Band keratopathy can be seen in this disease also. It is present in the picture.

57. c. Behçet's disease is much more common among Japanese and individuals from eastern Mediterranean countries. Posterior uveitis, which can include retinal vasculitis, retinal hemorrhages, and retinal necrosis, is more common than anterior uveitis in Behçet's disease. Oral lesions are the most common finding in Behçet's disease. These are recurrent in nature.

58. c. The hypopyon can shift as the patient tilts their head. Behçet's disease is generally recurrent disease. Patients suffer relapses frequently. Some of the cardiac issues include endocarditis, coronary arteritis, pericarditis, myocarditis, endocardial fibrosis. In addition, pulmonary arteritis can occur as well as GI ulcers. Corticosteroids are used to treat Behçet's disease. Other immunomodulatory medications such as chlorambucil and azathioprine have been shown to preserve vision.

59. d. Scleromalacia perforans is a type of scleritis. The sclera is severely thinned and the underlying uvea is protruding. It is usually associated with connective tissue diseases and workups are warranted by medicine or rheumatology.

7

60. **d.** Aspirin is the drug of choice for Kawasaki's disease. Although the vast majority of patients recover without complication, approximately 3% of children with Kawasaki's disease develop acute coronary arteritis, which may lead to myocardial infarction and death. Corticosteroids are contra-indicated in Kawasaki's because of the increased risk of coronary aneurysm formation.

61. **a.** The above child has pars planitis. It is an idio-pathic condition and the most common cause of intermediate uveitis. Pars planitis has bimodality in its age distribution. It has been associated with HLA-DR15 and HLA-DR51.

62. **b.** Classically, chronic CME is a major cause of decreased vision in pars planitis. Also in these patients, the following may occur to cause vision loss: retinal detachment, band keratopathy, PSC cataracts, ERM.

63. **d.** HLA-DR15 is also associated with MS. Patients with MS can present with a pars planitis type clinical picture.

64. **c.** Corticosteroids are first line therapy for pars planitis. These can be periocular/topical/sys-temic/intravitreal. Laser or cryo-ablation can be applied if corticosteroid therapy does not control the disease. Vitrectomy and systemic immuno-therapy are other options.

65. **d.** Ocular manifestations of SLE include all of the choices except for retinitis. Also patients may present with retinal vascular occlusions and sub-sequent development of neovascularization.

66. **b.** p-ANCA aids in the diagnosis of polyar-teritis nodosa. c-ANCA is highly diagnostic for Wegner's granulomatosis.

67. **b.** The oral lesions seen are aphthous ulcers seen in Behcet's disease. These can occur on all mucosal surfaces and are painful. Major criteria for diagnosis of Behcet's disease include recurrent oral aphthous ulcers, skin lesions, ocular inflam-mation, and genital ulcers.

68. **a.** Birdshot is typically seen in Caucasian women over 40. The ERG can be reduced and the lesions generally do not pigment over time.

69. **b.** HLA A-29 is present in 7% of the general population. This test is confirmatory in birdshot chorioretinopathy with positivity in >90%.

70. **c.** The other answers listed can cause vision loss late in the disease.

71. **b.** Visual field loss can be progressive. Optic nerve edema can be present during the acute phase. Color vision can be decreased, as well as night vision. ICG angiography shows more hypo-fluorescent lesions than on clinical exam or fluo-rescein angiography.

72. **a.** Posterior and anterior synechiae can be exten-sive in sarcoidosis. Although the iridocyclitis in sarcoidosis is classically granulomatous, it also can be nongranulomatous.

73. **d.** An elevated angiotension-converting enzyme (ACE) level occurs in approximately two-thirds of patients with sarcoidosis, and an abnormal chest x-ray (hilar and/or mediastinal adenopathy) is very likely to be found. Elevated serum lysozyme is more sensitive but less specific. Gallium scan also may be helpful in the diagnosis. The anti-neutrophil cytoplasmic antibody (ANCA) assay is useful in diagnosing Wegener granulomatosis, not sarcoidosis.

74. **b.** Caseation is the hallmark of tuberculosis. Sarcoidosis features noncaseating granulomas.

75. **d.** Parotid gland infiltration compresses the facial nerve as an innocent bystander (remember that the terminal branches of the facial nerve splits within the substance of the parotid gland). Palsy can be bilateral. The Heerfordt-Waldenström syndrome describes fever, parotid enlargement, anterior uveitis, and facial nerve palsy secondary to sarcoidosis.

76. c. There is a potential association with cerebral vasculitis. In addition, APMPPE has also been associated with other inflammatory and infectious conditions.

77. a. This is the classic finding regarding APMPPE lesions.

78. c. Interstitial keratitis (IK) usually produces intense pain and photophobia. The immune response in interstitial keratitis is felt to be an immune response to treponemal antigens (and not live organisms). Standard regimens for neurosyphilis are sufficient to treat luetic IK. Although results of the RPR and Venereal Disease Research Laboratory (VDRL) tests may be negative in congenital syphilis, those of the FTA-Abs are usually positive.

79. a. Although nontreponemal tests such as the VDRL and rapid plasma reagin (RPR) titers decrease with successful syphilis treatment, the FTA-Abs titer usually does not decrease after treatment. Ocular inflammation (e.g., uveitis, chorioretinitis) secondary to syphilis should be treated as neurosyphilis.

80. c. Lyme immunofluorescent antibody titers and ELISA for IgM and IgG are positive in only 40% to 60% of cases.

81. c. Tuberculosis is an uncommon, but increasingly frequent, cause of uveitis in the United States. Tuberculous bacilli may be found histopathologically in eyes with tuberculous uveitis. Tuberculous uveitis may be present even with a normal PPD and normal chest x-ray. For these cases, a second strength (250 tuberculin units) skin test may be positive. Systemic corticosteroids may cause a dangerous flare-up in otherwise quiescent tuberculosis. Tuberculosis may cause a severe scleritis as well.

82. a. Eighty percent of cases of "peripheral" or intermediate uveitis are bilateral. Vitrectomy may be helpful in clearing media opacities and alleviating vitreous traction, but chronic cystoid macular edema often limits vision. Hypotony due to chronic ciliary body inflammation may also occur.

83. d. PIC is commonly seen in young, myopic, mostly Caucasian women. It is localized to the macular area and has no vitritis. CNVM formation can cause severe vision loss in these patients.

84. b. MEWDS, multiple evanescent white dot syndrome, has classic findings including foveal granularity and white spots that resolve.

85. d. Acute bleb-associated endophthalmitis can occur at any time following filtration surgery. Pneumococcus (*S. pneumoniae*) and *H. influenzae* are the most frequent pathogens. This tends to be a very aggressive infection.

86. b. Although prolonged, complicated, invasive surgeries have a higher incidence of postoperative endophthalmitis, even surgeries that do not include ocular penetration, such as pterygium excision and strabismus surgeries may be associated with endophthalmitis.

87. c. Serratia species produce severe acute postoperative endophthalmitis. Certain organisms are clearly implicated in chronic postoperative endophthalmitis and are associated with typical time courses:
Staphylococcus epidermidis, within 6 weeks.
Candida species, 1 to 3 months.
Propionibacterium acnes, 2 months to 2 years.

88. c. Posttraumatic endophthalmitis incurs a poor prognosis, with <10% retaining vision better than 20/400.

89. d. Posttraumatic endophthalmitis has a uniquely high percentage of Bacillus species, especially *Bacillus cereus*, represented etiologically. Estimates have ranged from 20% to 25%, and the organisms seem to be particularly associated

7

with retained metallic foreign bodies, as well as farm or soil-related injuries. *Bacillus cereus* endophthalmitis can be extremely fulminant. Of slightly greater incidence is *Staphylococcus epidermidis* (about 30% of posttraumatic endophthalmitis).

90. **d.** *Bacillus cereus* may be the single most destructive organism encountered in ocular infections. The organism's enzymes and exotoxins can produce unsalvageable destruction within 24 hours. Of interest, *Bacillus cereus* and Clostridium are two organisms capable of producing systemic, constitutional symptoms from endophthalmitis.

91. **b.** AZOOR is the diagnosis. The classic curvilinear area is seen that separates normal retina and damaged retina. Patients are usually young myopic females. Vitritis may be present. Patients develop bilateral disease. Most patient's visual acuity remain in the 20/40 range. Visual field also stabilizes over time.

92. **c.** The majority of fungal endogenous endophthalmitis occurs without evidence of fungemia.

93. **b.** Sympathetic ophthalmia characteristically spares the choriocapillaris.

94. **a.** Ocular and CNS findings precede skin changes in this disease. The differential diagnosis for VKH includes sympathetic ophthalmia and posterior scleritis.

95. **c.** Granulomatous inflammation of the anterior segment can occur in toxoplasmosis. High IOP can also occur. Perivasculitis near active retinal lesions is common (Kyrieleis arteriolitis). The classic lesion of toxoplasmosis is exudative focal retinitis. The definitive host for *Toxoplasma gondii* is the cat, where it is found as an intestinal parasite. (The gondi is a small South American rodent, which is an important intermediate host in that region of the world.)

96. **d.** Clindamycin is clearly associated with pseudomembranous colitis. Sulfa drugs can cause Stevens-Johnson syndrome, as well as either hemolytic or aplastic anemia. Pyrimethamine can cause aplastic anemia (hence the concurrent use of folinic acid). Steroid therapy can aggravate diabetes.

97. **b.** The larvae of *Onchocerca volvulus* form subcutaneous nodules when they develop into mature worms. This is one manifestation of onchodermatitis.

98. **d.** The nodules pictured are classic for ocular sarcoid. Sarcoidosis can involve all areas of the eye. The orbit, cranial nerves, and glands can also be affected by sarcoid. These nodules may be easily biopsied for tissue diagnosis.

99. **c.** This is a classic picture of CMV retinitis. The white areas are active with viral infections. This is a serious disease and potentially may cause blindness from necrosis of the retina and retinal detachment. Patients are treated with a combination of antiviral medications such as ganciclovir and foscarnet, systemically and intravitreally.

100. **c.** Ocular infection by CMV may cause exudative or rhegmatogenous retinal detachments, with holes in the area of retinal necrosis.

101. **b.** IV gangciclovir, IV foscarnet, IV cidofovir, oral valganciclovir, and intravitreal ganciclovir/foscarnet are treatment options. IV acyclovir is generally not used in CMV retinitis.

102. **d.** Iatrogenic immunosuppression, intravenous drug abuse, and indwelling intravenous catheters for hyperalimentation are risk factors for candidal infections. Candida endophthalmitis is less common in AIDS (mucocutaneous candidiasis is common).

103. **d.** Patients with necrotizing herpetic retinitis/acute retinal necrosis (ARN) are usually

otherwise healthy and not debilitated, as opposed to the typical patient with viral (CMV) retinitis. (Severe, bilateral ARN has been described in patients with AIDS.)

104. **b.** Ocular histoplasmosis syndrome has NO vitreous cells. The other conditions are masquerade syndromes that may produce a chronic vitreous cellular reaction. Primary CNS lymphoma is also on this differential and critically important to consider.

105. **b.** Systemic infection with Nocardia is characterized by pneumonia and disseminated abscesses. Nocardia is a filamentary bacterium. Ocular involvement results from hematogenous spread and is rare. It may cause a range of ocular inflammation from a focal mass to disseminated inflammation.

106. **d.** *Toxocara canis* is an intestinal parasite of dogs and cats. Dogs are more commonly implicated in human infections. After ingestion of ova, larvae are spawned that will penetrate the intestinal wall and take up residence in the liver and lungs. From there, larvae can disseminate to any organ, including the eye. Eye involvement is usually unilateral. Dragging of the retina may occur.

107. **d.** Peripheral histo spots begin to appear around adolescence. The maculopathy usually does not appear until the 20s. The early stage of the disease is thought to be a choroiditis. Vitreous cells are not seen in POHS. Visual complaints are caused by the maculopathy and development of CNVM.

108. **c.** The presentation shown is that of APMPPE. This disorder is seen in healthy young adults after a flu-like illness. It is seen equal in males and females. Scotomas are acute in presentation. In the fundus, there are several large, flat lesions at the level of the RPE. On angiography, these lesions classically show early hypofluorescence and late hyperfluorescent staining. The majority of these patients return to good visual acuity within 6 months. The condition is self-limited. Rarely, it may be associated with cerebral vasculitis.

109. **d.** Berlin's nodules are located in the angle. Koeppe nodules are present on the pupillary border, and Busacca nodules are located in the mid-iris. Iris atrophy and anterior and posteror synechaie may also occur in uveitis.

110. **b.** Periocular steroid injection should not be used in cases of infectious uveitis. They can also lead to further melting and perforation in necrotizing scleritis. Longer-acting steroids (e.g., triamcinolone) given via periocular injection have the potential for raising IOP for an extended period of time.

111. **b.** The worms typically affect unilaterally, (hence the name). Laser photocoagulation of the subretinal worm is highly effective. Systemic therapy with thiabendazole and albendazole has also been implemented in some cases. Reinfection is possible with this disease with a second worm.

112. **c.** This is an example of band keratopathy. It can be seen in eyes with history of previous surgery (including vitrectomy and use of silicone oil), ocular tumors, phthisis, and chronic inflammatory conditions. It is related to the deposition of calcium in the cornea.

113. **d.** HIV retinopathy is the most common ocular manifestation of patients with AIDS. It is characterized by microaneurysms, cotton-wool spots, and retinal hemorrhages. Fifty to seventy percent of patients with AIDS develop some ocular abnormality. One series reported that up to 92% of patients with AIDS would develop cotton-wool spots.

114. **d.** CMV retinitis, along with *Pneumocystis carinii* pneumonia and Kaposi's sarcoma, was one of the infections recognized early in the course of the epidemic as a defining feature of the disease.

115. **b.** Pneumocystis choroiditis is seen particularly in patients receiving aerosolized pentamidine. Histopathologically, the lesions in the choroid

7

contain cysts or trophozoites of *Pneumocystis carinii*. IV TMP–SMX therapy is the treatment of choice for PCP choroiditis. APMPPE can resemble this clinical disease.

116. **c.** Kaposi's sarcoma may be noted on the eyelid skin or conjunctiva. Skin lesions usually appear as nontender, elevated, purple nodules. Conjunctival involvement is manifested by red subconjunctival masses.

117. **b.** Herpetic uveitis, HSV and HZV, may cause stromal atrophy of the iris. This is a clue to diagnosis. The other conditions tend not to cause atrophy. Transillumation allows for best visualization of iris stromal atrophy.

118. **c.** The picture in question 118 is classic punctate inner choroidopathy. The patient is in the classic demographic as she is a young, myopic woman.

119. **c.** Chorioretinits from documented candidemia can occur in 9% to 10% of patients.

120. **a.** Most patients develop an intermediate uveitis (pars planitis) or panuveitis. Macular edema is less common. HLA-DR15 is associated with MS and uveitis. The uveitis is usually less aggressive than the idiopathic form.

121. **d.** Both PORN and ARN are manifestations of severe posterior segment infection by the herpes family of viruses. ARN, particularly in immunocompetent hosts, responds to intravenous acyclovir more reliably than PORN. Up to two-thirds of PORN eyes will end up with no light perception (NLP), despite treatment. The vision outcomes in PORN are poor.

122. **d.** Laser photocoagulation may have the same salutary effect on resistant pars planitis as cryotherapy, but without the risk of RD.

123. **d.** Systemic corticosteroids are generally used initially, followed by cyclosporine or cytotoxic drugs as second-line options.

124. **b.** The choroid has the highest amount of blood flow in the entire body.

125. **c.** Up to 25% of patients with PCNSL will have ocular involvement.

126. **c.** Ninety-eight percent are non-Hodgkin B-lymphocyte lymphomas. Two percent are T-lymphocyte lymphomas.

127. **a.** Steroids may initially improve the inflammation but will eventually fail as a therapy. Most cases are B cell derived. Vitreous biopsy/retinal biopsy/CSF histology may lead to a diagnosis. Vitreous biopsy is not the only way for tissue diagnosis. The current therapy is combination chemotherapy and radiotherapy. Surgery alone is associated with a poor prognosis.

128. **a.** Choroidal metastases are most commonly from a primary lung tumor in men.

129. **b.** Choroidal metastases are most commonly from a primary breast tumor in women.

130. **d.** Retinal metastases are rare. Cutaneous melanoma is the most common primary tumor.

CHAPTER 8

Glaucoma, Lens, and Anterior Segment Trauma

Questions

1. Which of the following factors does not play a role in determining IOP?
   a. rate of aqueous humor production by the ciliary body.
   b. resistance to aqueous outflow across the trabecular meshwork-Schlemm's canal system.
   c. level of intracranial pressure.
   d. level of episcleral venous pressure.

2. Glaucoma is defined as
   a. a group of diseases that have in common a characteristic optic neuropathy associated with increased intraocular pressure.
   b. a group of diseases that have in common a characteristic optic neuropathy with associated visual function loss.
   c. a group of diseases that have in common high intraocular pressure with or without optic neuropathy.
   d. a group of diseases that have in common a characteristic optic neuropathy with poor visual acuity.

3. Which of the following epidemiologic statistics is true regarding primary open angle glaucoma?
   a. In the United States, it is the most frequent cause of nonreversible blindness in African Americans.
   b. By the year 2020, it is estimated that 2.2 million Americans will be affected.

   c. It is estimated that 10% have become bilaterally blind (best-corrected visual acuity ≤20/200 or visual field <20°).
   d. Data from meta-analysis tends to overestimate the prevalence.

4. Which of the following is true in regard to worldwide racial disparity and primary open angle glaucoma?
   a. Prevalence among blacks is three to four times higher than whites.
   b. The racial disparity decreases with age.
   c. In general, blacks have been found to have fewer nerve fibers at baseline.
   d. Despite the higher prevalence in blacks, the likelihood of blindness is four times lower when compared to whites.

5. Which of the following is not a risk factor for the development of primary open angle glaucoma?
   a. positive family history.
   b. advanced age.
   c. increased IOP.
   d. increased corneal thickness.

6. Intraocular pressure can fluctuate throughout the day. Peak IOP occurs
   a. upon awakening.
   b. midday.
   c. late evening.
   d. during the night.

7. With respect to angle-closure glaucoma, which of the following is true?
   a. Men are at increased risk.
   b. The anterior chamber depth increases with age, predisposing to pupillary-block- induced angle-closure glaucoma.
   c. Primary angle-closure glaucoma may occur in eyes with any type of refractive error.
   d. Family history, while important in open-angle glaucoma, does not play a role in angle-closure glaucoma.

8. Which of the following gene mutation-phenotype pairings is incorrect?
   a. GLC1A—associated with myocilin production in the trabecular meshwork after treatment with dexamethasone in both juvenile and adult forms of glaucoma.
   b. GLC1B—associated with normal-tension forms of open-angle glaucoma.
   c. GLC1C—associated with high pressure, late onset forms of glaucoma.
   d. GLC1D—associated with a protein that catalyzes the formation of elastin fibers in exfoliation syndrome.

9. Several investigators have provided evidence that a gene responsible for some cases of juvenile-onset primary open-angle glaucoma resides on chromosome
   a. 1.
   b. 3.
   c. 8.
   d. X.

10. Which of the following is true in regard to aqueous humor dynamics?
    a. Aqueous humor is produced in the anterior chamber and flows through the pupil.
    b. Aqueous humor is produced by the inner nonpigmented cells of the ciliary processes.
    c. Aqueous humor exits the eye by passing through the trabecular meshwork and into Schlemm's canal before draining into the suprachoroidal spaces.
    d. Aqueous humor exits the eye by passing through the uveoscleral pathway that ultimately drains into the venous system through a plexus of collector channels.

11. Aqueous humor is not formed or secreted as a result of
    a. facilitated diffusion.
    b. simple diffusion.
    c. active secretion.
    d. ultrafiltration.

12. Relative to plasma, aqueous has all of the following except
    a. excess hydrogen ions.
    b. excess chloride ions.
    c. excess ascorbate.
    d. excess bicarbonate.

13. All of the following can decrease aqueous humor production except
    a. trauma.
    b. intraocular inflammation.
    c. general anesthetics such as Ketamine.
    d. carotid occlusive disease.

14. Which of the following is not true in regard to trabecular outflow?
    a. It is increased by cycloplegia.
    b. It is the site of pressure-dependent outflow.
    c. The juxtacanalicular meshwork is likely the major site of outflow resistance.
    d. The trabecular meshwork functions as a one-way valve, permitting aqueous to leave and limiting flow in the other direction.

15. Uveoscleral outflow accounts for what percentage of total aqueous outflow facility?
    a. <5%.
    b. 5% to 10%.
    c. 10% to 50%.
    d. 75% to 90%.

16. The mean value for outflow facility in normal eyes is
    a. 0.05 μL/min/mm Hg.
    b. 0.15 μL/min/mm Hg.
    c. 0.28 μL/min/mm Hg.
    d. 0.48 μL/min/mm Hg.

8

17. Episcleral venous pressure
    a. is not affected by alterations in body position.
    b. normally ranges from 10 to 12 mm Hg.
    c. can be altered by certain diseases of the orbit, the head, and the neck that obstruct venous return to the heart or shunt blood from the arterial to the venous system.
    d. is associated with a rise in IOP in a 1:1 fashion in chronic conditions.

18. Data from large western epidemiologic studies demonstrate that intraocular pressure has a
    a. non-Gaussian distribution with a skew toward lower pressures.
    b. non-Gaussian distribution with a skew toward higher pressures.
    c. gaussian distribution centered at 16 mm Hg.
    d. gaussian distribution centered at 22 mm Hg.

19. Which of the following regarding intraocular pressure is false?
    a. Screening for glaucoma based on IOP > 21 misses half of people with glaucoma and optic nerve damage.
    b. There is no clear IOP level below which IOP can be considered safe and above which IOP can be considered elevated.
    c. IOP is no longer considered a risk factor for the development of glaucoma.
    d. IOP varies with heartbeat, respiration, and exercise.

20. Regarding Goldmann applanation tonometry:
    a. The tonometer measures the force necessary to flatten a 3.06 mm² area of cornea.
    b. Measurements are most accurate with a central corneal thickness of 520 μm.
    c. Excessive amounts of fluorescein result in inaccurately low IOP readings.
    d. Corneal edema predisposes to inaccurately high IOP readings.

21. Which of the following findings was not reported in the Ocular Hypertension Treatment Study (OHTS)?
    a. A thinner central cornea was a strong predictive factor for the development of glaucoma in subjects with ocular hypertension.
    b. Subjects with a corneal thickness of 555 μm or less had a threefold greater risk of developing POAG when compared to those measuring >588 μm.
    c. Central corneal thickness was found to be a risk factor for progression independent of IOP level.
    d. More than four times as many subjects progressed to glaucoma in the observation group compared to those that were treated.

22. Current recommendations for cleaning Goldman-type tonometry tips between patients include all of the following except
    a. 5 minutes soak in 40% isopropyl alcohol.
    b. 5 minutes soak in 1:10 sodium hypochlorite solution (household bleach).
    c. 5 minutes soak in 3% hydrogen peroxide.
    d. Thorough wipe with an alcohol sponge.

23. Which of the following is incorrect in regard to gonioscopy?
    a. Under normal conditions light reflected from the angle structures undergoes total internal reflection at the tear–air interface.
    b. All gonioscopy lenses eliminate tear-air interface by placing a plastic or glass surface on the front surface of the eye while the space between the lens and cornea is filled by tears, saline, or a clear viscous substance.
    c. The Goldmann lens is a type of direct viewing system.
    d. The Zeiss lens is a type of mirrored, indirect viewing system.

24. Which of the following gonioscopy lenses would most likely narrow the angle on indentation gonioscopy?
    a. Goldmann.
    b. Posner.
    c. Sussman.
    d. Zeiss.

25. Which method of gonioscopy is considered best for evaluating a patient with potential traumatic (angle-recession) glaucoma?
    a. Goldmann.
    b. Koeppe.
    c. Zeiss.
    d. Sussman.

8

26. Which of the following is least likely to undergo spontaneous closure?
    a. grade I angle.
    b. grade II angle.
    c. grade III angle.
    d. grade IV angle.

27. The gonioscopic criteria for posttraumatic angle recession include all of the following except
    a. an abnormally wide ciliary body band.
    b. decreased prominence of the scleral spur.
    c. torn iris processes.
    d. marked variation of ciliary face width and angle depth in different quadrants of the same eye.

28. The adult optic nerve
    a. is composed of neural tissue, glial tissue, extracellular matrix, and blood vessels.
    b. consists of approximately 6 million axons.
    c. has axons with cell bodies that lie in the bipolar layer of the retina.
    d. expands from 1 to 2 mm in diameter upon exiting the globe.

29. The lamina cribrosa is made up of fenestrated sheets of connective tissue. Which of the following is incorrect regarding this structure?
    a. It provides the main support for the optic nerve as it exits the eye.
    b. The connective tissue is composed primarily of collagen.
    c. The fenestrations within the lamina are larger temporally and nasally as compared with superior and inferior aspects.
    d. The fenestrations may be seen on exam at the base of the optic nerve head cup.

30. There is a rich vascular supply to the optic nerve, retina, and choroid. Which of the following is a true statement?
    a. The long posterior ciliary arteries penetrate the perineural sclera of the posterior globe to supply the peripapillary choroid, as well as most of the anterior optic nerve.

    b. Some long posterior ciliary arteries course, without branching, through the sclera directly into the choroid; others divide within the sclera to provide branches to both the choroid and the optic nerve.
    c. The central retinal artery penetrates the globe 3 to 5 mm behind the globe.
    d. A noncontinuous arterial circle exists within the perineural sclera, known as the circle of Zinn-Haller, and is not found in all eyes.

31. There are four anatomic regions of the anterior optic nerve. Which of the following regions is incorrectly associated with a blood supply?
    a. Superficial nerve fiber layer—supplied principally by recurrent retinal arterioles from the central retinal artery.
    b. Prelaminar region—supplied by branches of short posterior ciliary arteries and branches of the circle of Zinn-Haller.
    c. Lamina cribrosa region—supplied by branches of short posterior ciliary arteries and branches of the circle of Zinn-Haller.
    d. Retrolaminar region—supplied solely by branches of short posterior ciliary arteries.

32. The mechanical theory of glaucomatous optic neuropathy emphasizes all of the following concepts except
    a. direct compression of axonal fibers and support structures of the anterior optic nerve.
    b. distortion of the lamina cribrosa plates and axoplasmic flow.
    c. intraneural ischemia from decreased optic nerve perfusion.
    d. cell death of the retinal ganglion cells from compression of axons.

33. What percentage of normal individuals will have cup–disc ratios of larger than 0.6?
    a. <1%.
    b. 5%.
    c. 10%.
    d. 25%.

34. Asymmetry of cup–disc ratio of more than 0.2 occurs in what percentage of the normal population?
    a. <1%.
    b. 5%.
    c. 10%.
    d. 25%.

35. In normal eyes, on average, _____ neuroretinal rim is thickest, while _____ rim is thinnest.
    a. inferior, superior.
    b. inferior, temporal.
    c. temporal, inferior.
    d. superior, inferior.

36. Which of the following is true with regard to splinter, or nerve fiber layer, hemorrhages near the optic nerve?
    a. They may occur in as many as half of glaucoma patients at some time during the course of their disease.
    b. Hemorrhages clear over weeks to months but are often followed by localized notching of the rim and visual field loss.
    c. Individuals with normal-tension glaucoma are less likely to have disc hemorrhages.
    d. They are pathognomonic for glaucoma.

37. Which of the following is not a characteristic of short-wavelength automated perimetry (SWAP)?
    a. A blue stimulus is projected onto a yellow background.
    b. This method is sensitive in early identification of glaucomatous damage.
    c. The rate of perimetric change from early glaucoma may be higher than with conventional white-on-white visual fields.
    d. The stimuli employed activate the M cells.

38. Which of the following is not true regarding visual field testing?
    a. A cluster of two or more points depressed ≥5 dB compared with surrounding points is suspicious.
    b. A single point depressed >10 dB is very unusual but is of less value on a single visual field than a cluster, because cluster points confirm one another.
    c. Corresponding points above and below the horizontal midline should not vary markedly.
    d. Normally the inferior field is depressed 1 to 2 dB compared with the superior field.

39. Which one of the following statements concerning perimetry is true?
    a. In static perimetry, the stimulus intensity is held constant (static) and moved centrally until it is detected.
    b. Kinetic perimetry is most useful for quantifying and tracking visual field changes in a patient with established glaucoma.
    c. Early, specific signs of glaucoma include generalized constriction of isopters and baring of the blind spot.
    d. For a visual field defect to be classified as glaucomatous, it should have corresponding optic nerve head abnormalities.

40. A 64-year-old African American man with a history of open-angle glaucoma presents with a Goldmann visual field documenting a superior nasal step to the I4e isopter in the right eye. When he returns with a deteriorated visual field 1 year later, the most likely form of deterioration is
    a. an inferior Bjerrum scotoma.
    b. a superior paracentral scotoma.
    c. an inferior nasal step.
    d. encroachment of his superior nasal step toward fixation.

41. Which one of the following visual field patterns will most quickly progress to loss of fixation?
    a. split fixation to the I4e isopter.
    b. central 5° island.
    c. a large superior nasal step encroaching on fixation (<10°).
    d. superior and inferior nasal steps encroaching to 20°.

8

42. When should other neurologic etiologies, other than glaucoma, be strongly considered?
    a. The patient's optic disc cupping is proportional to visual field loss.
    b. The cupping of the nerve is more impressive than the pallor.
    c. The progression of the visual field loss seems excessive.
    d. The pattern of visual field loss respects the horizontal midline.

43. What percent of individuals in the general population who have glaucomatous optic neuropathy and/or visual field loss have an initial screening IOP of below 22 mm Hg?
    a. 70% to 80%.
    b. 30% to 50%.
    c. 10% to 30%.
    d. <10%.

44. Which of the following was not a finding in the Ocular Hypertension Treatment Study (OHTS)?
    a. The purpose of the study was to evaluate the safety and efficacy of topical ocular hypotensive medications in preventing or delaying the onset of visual field loss and/or optic nerve damage in subjects with ocular hypertension.
    b. Topical ocular hypotensive medication was effective in delaying or preventing the onset of POAG: a 22.5% decrease in IOP in the treatment group (vs. 4.0% in controls) was associated with a reduction of the development of POAG from 9.5% in controls to 4.4% in treated patients at 60 months' follow-up.
    c. OHTS subjects had thinner corneas than the general population, with black subjects having thinner corneas than white subjects.
    d. Increased risk of onset of POAG was associated with increases in age, vertical and horizontal cup–disc ratio, pattern standard deviation, and IOP at baseline.

45. Which of the following was a finding in the Early Manifest Glaucoma Trial (EMGT)?
    a. Treatment reduced IOP by 30%.
    b. In multivariate analyses, progression risk was halved by treatment.
    c. Progression risk decreased by 20% with each millimeter of mercury of IOP reduction from baseline to the first follow-up visit.
    d. At 6 years, 62% of untreated patients showed progression, whereas 30% of treated patients progressed.

46. The Collaborative Initial Glaucoma Treatment Study compared medical and surgical approaches to newly diagnosed open-angle glaucoma patients and demonstrated that
    a. Early visual loss was greater in the medically treated group.
    b. After 5 years, the surgically managed group had worse visual field outcomes.
    c. IOP reduction in the surgical group averaged 17 to 18 mm Hg, whereas that in the medically treated group was 14 to 15 mm Hg.
    d. The rate of cataract removal was greater in the surgically treated group.

47. Which of the following is true in regard to low-tension or normal-tension glaucoma?
    a. Authorities have separated normal-tension glaucoma into two groups based on disc appearance: a senile sclerotic group and a focal ischemic group.
    b. Visual field defects in POAG tend to be more focal, deeper, and closer to fixation, especially early in the course, compared with those commonly seen in normal-tension glaucoma.
    c. When compared to those with POAG, the neuroretinal rim has been reported to be thinner, especially superiorly, in persons with normal-tension glaucoma.
    d. The Collaborative Normal-Tension Glaucoma Study (CNTGS) found that lowering IOP by at least 20% reduced the rate of visual field progression from 35% to 12% in subjects with normal-tension glaucoma.

48. A 54-year-old white woman presents with glaucomatous optic nerve head changes in each eye and split fixation in her right eye, consistent with her disc findings. Review of her record documents that she has progressively lost visual field and neural rim tissue while running IOPs in the low teens. Gonioscopy has been documented as normal repeatedly. She is currently on maximal tolerated medical therapy and reports subjective decrease in vision in her right eye. A surgical intervention in the right eye is felt to be the next indicated maneuver. Which procedure might be the one of choice?

   a. iridoplasty.

   b. surgical peripheral iridectomy.

   c. trabeculectomy.

   e. cyclocryotherapy or cyclophotocoagulation.

49. A 75-year-old Scandinavian woman presents for routine eye examination. She has no complaints. Her examination is significant for IOP of 23 in both eyes, anterior segment exam significant for findings as indicated by photograph below, and cup:disc ratio of 0.7 in both eyes. Which of the following is most likely true in regard to the remainder of her examination?

   a. On gonioscopy, the trabecular meshwork is heavily pigmented with pigment deposition anterior to the Schwalbe line.

   b. On gonioscopy, the chamber angle is narrow due to formation of synechiae.

   c. On retroillumination, peripheral transillumination defects are seen.

   d. On examination of the lens, she is noted to dilate widely with pigment visible on zonules.

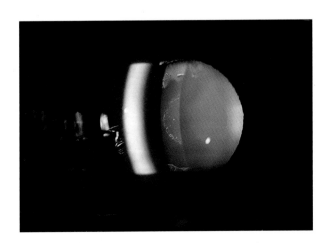

50. In regard to the patient described in question 49, which of the following is least likely true?

   a. The open-angle glaucoma associated with this condition is thought to be caused by material obstructing flow through, and causing damage to, the trabecular meshwork.

   b. In this condition, IOP is often higher, with greater diurnal fluctuations than in POAG, and the overall prognosis is worse.

   c. Laser trabeculoplasty can be very effective, but the response may not last as long as with POAG.

   d. Lens extraction has a high likelihood of alleviating the condition.

51. Features that distinguish pseudoexfoliation glaucoma from primary open-angle glaucoma include all of the following except

   a. greater sensitivity to laser therapy.

   b. greater degree of interocular asymmetry.

   c. the age of affected patients.

   d. degree of trabecular meshwork (TM) pigmentation.

52. Which of the following glaucomas is least likely to respond to medical therapy alone?

   a. pseudoexfoliation.

   b. pigmentary glaucoma.

   c. phacolytic glaucoma.

   d. lens particle glaucoma.

53. A patient presents with clinical findings as shown in the photographs A and B in the left column at the top of the next page. Which of the following statements is most applicable to this patient?

   a. The risk of developing glaucoma is approximately 50% to 75%.

   b. Glaucoma associated with these findings occurs most commonly in young black males who have high myopia.

   c. Glaucoma associated with these findings is characterized by wide fluctuations in IOP which can exceed 50 mm Hg.

   d. The presence of a Krukenberg's spindle is necessary to make the diagnosis.

8

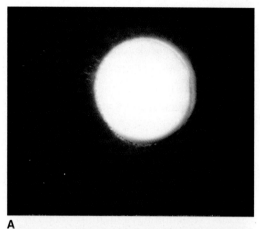

A

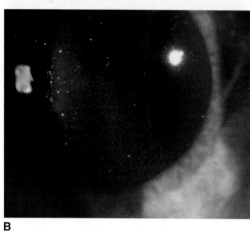

B

b. Cellular debris may be seen layering in the anterior chamber, leading to a pseudohypopyon.

c. Definitive therapy requires laser iridotomy.

d. Leakage of lens protein occurs through large defects in the lens capsule.

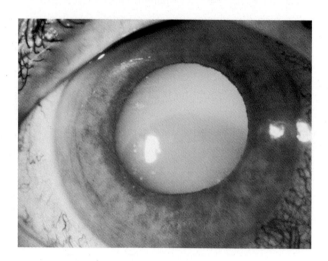

54. In regard to treatment options for the patient in question 53, which of the following is not true?
    a. Medical treatment is often successful in reducing IOP.
    b. Patients respond well to laser trabeculoplasty, although the effect may be short-lived.
    c. Laser iridectomy has been proposed as a means of minimizing posterior bowing of the iris.
    d. Filtering surgery is usually unsuccessful in these patients.

55. A 73-year-old male presents with sudden onset pain and redness in his right eye (see image in next column). His vision has been poor in the eye for 3 years. His only significant history is that he had cataract surgery in the fellow eye 4 years ago. There is no history of trauma. Clinical examination demonstrates markedly elevated IOP and an open angle. Which of the following is most likely true?
    a. Keratic precipitates are often present in this condition.

56. The most common cause of glaucoma in primary or metastatic tumors of the ciliary body is
    a. direct tumor invasion of the anterior chamber angle.
    b. angle closure by rotation of the ciliary body.
    c. angle closure by anterior displacement of the lens-iris diaphragm.
    d. neovascularization of the angle.

57. Which of the following regarding glaucomatocyclitic crisis is not true?
    a. The iritis associated with this entity is mild, with few small, round keratic precipitates (KP).
    b. Chronic suppressive therapy with topical nonsteroidal anti-inflammatory agents or mild steroids is effective in preventing attacks.
    c. KP may be seen on the trabecular meshwork, suggesting trabeculitis.
    d. Intraocular pressure is usually markedly elevated, in the 40 to 50 mm Hg range, and corneal edema may be present.

58. What percent of patients with Fuchs heterochromic iridocyclitis will have a secondary open-angle glaucoma?
    a. 15%.
    b. 30%.
    c. 50%.
    d. 90%.

59. Which of the following is true in regard to treating glaucoma secondary to elevated episcleral venous pressure.
    a. Medications that increase trabecular outflow are more effective than drugs that reduce aqueous humor formation.
    b. Glaucoma filtering surgery may be complicated by a ciliochoroidal effusion or a suprachoroidal hemorrhage.
    c. Prostaglandin analogs are not effective in any patients.
    d. Laser trabeculoplasty is effective unless there are secondary changes in the outflow channels.

60. In a patient who presents with traumatic hyphema, elevated IOP, and a history of sickle cell disease, which of the following is safest to use for IOP reduction?
    a. apraclonidine.
    b. brimonidine.
    c. epinephrine.
    d. dipivefrin.

61. Which of the following is not true in regard to ghost cell glaucoma?
    a. It is considered a secondary open-angle glaucoma caused by degenerated red blood cells blocking the trabecular meshwork.
    b. The cells develop within 1 to 3 weeks of a vitreous hemorrhage.
    c. The cells gain access to the anterior chamber through a disrupted hyaloids face.
    d. Medical therapy with aqueous suppressants is the preferred initial approach.

62. The cells that are postulated to cause increased IOP in cases of retinal detachment (Schwartz-Matsuo syndrome) are
    a. pigment.
    b. inflammatory cells.

c. retinal pigment epithelium.
    d. photoreceptor outer segments.

63. Which of the following ocular biometrics does not predispose to primary angle closure?
    a. shallow anterior chamber.
    b. thick lens.
    c. increased anterior curvature of the lens.
    d. large corneal diameter.

64. A 60-year-old Chinese woman presents with sudden onset pain, headache, blurred right eye vision, nausea, and vomiting. She reports that she had been watching a movie with her husband when these symptoms started and now describes rainbow-colored halos around lights. On examination of her right eye she has hand motions vision, intraocular pressure of 50, iris bombé, mid-dilated pupil, and corneal edema. Which of the following findings is least likely to be found on further evaluation of the eye?
    a. mild aqueous cell and flare.
    b. congested episcleral vessels.
    c. retinal vascular occlusion.
    d. anterior chamber depth of 2.6 mm.

65. In patient referenced in question 64, what is the best course of action at this time?
    a. argon laser trabeculoplasty.
    b. selective laser trabeculoplasty.
    c. peripheral iridectomy.
    d. trabeculectomy.

66. An untreated fellow eye in a patient who has had an acute angle-closure attack has a _____ chance of developing an acute attack of angle closure over the next 5 to 10 years.
    a. 5% to 10%.
    b. 15% to 35%.
    c. 40% to 80%.
    d. >90%.

67. Which of the following medications is least likely to be associated with the induction or aggravation of angle-closure glaucoma?
    a. pilocarpine.
    b. oral antihistamines.
    c. cyclopentolate.
    d. aspirin

8

68. A patient with bilaterally narrow anterior chamber angles and normal IOP should probably undergo which of the following tests?
    a. the prone-dark room test.
    b. topical steroid challenge.
    c. thymoxamine test.
    e. careful, depressed dilated examination.

69. A patient with bilaterally narrow anterior chamber angles and elevated IOP should probably undergo which of the following tests?
    a. the prone-dark room test.
    b. topical steroid challenge.
    c. thymoxamine test.
    e. careful, depressed dilated examination.

70. Which of the following clinical features is least likely to lead to a suspicion of plateau iris in a patient with angle closure?
    a. deep anterior chamber centrally.
    b. a young, myopic patient.
    c. a flat iris plane.
    d. a small anterior segment.

71. A 24-year-old myope presents with acute angle closure glaucoma. Examination reveals that the central anterior chamber appears to be of normal depth and the iris plane appears to be rather flat for an eye with angle closure. What entity is most likely to be found on gonioscopy?
    a. plateau iris.
    b. blood in Schlemm's canal.
    c. heavily pigmented trabecular mesh work.
    d. neovascularization of the angle.

72. Angle closure secondary to plateau iris is most often secondary to what primary underlying anatomic derangement?
    a. abnormally concave corneoscleral limbus.
    b. abnormally thickened peripheral iris stroma.

c. forward displacement of the ciliary processes.
d. increased relative pupillary block.

73. Which of the following is true in regard to microspherophakia?
    a. It is often familial and may occur as part of either Weill-Marchesani or Down's syndrome.
    b. It can lead to ectopia lentis.
    c. Treatment with miotics may tighten zonules, flatten the lens, and pull it posteriorly, breaking pupillary block.
    d. Cycloplegics may make pupillary block worse by rotating the ciliary body forward, loosening the zonule, and allowing the lens to become more globular.

74. What is the treatment of choice for neovascularization of the iris due to retinal ischemia in a patient with clear media?
    a. observation.
    b. panretinal photocoagulation.
    c. panretinal cryotherapy.
    d. vitrectomy with endophotocoagulation.

75. A 65-year old female with history of angle closure glaucoma in the past and pseudophakia presents 1 week after trabeculectomy. Her vision is hand motions, intraocular pressure is 50 and on exam she has a cloudy cornea and uniformly shallow anterior chamber. Of the following pathologies, which is least likely?
    a. aqueous misdirection.
    b. choroidal detachment.
    c. acute angel-closure glaucoma.
    d. suprachoroidal hemorrhage

76. In reference to the patient in question 75, her B-scan ultrasound demonstrates no choroidal pathology. What is the optimal management at this time if the patient has a patent peripheral iridotomy?
    a. surgical iridectomy.
    b. vitrectomy.
    c. mydriatic and IOP lowering agents.
    d. lensectomy.

77. Which of the following is true in regard to epithelial and fibrous downgrowth?
    a. Epithelial downgrowth is more prevalent than fibrous ingrowth and progresses more rapidly.
    b. The YAG laser produces characteristic white burns on the epithelial membrane on the iris surface that can help confirm the diagnosis of epithelial downgrowth as well as demarcate the extent of involvement.
    c. The growth of epithelium or fibrovascular tissue into the angle can cause a secondary angle-closure glaucoma for which surgery is the preferred treatment.
    d. Epithelial proliferation can be present in three forms: pearl tumors of the iris, epithelial cysts, and epithelial ingrowth.

78. A 46-year-old female with no prior ocular history presents with bilateral ocular pain, headaches, and worsening of vision. On examination she is noted to have a six diopter myopic shift, IOP of 60, and uniformly shallow anterior chamber in both eyes. What oral medication was she most likely started on recently?
    a. isoniazid.
    b. ethambutol.
    c. topiramate.
    d. clonazepam.

79. For the patient in question 78 what is the best initial treatment?
    a. discontinuation of offending oral medication, IOP lowering agents, and laser peripheral iridotomy.
    b. discontinuation of offending oral medication, IOP lowering agents, and surgical peripheral iridectomy.
    c. discontinuation of offending oral medication, IOP lowering agents, and miotics.
    d. discontinuation of offending oral medication, IOP lowering agents, and cycloplegics.

80. The underlying mechanism of the syndrome above is
    a. ciliochoroidal effusion or detachment.
    b. central serous retinopathy.

    c. acute elongation of the globes.
    d. pupillary block.

81. A mother states that her 6-month-old child has been tearing for the past month and feels that he may not see well with his right eye. Given the findings in the image below, what is the most likely diagnosis?
    a. retinoblastoma.
    b. congenital glaucoma.
    c. nasolacrimal duct obstruction.
    d. congenital hereditary endothelial dystrophy.

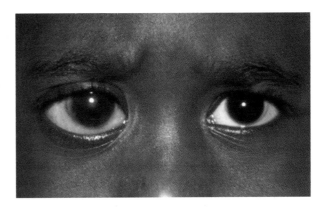

82. What is the optimal management for lowering IOP in a child with congenital glaucoma and a hazy cornea?
    a. topical IOP lowering agents.
    b. goniotomy.
    c. trabeculotomy ab externo.
    d. trabeculectomy or shunt procedure.

83. Which of the following IOP lowering agents should be avoided in children <3 years of age?
    a. topical brimonidine.
    b. topical timolol.
    c. topical dorzolamide.
    d. oral acetazolamide.

84. The infant pictured at the top of the next page presents with glaucoma; the mechanism leading to elevated IOP is most likely which of the following?
    a. increased aqueous production.
    b. elevated episcleral venous pressure.
    c. congenital anterior chamber anomalies.
    d. choroidal hemangioma leading to optic nerve cupping.

8

189

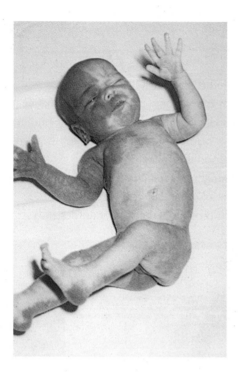

85. Which of the following syndromes is not associated with glaucoma?
    a. Axenfeld-Rieger syndrome.
    b. Sturge-Weber syndrome.
    c. neurofibromatosis 1.
    d. neurofibromatosis 2.

86. Which of the following pairings of medication and method of action is incorrect?
    a. latanoprost: increase uveoscleral outflow.
    b. timolol: decrease aqueous production.
    c. brimonidine: decrease aqueous production, increase trabecular outflow.
    d. dorzolamide: decrease aqueous production.

87. Which of the following pairings of medication and ocular side effects is incorrect?
    a. latanoprost: increased pigmentation of iris, lashes, hypertrichosis.
    b. timolol: corneal anesthesia, punctate keratitis.
    c. brimonidine: blurring, dryness, eyelid edema.
    d. dorzolamide: induced hyperopia, keratitis, dermatitis.

88. Which of the following pairings of medication and systemic side effects is incorrect?
    a. latanoprost: flulike symptoms, joint or muscle pain, headache.

    b. timolol: bradycardia, heart block, bronchospasm, decreased libido, mood swings, reduced exercise tolerance.
    c. brimonidine: fatigue, hypertension, syncope, dizziness, anxiety.
    d. dorzolamide: depression, malaise, bitter taste.

89. Which of these is not a concern when using echothiophate iodide?
    a. intense miosis.
    b. retinal detachment.
    c. angle closure.
    d. dry mouth.

90. All glaucoma agents are considered class C during pregnancy except for one agent. Which of the following is considered a class B agent during pregnancy?
    a. brimonidine.
    b. pilocarpine.
    c. timolol.
    d. dorzolamide.

91. The proper pediatric dose of acetazolamide (Diamox) is
    a. 15 mg/kg/day in one dose.
    b. 15 mg/kg/day in three or four divided doses.
    c. 5 mg/kg/day in one dose.
    d. 5 mg/kg/day in three or four divided doses.

92. The agent most likely to cause topical sensitization and medicamentosa is
    a. timolol.
    b. betaxolol.
    c. epinephrine.
    d. pilocarpine.

93. Which of the following miotics is a direct-acting agent?
    a. echothiophate.
    b. carbachol.
    c. demecarium.
    d. pilocarpine.

94. Which of the following complications of miotic administration is least likely with the indirect agents?
    a. cataractogenesis.
    b. bradycardia.
    c. punctal stenosis.
    d. retinal tears and detachment.

95. The side effect of carbonic anhydrase inhibitors that is most commonly encountered is
    a. paresthesias.
    b. gastrointestinal distress.
    c. kidney stones.
    d. anemia.

96. A 73-year-old man reports to the office on his first day following a cataract extraction complaining of severe eye pain. Visual acuity is counting fingers at 3 ft in the involved eye. Slit-lamp examination reveals a diffusely shallow anterior chamber and corneal edema without hypopyon. The *next* step should be
    a. dilated fundus examination.
    b. tonometry.
    c. gonioscopy.
    d. B-mode ultrasonography.

97. In the patient referenced in question 96, after obtaining an applanation IOP of 42 mm Hg and attempting to examine the fundus unsuccessfully, ultrasonography is performed and reveals a normal posterior segment. Gonioscopy reveals a completely closed angle. The next intervention should be
    a. surgical revision of the wound.
    b. peripheral iridotomy.
    c. dilation with potent cycloplegics.
    d. medical treatment with potent miotics.

98. The intervention in question 97 fails. What is the next step?
    a. surgical revision of the wound.
    b. peripheral iridotomy.
    c. dilation with potent cycloplegics.
    d. medical treatment with potent miotics.

99. During initial laser trabeculoplasty for open angle glaucoma, what circumference of the trabecular meshwork is usually treated?
    a. 90°.
    b. 180°.
    c. 270°.
    d. 360°.

100. The correct spot size for argon laser trabeculoplasty (ALT) is
    a. 50 μm.
    b. 100 μm.
    c. 200 μm.
    d. 500 μm.

101. When effective, laser trabeculoplasty is expected to lower intraocular pressure by what percent?
    a. 10% to 15%.
    b. 20% to 25%.
    c. 30% to 40%.
    d. 50%.

102. In which of the following patients is laser trabeculoplasty contraindicated?
    a. primary open angle glaucoma.
    b. pigmentary glaucoma.
    c. exfoliation syndrome.
    d. synechial angle closure.

103. What percentage of patients who undergo laser trabeculoplasty have a transient rise in intraocular pressure?
    a. <1%.
    b. 5%.
    c. 10%.
    d. 20%.

104. In regard to iridocorneoendothelial (ICE) syndromes, which of the following is not true?
    a. They are almost always unilateral and affect women more frequently than men.
    b. The degree of IOP elevation directly reflects the amount of angle synechialization.
    c. In Chandler's syndrome, there may be corneal edema with only modestly elevated or normal IOP.
    d. Essential iris atrophy features stretch and atrophic iris holes with corectopia.

8

105. A 37-year-old man presents with gradual loss of vision affecting his right eye. His past medical and ocular histories are unremarkable. Visual acuity is 20/400 in the right eye and 20/15 in the left eye. The neuromuscular examination is normal. Slit-lamp examination reveals stellate keratic precipitates on the right corneal endothelium, along with a dense white cataract and "washed-out" appearing iris stroma, as shown in image A. There are trace cells in the aqueous. The left eye is normal (image B). IOPs are 32 in the right eye and 12 in the left eye. Gonioscopy of the right eye reveals prominent, engorged vessels that bridge the angle without synechiae. Gonioscopy of the left eye is normal. The right fundus cannot be clearly seen due to the cataract. Which one of the following is true regarding this patient?

a. There was probably an episode of intense intraocular inflammation affecting the right eye in the past.

b. Antibody titers to herpes zoster virus are likely to be elevated in serum and aqueous humor.

c. A classic sign of this disorder is hyphema occurring at the beginning of filtration surgery.

d. The glaucoma is due to typical rubeosis and secondary angle closure.

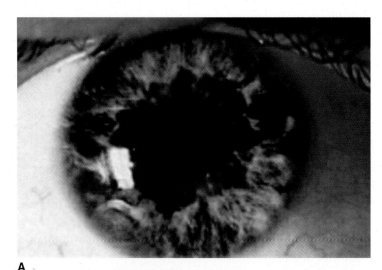

A

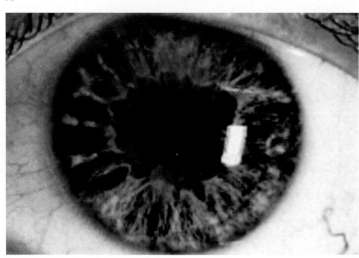

B

192

106. A 48-year-old man presents complaining of difficulty reading. Subjective refraction reveals +0.25 in both eyes, giving 20/15 in both eyes. During the completion of the routine examination, IOP is measured as 34 mm Hg in the right eye and 16 mm Hg in the left eye. Gonioscopy of the right eye is shown in image A and the left eye is shown in image B. The right optic nerve shows evidence of inferior rim excavation. Which one of the following regarding these findings is false?

a. This entity is more common in men.

b. The incidence and severity of the glaucoma in this condition are correlated with the extent of angle abnormalities.

c. Careful slit-lamp examination may reveal iris abnormalities in the right eye.

d. The same pathophysiologic process will usually affect the left eye within the next 3 to 5 years.

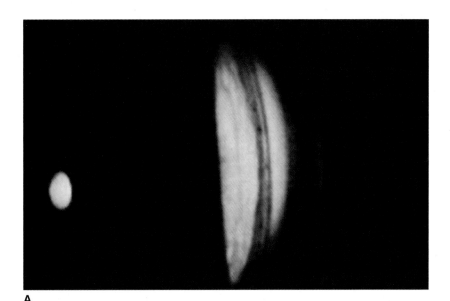

A

8

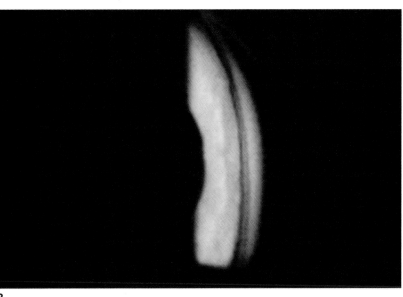

B

107. Which one of the following regarding antimetabolite glaucoma therapy is false?
    a. Mitomycin-C (MMC) directly interacts with DNA, blocking RNA and subsequent protein synthesis in all metabolically active cells.
    b. The antiproliferative effects of MMC are generally more potent and longer-lasting than those of a comparable dose of 5-fluorouracil (5-FU).
    c. Great care should be taken to ensure adequate exposure of the bleb wound edges to MMC in order to gain the maximal antifibrotic effect.
    d. 5-FU is associated with a greater incidence of postoperative hypotony and surface-related complications than MMC.

108. Which of the following is not a risk factor for bleb-related endophthalmitis?
    a. old age.
    b. blepharitis.
    c. male gender.
    d. nasolacrimal duct obstruction.

109. Which of the following is true in regard to the adult lens?
    a. It typically measures 9 mm equatorially and 5 mm anteroposteriorly.
    b. The relative thickness of the cortex decreases with age.
    c. The lens adopts an increasingly flat shape with age.
    d. The index of refraction increases with age.

110. The lens capsule is made of a transparent basement membrane composed of what type of collagen?
    a. type I.
    b. type II.
    c. type III.
    d. type IV.

111. What is the thickness of the lens capsule at the central posterior pole?
    a. 2 to 4 μm.
    b. 8 to 10 μm.
    c. 12 to 15 μm.
    d. 18 to 20 μm.

112. What enzyme has been found to play a pivotal role in the development of "sugar" cataracts that can occur in diabetics?
    a. hexokinase.
    b. polyol dehydrogenase.
    c. aldose reductase.
    d. glucose-6-phosphatase.

113. When the ciliary muscle contracts, the diameter of the muscle ring is
    a. reduced, relaxing tension on the zonules, allowing the lens to become more spherical.
    b. increased, relaxing tension on the zonules, allowing the lens to become more spherical.
    c. reduced, increasing tension on the zonules, allowing the lens to become less spherical.
    d. increased, increasing tension on the zonules, allowing the lens to become less spherical.

114. Anterior lenticonus can be found in association with what syndrome?
    a. Alport's syndrome.
    b. Down's syndrome.
    c. Edwards' syndrome.
    d. Patau's syndrome.

115. Lens colobomas are typically located in which quadrant?
    a. superior.
    b. inferior.
    c. nasal.
    d. temporal.

116. Patients with Peters' anomaly may display which of the following lens anomalies?
    a. posterior cortical or polar cataract.
    b. adhesion between the lens and retina.
    c. a misshapen lens displaced anteriorly into the pupillary space.
    d. macrospherophakia.

117. Approximately what percentage of congenital cataracts are a component of a more extensive syndrome or disease?
    a. 10%.
    b. 33%.
    c. 50%.
    d. 75%.

118. Of the congenital and infantile cataracts, which type is the most common?
    a. lamellar.
    b. anterior polar.
    c. posterior polar.
    d. cerulean.

119. Which of the following statements is true in regard to congenital rubella syndrome and lens changes?
    a. Cataract and glaucoma are often found simultaneously.
    b. Live virus particles may be recovered from the lens as late as 3 years after the patient's birth.
    c. Excessive postoperative inflammation is very rare after cataract removal.
    d. Lens changes are most often characterized by blue nuclear opacifications.

120. Dilated examination reveals a dense white spot on the vitreal surface of the posterior capsule just inferonasal to the center of the posterior capsule. The patient should be advised that
    a. Cataract formation with visual loss is imminent.
    b. The patient should have a glucose tolerance test immediately.
    c. The patient should have urinalysis performed to detect hematuria and proteinuria.
    d. The patient has a benign finding with no significant implications.

121. Which of the following is the histopathological description of the cataract shown at the top of next column?
    a. increased number of lamellar membrane whorls.
    b. local swelling and disruption of lens fiber cells.
    c. collection of crystals on the inner surface of the posterior capsule.
    d. posterior migration of the lens epithelial cells from the lens equator.

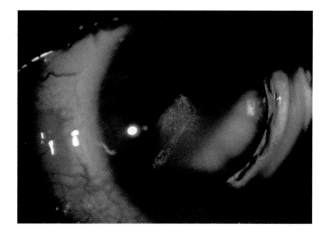

122. Which of the following drugs is correctly matched with the lens changes it classically causes?
    a. phenothiazines: small vacuoles within the anterior lens capsule and epithelium.
    b. miotics: pigmented deposition in the anterior lens epithelium.
    c. amiodarone: stellate anterior axial pigment deposition.
    d. statins: posterior subcapsular cataracts.

123. An infant presents to clinic with bilateral oil droplet cataracts. Mom notes that the child has appeared yellow and is not feeding well. Once the diagnosis is confirmed, how should this child be systemically managed?
    a. elimination of milk and milk products from the diet.
    b. enzyme replacement therapy.
    c. penicillamine.
    d. liver transplant.

124. A patient presents with red, painful eye 2 weeks after significant blunt trauma. On exam, significant cell and flare with keratic precipitates are noted along with increased intraocular pressure, cataract, and disruption of the capsular surface. These findings are most likely representative of
    a. phacoantigenic uveitis.
    b. phacolytic glaucoma.
    c. phacomorphic glaucoma.
    d. Posner-Schlossman syndrome.

8

195

125. For the patient in question 124, histopathologic examination would demonstrate
    a. rare white blood cells.
    b. pigmented debris but no white blood cells.
    c. macrophages with ingested lens proteins.
    d. zonal granulomatous inflammation surrounding a breach of the lens capsule

126. For the patient in question 124, what is the definitive therapy for this condition?
    a. topical or periocular steroids.
    b. lens extraction.
    c. systemic steroids.
    d. topical intraocular pressure lowering agents.

127. What is the most common indication for cataract surgery?
    a. glare.
    b. visual acuity worse than 20/50.
    c. patient's desire for improved vision.
    d. mature cataract.

128. After cataract surgery, corneal edema may occur in the immediate postoperative period. Epithelial edema in the face of a compact stroma immediately after surgery is likely due to which of the following?
    a. prolonged surgery.
    b. inflammation.
    c. small retained nuclear fragments in the angle.
    d. elevated IOP with an intact endothelium.

129. Epithelial downgrowth is a rare complication of intraocular surgery, occurring less frequently with modern cataract surgery techniques. How should diagnosis be confirmed?
    a. surgical sampling of membrane.
    b. anterior segment OCT.
    c. ultrasound biomicroscopy.
    d. Argon laser application to demonstrate white burn formation.

130. A 77-year-old female presents 12 hours after cataract surgery with pain, redness, and photophobia in the operated eye. On exam she is found to have 20/400 vision with marked anterior chamber reaction and trace hypopyon. Which detail in the history above favors a diagnosis of Toxic Anterior Segment Syndrome (TASS) over infectious endophthalmitis?
    a. the age of the patient.
    b. the timing of the findings.
    c. the level of vision.
    d. the amount of anterior chamber reaction.

131. During cataract surgery, the surgeon notices that the patient's pupil dilates poorly and undulates in response to intraocular irrigation. What medication is this patient likely on?
    a. tamoxifen.
    b. tamsulosin.
    c. tacrolimus.
    d. flonase.

132. Which is not recommended in the event of posterior capsular rupture during cataract surgery?
    a. anterior vitrectomy to avoid vitreous prolapse.
    b. insertion of IOL when safe and indicated.
    c. careful removal of fragments that are not visible.
    d. watertight closure of incisions.

133. Which of the following lenses has the lowest likelihood of posterior capsular opacification (PCO)?
    a. silicone lens with round edge.
    b. silicone lens with square edge.
    c. acrylic lens with round edge.
    d. acrylic lens with square edge.

134. A patient with history significant for deep vein thrombosis is brought to the operating room in preparation for cataract surgery. A retrobulbar injection is performed, and soon after the injection the orbit is taut with marked proptosis, elevated IOP, and significant ecchymosis of the lids and conjunctiva. What is the most likely complication of the retrobulbar injection at this time?
    a. globe penetration.
    b. retrobulbar hemorrhage.
    c. inadvertent intradural injection.
    d. inadvertent intravenous injection.

135. In the patient described in question 134, which of the following is not considered a potential maneuver to counteract the complication described?
    a. topical IOP lowering agents.
    b. anterior chamber paracentesis.
    c. lateral canthotomy and cantholysis.
    d. extracapsular cataract extraction.

136. Which of the following is not a risk factor for the development of suprachoroidal hemorrhage during cataract surgery?
    a. hyperopia.
    b. hypertension.
    c. glaucoma.
    d. chronic intraocular inflammation.

137. A 75-year-old gentleman presents with pain, photophobia, and worsening vision 3 days after uneventful cataract surgery. His vision is found to be light perception and clinical findings as depicted in the image below. Which of the following is indicated for this patient?
    a. management with topical antibiotics and steroids.
    b. systemic fourth generation fluoroquinolones.
    c. vitreous tap with injection of intravitreal antibiotics.
    d. pars plana vitrectomy with intravitreal antibiotics.

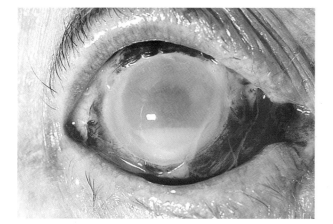

138. The crystalline lens is derived from which embryonic tissue?
    a. ectoderm.
    b. endoderm.
    c. mesoderm.
    d. neural crest.

139. A patient presents after filtering surgery with a large filtering bleb and a shallow anterior chamber. Which of the following is the most likely diagnosis?
    a. bleb leak.
    b. overfiltration.
    c. pupillary block.
    d. aqueous misdirection.

140. Which of the following organisms is the most common cause of bleb-associated endophthalmitis?
    a. *Bacillus cereus*.
    b. *Streptococcus* species.
    c. Coagulase negative *Staphylococcus*.
    d. *Haemophilus influenzae*.

8

■ Answers

1. c. The Goldmann equation summarizes the relationship between many of these factors and the intraocular pressure (IOP) in the undisturbed eye:

$$P_o = (F / C) + P_v$$

where P_0 is the IOP in millimeters of mercury (mm Hg), F is the rate of aqueous formation in microliters per minute (μL/min), C is the facility of outflow in microliters per minute per millimeter of mercury (μL/min/mm Hg), and P_v is the episcleral venous pressure in millimeters of mercury. Resistance to outflow (R) is the inverse of facility (C).

2. b. While intraocular pressure is one of the primary risk factors for glaucoma, its presence or absence does not have a role in the definition of the disease.

3. a. The estimated prevalence of POAG in the United States in individuals older than 40 years is 1.86%. This translates to nearly 2.22 million Americans affected in the year 2000. Three to five percent have become bilaterally blind. The number of POAG patients is estimated to increase by 50% to 3.36 million in 2020. This number may be an underestimate, since visual field loss is required in the definition of POAG, and many individuals have glaucoma without documented visual field loss. POAG is the most frequent cause of nonreversible blindness in African Americans.

4. a. Among whites aged 40 years and older, a prevalence of between 1.1% and 2.1% has been reported based on population-based studies performed throughout the world. The prevalence among blacks is three to four times higher, with at least four times the likelihood of blindness. This racial disparity increases with age, with the likelihood of blindness from POAG increasing to 15 times higher for blacks in the age group 46 to 65 years. Blacks have larger discs and more nerve

fibers; it has been hypothesized that the increased disc size is associated with increased mechanical strain in the region of the optic nerve.

5. d. Besides increased IOP, factors known to be associated with an increased risk for the development of glaucoma include advanced age, decreased corneal thickness, racial background, and a positive family history.

6. d. Current evidence suggests that peak IOP occurs during the night and is therefore, not caught on routine diurnal testing. The nocturnal rise may be due to variations in body position, and it has been suggested that measurement of supine IOP during office visits may approximate this nocturnal peak.

7. c. Women are at higher risk, likely due to shallower anterior chambers when compared to men. The anterior chamber decreases in depth and volume with age, which predisposes to pupillary block. Anterior chamber depth and volume are smaller in hyperopic eyes. Although PACG may occur in eyes with any type of refractive error, it is typically associated with hyperopia. Some of the anatomic features of the eye that predispose to pupillary block, such as more forward position of the lens and greater than average lens thickness, are inherited. Thus, relatives of subjects with angle-closure glaucoma are at greater risk of developing angle closure than is the general population.

8. d. Exfoliation syndrome is associated with the LOXL1 gene. The glaucoma associated with GLC1D resembles high-pressure POAG. The other associations are correct.

9. a. This form of the disease is characterized by markedly elevated pressures, often greater than 40 mm Hg, and poor response to medication. Other cloned genes known to be associated with glaucoma include PAX6 (11p13, aniridia), CYP1B1 (2p21, congenital glaucoma), PITX2 (4q25, Axenfeld-Rieger syndrome), LMX1B (9q34, glaucoma associated with nail-patella syndrome).

10. **b.** Aqueous humor is produced in the posterior chamber and flows through the pupil into the anterior chamber. Aqueous exits the eye by passing through the trabecular meshwork and into Schlemm's canal before draining into the venous system through a plexus of collector channels, as well as through the uveoscleral pathway, which is proposed to exit through the root of the iris and the ciliary muscle, into the suprachoroidal spaces and through the sclera. The inner nonpigmented epithelial cells, which protrude into the posterior chamber, contain numerous mitochondria and microvilli; these cells are thought to be the actual site of aqueous production.

11. **a.** Active secretion, or transport, consumes energy to move substances against an electro-chemical gradient and is *independent* of pressure; it accounts for the majority of aqueous production and involves, at least in part, activity of the enzyme carbonic anhydrase II. Ultrafiltration refers to a *pressure-dependent* movement along a pressure gradient. In the ciliary processes, the hydrostatic pressure difference between capillary pressure and IOP favors fluid movement into the eye, whereas the oncotic gradient between the two resists fluid movement. Diffusion is the passive movement of ions across a membrane related to charge and concentration.

12. **d.** Aqueous humor has an excess of hydrogen and chloride ions, an excess of ascorbate, and a deficit of bicarbonate relative to plasma.

13. **c.** Aqueous humor production may decrease following trauma or intraocular inflammation and following the administration of certain drugs, such as general anesthetics and some systemic hypotensive agents. Ketamine is a general anesthetic that is associated with a rise in intraocular pressure. Carotid occlusive disease may also decrease aqueous humor production.

14. **a.** Uveoscleral outflow, not trabecular outflow, is increased by cycloplegia. Trabecular outflow is increased by miotics.

15. **c.** Estimates of this value vary significantly. Most widely accepted estimates range from 15% to 20% with some being as low as 10%, and some as high as 50%. Uveoscleral outflow is pressure-independent.

16. **c.** Outflow facility in normal eyes ranges from 0.22 to 0.28 μL/min/mm Hg, and decreases with age, ocular surgery, and trauma. Glaucoma patients often have decreased outflow facility.

17. **c.** Episcleral venous pressure changes are associated with alterations in body position and with certain diseases of the orbit, the head, and the neck that obstruct venous return to the heart or shunt blood from the arterial to the venous system. The usual range of values is 8 to 10 mm Hg. In acute conditions, according to the Goldmann equation, IOP rises approximately 1 mm Hg for every 1 mm Hg increase in episcleral venous pressure. The relationship is more complex and less well understood, however, in chronic conditions. Chronic elevations of episcleral venous pressure may be accompanied by changes in IOP that are of greater or less magnitude than predicted by the Goldmann equation.

18. **b.** Data from these studies demonstrated a mean IOP of 16 mm Hg, with a standard deviation of 3 mm Hg. IOP had a non-Gaussian distribution with a skew toward higher pressures, especially in individuals older than age 40.

19. **c.** Elevation of IOP is still seen as an important risk factor for the development of glaucoma. Although other risk factors affect an individual's susceptibility to glaucomatous damage, IOP is the only one that can be effectively altered. IOP can vary with time of day, heartbeat, respiration, exercise, fluid intake, systemic medication, and topical medications.

8

20. **b.** The Goldmann applanation tonometer measures the force necessary to flatten an area of the cornea of 3.06 mm diameter. An excessive amount of fluorescein results in wide mires and an inaccurately high reading. Measurements are most accurate with a central corneal thickness of 520 μm; however, the accepted range of normal is between 537 and 554 μm. Increased corneal thickness may give an artificially high IOP measurement; decreased corneal thickness, an artificially low reading. Corneal edema predisposes to inaccurate low readings, whereas pressure measurements taken over a corneal scar will be falsely high.

21. **d.** The last statement is false. OHTS included patients with IOP 24 to 32 mm Hg and randomized patients to observation or to the reduction of IOP by at least 20% by topical medications. 4.4% of patients that were treated progressed to optic nerve or visual field loss during a 5-year period. More than twice as many of the untreated observation group (9.5%) progressed.

22. **a.** A 5-minute soak of 70% isopropyl alcohol should be used.

23. **c.** Direct gonioscopy is performed with a binocular microscope, a fiber-optic illuminator or slit-pen light, and a direct goniolens, such as the Koeppe, Barkan, Wurst, Swan-Jacob, or Richardson lens. Indirect gonioscopy is more frequently used and utilizes Posner, Sussman, Zeiss, and Goldmann-type lenses.

24. **a.** The Posner, Sussman, and Zeiss lenses have a smaller area of contact than the Goldmann lens and about the same radius of curvature; pressure on the cornea may falsely open the angle with the first three lenses while narrowing the angle with the Goldmann-type lenses.

25. **b.** Koeppe gonioscopy is considered best for evaluating a patient with potential angle recession because this system allows easier comparison of one eye with the fellow eye, or one portion of the angle with another.

26. **d.** Grade IV describes a 45° angle between the surface of the trabecular meshwork and the iris while grade I describes a 10° angle. Thus, a grade IV angle is less likely to undergo spontaneous closure.

27. **b.** The criteria include an increased prominence of the scleral spur. Other findings on gonioscopy may include microhyphema, hypopyon, retained foreign body, iridodialysis, precipitates, pigmentation of lens equator, IOL haptics, ciliary body tumors.

28. **a.** The adult optic nerve consists of 1.2 to 1.5 million axons that have cell bodies located in the ganglion cell layer. The optic nerve head is 1.5 mm in diameter, and expands to 3 to 4 mm upon exiting the globe as the fibers become myelinated.

29. **c.** The fenestrations within the lamina are larger superiorly and inferiorly as compared with the temporal and nasal aspects of the optic nerve. It is possible that these differences play a role in the development of glaucoma.

30. **d.** The first two statements are true for the short posterior ciliary arteries, not the long posterior ciliary arteries. The central retinal artery penetrates the optic nerve at 10 to 15 mm behind the globe.

31. **d.** The prelaminar and laminar regions have similar blood supplies. The retrolaminar region is supplied by the short posterior ciliary arteries as well as the pial arterial branches coursing adjacent to the retrolaminar optic nerve region.

32. **c.** Two hypotheses have emerged to explain the development of glaucomatous optic neuropathy, the mechanical and ischemic theories. The mechanical theory stresses the importance of direct compression of the axonal fibers, distortion of the lamina cribrosa plates, and interruption of axoplasmic flow, resulting in the death of the RGCs. The ischemic theory focuses on intraneural ischemia resulting from decreased optic nerve

8

perfusion. This perfusion may result from the stress of IOP on the blood supply to the nerve or from processes intrinsic to the optic nerve.

33. **b.** Five percent of normal individuals will have cup–disc ratios of greater than 0.6.

34. **a.** Less than 1% of normal individuals have an asymmetry of >0.2.

35. **b.** A convention referred to as the ISNT rule may be useful in identifying thinning of the neuroretinal rim. In general, the Inferior neuroretinal rim is the thickest, followed by the Superior rim, the Nasal rim, and finally the Temporal rim. If the rim widths do not follow this progression, there should be increased concern for the presence of focal loss of rim tissue.

36. **b.** Disc hemorrhages may occur in as many as one-third of glaucoma patients at some time during the course of their disease. Individuals with normal-tension glaucoma are more likely to have disc hemorrhages. Optic disc hemorrhage is an important prognostic sign for the development or progression of visual field loss, and any patient with a splinter hemorrhage requires detailed evaluation and follow-up. These hemorrhages are not pathognomonic as they may be caused by posterior vitreous detachments, diabetes mellitus, branch retinal vein occlusions, and anticoagulation therapy.

37. **d.** Frequency-doubling technology (FDT) is believed to activate M cells.

38. **d.** Normally the superior field is depressed 1 to 2 dB compared with the inferior field.

39. **d.** If a patient has glaucomatous visual field–type defects, corresponding optic nerve head abnormalities should exist. Otherwise, alternative etiologies should be considered. In static perimetry, the stimulus is of variable intensity and is kept stationary (static) until it is noticed by the patient. Baring of the blind spot and generalized

constriction are not very specific and can be produced by miosis, uncorrected refractive error, aging, and cataract.

40. **d.** Areas of retina and/or optic nerve damaged by glaucoma are believed to be more vulnerable to ongoing damage at lower IOPs. Thus, field defects tend to become more severe with time. New defects also may appear, of course, but generally accompany progression of previous defects.

41. **a.** Split fixation is the presence of visual field loss that comes close to fixation. A typical pattern of progression is (a) loss near fixation (paracentral scotoma) to (b) split fixation to (c) loss of fixation. Thus, the eye at greatest risk is not one with a 5° central field but one with split-fixation in the horizontal meridian.

42. **c.** Other neurologic etiologies of field loss should be explored when the patient's optic disc seems less cupped than would be expected for the degree of visual field loss; pallor of the disc is more impressive than cupping; progression of field loss seems excessive; pattern of field loss respects the vertical midline; and location of cupping or thinning does not correspond to proper location of field defect.

43. **b.** Several studies have indicated that as many as 30% to 50% of individuals in the general population who have glaucomatous optic neuropathy and/or visual field loss have initial screening IOPs below 22 mm Hg.

44. **c.** OHTS subjects had thicker corneas than the general population, with black subjects having thinner corneas than white subjects.

45. **b.** At 6 years, 62% of untreated patients showed progression, whereas 45% of treated patients progressed. Treatment reduced IOP by 25%. Risk factors for progression included no treatment, age, higher IOP, exfoliation, more severe visual field defect, and bilateral glaucoma. In multivariate analyses, progression risk was halved

8

by treatment. Progression risk decreased by 10% with each mm HG of IOP reduction from baseline to the first follow-up visit.

46. **d.** Early visual loss was greater in the surgically treated group, but after 5 years both groups had similar visual field outcomes. IOP reduction in the medical group averaged 17 to 18 mm Hg, whereas that in the surgically managed group was 14 to 15 mm Hg.

47. **a.** Visual field defects in normal-tension glaucoma tend to be more focal, deeper, and closer to fixation compared with those commonly seen in normal-tension glaucoma. When compared to those with POAG, the neuroretinal rim has been reported to be thinner, especially inferiorly and inferotemporally. CNTGS found that lowering IOP by 30% reduced the rate of visual field progression from 35% to 12% in subjects with normal-tension glaucoma.

48. **c.** Given the extent of the glaucomatous damage as indicated by split fixation and progression of both fields and disc at low-normal pressures, the maximal decrease in IOP is necessary. Primary filtration presents the best choice. Iridoplasty is usually reserved for eyes with plateau iris syndrome (or, sometimes angle closure). Peripheral iridectomy would not be appropriate because the angles appear normal, and the likelihood of excellent pressure control after combined procedure is not high enough. Cyclocryotherapy and cyclophotocoagulation are reserved for end-stage disease.

49. **a.** (see explanation for answer 50).

50. **d.** This patient has pseudoexfoliation syndrome, which is characterized by the deposition of fibrillar material in the anterior segment of the eye. The trabecular meshwork is often heavily pigmented with inferior pigmented deposition referred to as the Sampaolesi's line. On gonioscopy, the angle can be narrow, most likely the result of anterior movement of the lens–iris diaphragm related to zonular weakness.

On retroillumination, transillumination defects are seen at the pupillary margin. These patients dilate poorly and are predisposed to zonular dehiscence and complications during and after cataract surgery. Lens extraction does not alleviate the condition, and these patients often have increased ocular inflammation after any ocular surgery.

51. **c.** In pseudoexfoliation, fibrillar material is deposited in the anterior segment of the eye. Patients with this glaucoma are often resistant to medical therapy, but laser trabeculoplasty is often very effective. Pseudoexfoliation with glaucoma also differs from POAG in that it is often monocular or asymmetric and has greater pigmentation of the trabecular meshwork, as well as pigment deposited anterior to Schwalbe's line (Sampaolesi's line). There is considerable overlap in the age range of patients affected by each disorder.

52. **c.** Phacolytic glaucoma results when mature or hypermature cataracts leak high molecular weight proteins through microscopic defects in the capsule. A resultant macrophage response clogs the trabecular meshwork. Although medication is used for short-term IOP control, definitive therapy requires cataract extraction. Other lens-induced conditions may respond to topical steroid. Lens particle glaucoma occurs when lens cortex material deposits along the TM and can be seen after cataract surgery. Medical therapy to lower IOP and reduce inflammation can help.

53. **c.** (see explanation for answer 54).

54. **d.** This patient has signs of pigment dispersion syndrome. The syndrome does not universally lead to glaucoma as the risk is approximately 25% to 50%. Glaucoma associated with these findings occurs most commonly in young (20–50 years of age) white males who have high myopia. Affected females tend to be older than affected males. The presence of a Krukenberg's spindle is not necessary to make the diagnosis. Filtering surgery is usually successful; however, extra

care is warranted, because young patients with myopia may be at increased risk of hypotony maculopathy.

55. **b.** This is phacolytic glaucoma, an inflammatory glaucoma caused by leakage of lens protein through microscopic openings in the capsule of a mature or hypermature cataract. The lack of keratic precipitates helps distinguish phacolytic glaucoma from phacoantigenic glaucoma. Definitive therapy requires cataract extraction.

56. **a.** The most common cause of glaucoma in primary or metastatic tumors of the ciliary body is direct invasion of the anterior chamber angle.

57. **b.** The etiology of glaucomatocyclitic crisis, or Posner-Schlossman syndrome, remains unknown. There is no evidence that chronic suppressive therapy with topical nonsteroidal anti-inflammatory agents or mild steroids is effective in preventing attacks.

58. **a.** Fifteen percent of patients with Fuchs heterochromic iridocyclitis will have secondary open-angle glaucoma.

59. **b.** Medications that reduce aqueous humor formation are more effective than drugs that increase trabecular aqueous outflow. Prostaglandin analogs may be effective in some patients. Laser trabeculoplasty is not effective unless there are secondary changes in the outflow channels. Glaucoma filtering surgery may be complicated by a ciliochoroidal effusion or a suprachoroidal hemorrhage.

60. **b.** Adrenergic agonists with significant α1-agonist effects (apraclonidine, dipivefrin, epinephrine) should also be avoided in sickle cell disease because of concerns regarding anterior segment vasoconstriction.

61. **b.** Ghost cells develop within 1 to 3 months of a vitreous hemorrhage. While medical therapy is the preferred initial approach, these patients may require anterior chamber irrigation, pars plana

vitrectomy, and/or trabeculectomy to control the condition.

62. **d.** It has been suggested that a chronic rhegmatogenous retinal detachment leads to the liberation of photoreceptor outer segments, which, migrating through the retinal tear, reach the anterior chamber and impede aqueous outflow through the trabecular meshwork.

63. **d.** A small corneal diameter and radius of curvature are factors that predispose to primary angle closure.

64. **d.** This is a patient with an acute angle closure attack. Anterior chamber depth of <2.5 mm predisposes patients to primary angle closure. Retinal vascular occlusion may occur as a result of increased intraocular pressure.

65. **c.** The definitive treatment for acute angle closure is an iridectomy, laser or surgical. In this patient, it may be best to first lower the intraocular pressure (IOP) using agents such as β-adrenergic antagonists; α2-adrenergic agonists; prostaglandin analogs; and oral, topical, or intravenous carbonic anhydrase inhibitors. Miotics do not tend to work when IOP is elevated above 40 to 50 mm Hg, but can be helpful once IOP has been lowered beyond this threshold.

66. **c.** An untreated fellow eye in a patient who has had an acute angle-closure attack has a 40% to 80% chance of developing an acute attack of angle closure over the next 5 to 10 years.

67. **d.** Both mydriatics and miotics can precipitate angle-closure in eyes with shallow anterior chambers. This is true for both topical medications and systemic drugs that affect the pupil. Examples include antihistamines, which can have anticholinergic activity.

68. **a.** Angle-closure develops in only a small number of patients with narrow anterior chambers. A number of provocative tests exist to attempt

8

to cause angle closure in susceptible patients. Perhaps the most predictive is the prone–dark room test. IOP is measured before and after 30 to 60 minutes of total dark adaptation attained with the patient prone. Dark will induce pupillary dilation, and prone positioning will move the lens forward. Both tend to increase pupillary block. None of these tests, however, has been evaluated in a prospective study.

69. c. The patient with very narrow angles and elevated pressure may have "mixed mechanism" glaucoma with partial angle closure due to pupillary block superimposed on open-angle glaucoma. To determine if an angle-closure component is present, the effect of minimizing pupillary block on IOP must be determined. Cholinergic miotics (pilocarpine) will cause miosis and lessen pupillary block but also will exert traction on the trabecular meshwork and lower IOP by this unrelated mechanism. Thymoxamine, a selective alpha-adrenergic antagonist, causes miosis and lessens pupillary block, without affecting outflow facility. A decrease in pressure after thymoxamine (lessened pupillary block) implies partial angle closure, and iridotomy is indicated. No change in IOP after thymoxamine-induced miosis implies that an iridotomy may not be helpful.

70. d. A small anterior segment is not associated with plateau iris.

71. a. Angle closure in plateau iris is most often caused by anteriorly positioned ciliary processes that critically narrow the anterior chamber recess by pushing the peripheral iris forward. A component of pupillary block is often present. Plateau iris may be suspected if the central anterior chamber appears to be of normal depth and the iris plane appears to be rather flat for an eye with angle closure. Plateau iris should be considered in younger patients with myopia.

72. c. Anterior displacement of the ciliary processes pushes the peripheral iris forward, which subsequently narrows the anterior chamber and blocks the trabecular meshwork. This has been confirmed with anterior segment ultrasonography. Patients who have plateau iris syndrome (e.g., resistant to laser peripheral iridotomy) should be treated with long-term miotics and possibly iridoplasty.

73. b. Treatment with cycloplegia may tighten the zonule, flatten the lens, and pull it posteriorly, breaking the pupillary block. Miotics may make the condition worse by increasing the pupillary block and by rotating the ciliary body forward, loosening the zonule and allowing the lens to become more globular. Microspherophakia is often familial and may occur as an isolated condition or as part of either Weill-Marchesani or Marfan's syndrome.

74. b. While anti-VEGF therapy has become more widely used, the treatment of choice is still considered panretinal photocoagulation.

75. b. Choroidal detachment can present with shallow or flat anterior chamber, but the IOP is typically low. All of the other choices can present with high IOP.

76. c. Ultrasound is a critical step in evaluation of this patient. If no posterior pathology is found, then aqueous misdirection is suspected, especially in the setting of a patent iridotomy. Atropine and phenylephrine can help break the attack, along with IOP lowering agents. If these measures fail, then surgical options can be explored. These include YAG laser disruption of the anterior hyaloids face, vitrectomy, lensectomy, or ALT of the ciliary processes.

77. d. Fibrous ingrowth is more prevalent than epithelial downgrowth. Argon laser gives the characteristic white burns on the epithelial membrane surface, not YAG. Medication is the preferred treatment of the secondary glaucomas that present without a pupillary block mechanism, although surgical intervention may be required.

78. c. See answer 80 for explanation.

79. d. See answer 80 for explanation.

80. a. This patient likely started topiramate (Topamax) <1 month ago. She is experiencing an idiosyncratic reaction in which bilateral acute myopia (>6 D), bilateral ocular pain, headache, and bilateral angle-closure glaucoma can occur. The underlying mechanism is ciliochoroidal effusion, which causes relaxation of the zonules and anterior displacement of the lens-iris complex. Aggressive cycloplegia may relieve the attack and the secondary angle-closure glaucoma usually resolves within 24 to 48 hours with medical treatment. The myopia takes longer to resolve, often times up to 2 weeks. A PI is not indicated because pupillary block is not the underlying mechanism of angle-closure in these patients.

81. b. A child that presents with a large eye, or buphthalmos, and tearing has congenital glaucoma until proven otherwise. Other signs and symptoms of this condition include corneal edema, increased IOP, increased cup:disc ratio, photophobia, and blepharospasm. An exam under anesthesia should be performed if enough information cannot be obtained in a clinic setting. This condition can be mistaken for nasolacrimal duct obstruction because tearing is often the only presenting symptom.

82. c. While medications can be used to control IOP in children for a short period of time, they are not recommended for long-term IOP control. Surgical management is preferred in these patients. If the cornea is clear, both goniotomy and trabeculotomy ab externo are viable surgical options with comparable success rates. In a patient with a hazy cornea, however, goniotomy is difficult to perform and trabeculotomy ab externo is the preferred surgical option. Trabeculectomy and shunt procedures are reserved for patients in whom prior surgical options have failed.

83. a. α2-Adrenergic agents should be avoided in children <3 years because of the risk of apnea and other CNS adverse effects. β-Adrenergic antagonists can be used but parents should be alert for apnea, hypotension, and cough (which may be a sign of reactive airway disease exacerbation). Carbonic anhydrase inhibitors (CAIs) may be used, but children require assessment for possible acidosis, hypokalemia, and feeding problems if given oral CAIs. Topical CAIs are relatively safe.

84. c. While elevated episcleral venous pressure plays a role in the glaucoma of Sturge-Weber syndrome, it often is implicated after the first decade of life. In infants, it is the angle anomalies that play the largest role in elevated IOP.

85. d. The principle ocular finding in NF2 is posterior subcapsular cataract. NF2 is not associated with glaucoma.

86. c. Brimonidine decreases aqueous production and increases uveoscleral outflow.

87. d. Dorzolamide can cause induced myopia, blurred vision, stinging, keratitis, conjunctivitis, and dermatitis.

88. c. Brimonidine can lead to hypotension, not hypertension.

89. d. Echothiophate iodide can cause increased salivation, secretions, and gastrointestinal cramping. Other ophthalmologic side effects include iris cysts and punctual stenosis.

90. a. Brimonidine is considered a class B agent during pregnancy, although use of this agent should be avoided in nursing mothers because of the effects on infants.

91. b. Caution must be exercised in the use of carbonic anhydrase inhibitors for small children because of their susceptibility to weight loss, lethargy, and metabolic acidosis.

92. c. Epinephrine has a well-established tendency to provoke irritation and allergic responses. More than one-fifth of patients will eventually experience an adverse local reaction with prolonged use.

8

93. **d.** Direct-acting miotics interact directly with the acetylcholine receptor, whereas indirect-acting agents increase the activity of native acetylcholine at the synaptic junction (by blocking its enzymatic degradation). Pilocarpine is a purely direct agent, whereas carbachol is felt to exhibit both direct and indirect effects.

The only commercially available purely indirect parasympathomimetic currently is demecarium. Indirect parasympathomimetics can also be used against eyelid lice infestations because of their potent insecticidal effects.

94. **b.** Indirect agents, along with the strongest direct agents, tend to have the most pronounced systemic and ocular side effects. Bradycardia is never seen with any of the miotics.

95. **a.** Changes in urine pH secondary to carbonic anhydrase inhibitors can predispose a patient to calcium oxalate and calcium phosphate nephrolithiasis. Aplastic anemia is a rare, but potentially lethal side effect related to the sulfa derivation of the drugs. Gastrointestinal distress occurs, but not most commonly. Hypokalemia may occur as a result of the effects on renal ion transport, but hypocalcemia is not seen. Paresthesias are reported by most patients taking these potent agents.

96. **b.** High IOP secondary to angle closure may be causing severe eye pain and decreased visual acuity. Hypotony (wound leak, cyclodialysis) could precipitate painful choroidal hemorrhage.

97. **b.** Because pupillary block is probably present, an iridotomy should be performed. Miotics tend to increase postoperative inflammation and should be avoided here.

98. **c.** Failure to relieve postoperative angle closure with iridotomy suggests malignant glaucoma, which often responds to potent cycloplegics. If medical management fails, laser treatment to open the anterior hyaloid face, or even pars plana vitrectomy, is necessary.

99. **b.** Usually, one half of the circumference, or 180°, of the trabecular meshwork is treated during an initial laser trabeculoplasty.

100. **a.** Argon laser trabeculoplasty (ALT) uses a 50 μm beam with variable power to produce blanching or a tiny bubble at the anterior pigmented edge of the TM. This requires 180° of treatment, rather than 360°. Outflow facility typically improves following successful ALT.

101. **b.** When effective, laser trabeculoplasty is expected to lower IOP 20% to 25%.

102. **d.** Laser trabeculoplasty is contraindicated in patients with inflammatory glaucoma, iridocorneal endothelial (ICE) syndrome, neovascular glaucoma, and synechial angle closure.

103. **d.** Up to 20% of patients undergoing laser trabeculoplasty can have a transient rise in IOP, sometimes reaching up to 50 to 60 mm Hg. Topical apraclonidine 1% or brimonidine 0.2% has been shown to blunt postoperative IOP elevation.

104. **b.** The glaucoma associated with ICE syndrome is often worse than predicted by the extent of synechiae, likely due to clinically undetectable endothelialization of the angle.

105. **c.** The constellation of heterochromia iridis (compare the two images carefully), gelatinous–stellate keratic precipitates, mild anterior chamber reaction, distinctive rubeosis, and ipsilateral cataract and glaucoma is nearly pathognomonic for Fuchs' heterochromatic iridocyclitis. If inflammation is severe, another diagnosis should be considered. The iris atrophy in Fuchs' is generally diffuse and stromal, whereas that of herpes zoster iritis is typically sectoral with pigment epithelial involvement. The rubeosis is distinctive because the vessels are typically quite fine and rarely induce synechiae or angle closure. The vessels are also quite fragile and spontaneous or iatrogenic hyphema (as the

paracentesis is performed at filtration surgery) is a classic sign. The mechanism for the glaucoma is poorly understood. Cataract surgery is usually indicated for visual rehabilitation; it has little or no effect on the glaucoma. In fact, in many patients, IOP does not increase for many months or years after cataract extraction.

106. d. Assuming the left angle is normal, this patient can be diagnosed with angle recession (posttraumatic) glaucoma affecting the right eye. Because men are victims of ocular trauma far more frequently than women, this glaucoma is more common in men. The lifetime risk for developing glaucoma seems to be correlated with the amount of angle recession and is estimated to be approximately 10% in patients with 180° of involved angle. Iris sphincter tears, Vossius' ring, and posterior subcapsular cataract all may be seen in conjunction with the disorder. Retinal dialysis must be ruled out in the posttraumatic period by a dilated retinal examination with 360° scleral depression. Although the disorder may be bilateral if the contralateral eye is traumatized, it is much more commonly unilateral.

107. c. Typically, the surgeon should fastidiously avoid contact between the MMC-containing sponge and the wound edges to reduce the risk of postoperative wound leaks and hypotony. This is one of the main reasons why most MMC filters are performed with a limbus-based flap. MMC is associated with a lower incidence of hypotony and corneal-surface disorders than 5-FU.

108. a. Young age is a risk factor for bleb-related endophthalmitis. In addition, contact lens use and chronic bleb leak are also risk factors.

109. a. The lens increases in thickness and curvature and has a decreased index of refraction with age. The eye may become more hyperopic or myopic with age depending on the balance of these changes.

110. d. The lens capsule is made up of type IV collagen.

111. a. The lens capsule is thinnest at the posterior pole.

112. c. Aldose reductase is the key enzyme in the sorbitol pathway. When glucose increases in the lens, as in hyperglycemic states, the sorbitol pathway is activated relatively more than glycolysis. Sorbitol accumulates and is retained in the lens.

113. a. This is the process of accommodation. When the ciliary muscle contracts, the axial thickness of the lens increases, diameter decreases, and dioptric power increases.

114. a. Alport's syndrome is usually X-linked, but can be autosomal recessive. In addition to anterior lenticonus, it is associated with renal failure, deafness, cataract, and fleck retinopathy.

115. b. They may be associated with colobomas of the uvea as well.

116. c. In addition to this finding, patients can display adhesions between lens and cornea, anterior cortical or polar cataract, and microspherophakia.

117. b. Approximately one-third of congenital cataracts are a component of a more extensive syndrome or disease, one-third occur as an isolated inherited trait, and one-third result from undetermined causes.

118. a. Lamellar cataracts are the most common type of congenital and infantile cataracts.

119. b. The lens changes are often characterized by pearly white nuclear opacifications. After cataract surgery, there is often excessive inflammation from the release of live virus particles. Both glaucoma and cataract are not usually present simultaneously in the same eye, which likely has to do with timing of the exposure and maternal infection.

120. d. Mittendorf's dot is a remnant of the posterior tunica vasculosa lentis and results in a white

8

dot inferonasally on the posterior capsule of the lens. It is meaningless visually.

121. **d.** This is a posterior subcapsular cataract. Choice "a" describes nuclear cataracts. Choice "b" is a cortical cataract.

122. **c.** Phenothiazines can cause pigmented deposits in the anterior lens epithelium in an axial configuration. Miotics can lead to small vacuoles within and posterior to the anterior lens capsule and epithelium that can progress to posterior cortical and nuclear lens changes. Long-term human studies demonstrated that statins do not increase cataract risk and may actually reduce the risk of nuclear cataracts by 50% over 5 years. Amiodarone, in addition to cataracts, can cause deposits in the cornea and optic neuropathy.

123. **a.** The characteristic lens changes and systemic findings point to galactosemia. This is an inherited autosomal recessive inability to convert galactose to glucose. The disease is fatal if untreated and can present within the first few weeks of life with cataracts, malnutrition, hepatomegaly, jaundice, and mental deficiency. Diagnosis can be confirmed by demonstration of galactose in the urine.

124. **a.** (See answer 126 for explanation)

125. **d.** (See answer 126 for explanation)

126. **b.** This is phacoantigenic (or phacoanaphylactic) uveitis that occurs days to weeks after a large amount of lens protein is released through a ruptured lens capsule. A granulomatous response ensues and is difficult to control until the lens is removed. Phacolytic glaucoma occurs as a complication of a mature or hypermature cataract in which lens proteins leak through an intact but permeable lens capsule. The trabecular meshwork can become clogged with lens particles and engorged macrophages in this condition. Phacomorphic glaucoma occurs when an intumescent cataract causes pupillary block and induces a secondary angle-closure glaucoma.

127. **c.** The decision to operate is not based solely on a specific level of reduced acuity.

128. **d.** Decreasing IOP via aqueous release from paracentesis site often results in immediate resolution of edema.

129. **d.** Argon laser burns applied to the membrane or iris surface will appear white if epithelial cells are present.

130. **b.** TASS presents within 12 to 24 hours, whereas acute infectious endophthalmitis typically develops 2 to 7 days after surgery.

131. **b.** Tamsulosin, or Flomax, can be associated with intraoperative floppy iris syndrome (IFIS). It is used for the treatment of benign prostatic hypertrophy.

132. **c.** It is recommended that only removal of fragments that are visible and easily accessible be attempted. Referral for prompt vitreoretinal consultation is also indicated.

133. **d.** PCO formation is influenced by lens material (PMMA > silicone > acrylic) and edge design (round > square). Pooled data has found the overall PCO rate at 5 years to be 28%.

134. **b.** (See answer 135 for explanation)

135. **d.** Treatment of retrobulbar hemorrhage is targeted at lowering intraocular pressure as quickly as possible. Cataract surgery should not be performed when a serious hemorrhage has occurred as the risk of iris prolapse and expulsive choroidal hemorrhage increases. The patient's medical history must always be considered as this patient had a history of thrombosis for which he was anticoagulated, increasing his risk for retrobulbar hemorrhage.

8

136. a. Suprachoroidal hemorrhage is more common in patients with hypertension, tachycardia, obesity, high myopia, anticoagulation, glaucoma, advanced age, and chronic ocular inflammation.

137. d. This patient has acute postoperative endophthalmitis. The Endophthalmitis Vitrectomy Study (EVS) demonstrated that for with HM or better vision, vitrectomy and vitreous tap/inject were equally beneficial. For patients with LP or worse vision, vitrectomy was found to be better than vitreous tap/inject.

138. a. The crystalline lens is derived from ectoderm.

139. b. A bleb leak would cause a flat bleb. Pupillary block and aqueous misdirection would not change the size of the bleb.

140. b. Streptococcus species account for about half of all bleb-associated endophthalmitis, followed by coagulase negative *Staphylococcus* and *Haemophilus influenzae*.

8

CHAPTER 9

Cornea, External Disease, and Refractive Surgery

▌ Questions

1. A 29-year-old contact lens wearer presents with pain, photophobia, decreased vision, and clinical findings as indicated in the below photograph. Which clinical feature is nearly universal in this disease process?
   a. tearing.
   b. hypopyon.
   c. severe pain.
   d. ring infiltrate.

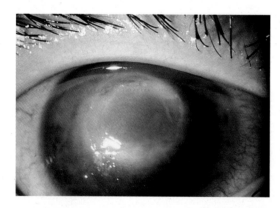

2. With regard to the patient in question 1, which of the following is least likely to be discovered in this patient's history?
   a. use of homemade contact lens solution.
   b. recent camping trip and exposure to open freshwater and soil.
   c. significant suppuration early in the disease course.
   d. recent treatment with topical antiviral and steroid.

3. Which of the following is TRUE regarding the condition in question 1?
   a. Epithelial dendrites may be found.
   b. Stromal infiltration should be primarily managed by debridement.
   c. Primary infection usually occurs on skin and mucosal tissues innervated by the trigeminal nerve.
   d. Gram-negative rods are seen on smears obtained by corneal scraping.

4. With regard to the patient in question 1, which of the following laboratory evaluations is LEAST useful in diagnosis?
   a. smear stained with Giemsa.
   b. smear stained with periodic acid-Schiff (PAS).
   c. smear stained with calcofluor white.
   d. nonnutrient agar with *Staphylococcus* overlay.

5. Which of the following is FALSE regarding the management of this disease described above?
   a. The risk of recurrent infection after penetrating keratoplasty is very high if performed within the first year of onset.
   b. Stromal infiltration often results in the need for prolonged treatment lasting 6 to 12 months.
   c. There is no consensus in optimal therapy as antimicrobial agents most commonly used against this organism are effective in killing cysts but have reduced efficacy against the free-living trophozoite form.
   d. Confocal microscopy is a useful adjuvant in detecting organisms in vivo.

6. A conjunctival inflammatory response characterized by multiple polygonal nodules with central fibrovascular cores is consistent with a
   a. follicular response.
   b. papillary response.
   c. phlyctenular response.
   d. ligneous response.

7. The least reliable location of a conjunctival papillary response for etiologic interpretation is the
   a. inferior fornix.
   b. superior fornix.
   c. superior edge of superior tarsus.
   d. inferior edge of superior tarsus.

8. The differential diagnosis of the patient in the photograph below includes all of the following except
   a. contact lens–related conjunctivitis.
   b. trachoma.
   c. atopic keratoconjunctivitis.
   d. ocular prosthesis–related conjunctivitis.

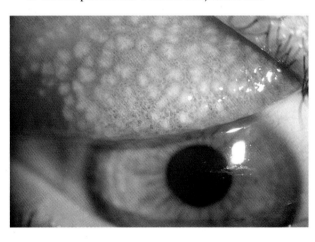

9. Clumps of calcific degeneration and eosinophils at the limbus are termed
   a. Herbert's pits.
   b. von Arlt's line.
   c. Fuchs' spots.
   d. Horner-Trantas dots.

10. Rounded, depressed regions of necrotic limbal follicles are termed
    a. Herbert's pits.
    b. von Arlt's line.

   c. Fuchs' spots.
   d. Horner-Trantas dots.

11. Mild contact lens–related GPC may be differentiated from an infectious follicular conjunctivitis by
    a. the presence of itching in the former.
    b. the presence of mucous and serous discharge in the latter.
    c. injection of bulbar conjunctiva in the latter.
    d. findings in the inferior conjunctival fornix of the latter.

12. Follicular conjunctivitides are typically more severe inferiorly than superiorly, except in
    a. adult inclusion conjunctivitis.
    b. epidemic keratoconjunctivitis (EKC).
    c. trachoma.
    d. medicamentosa.

13. The differential diagnosis for acute follicular conjunctivitis includes all of the following except
    a. epidemic keratoconjunctivitis (EKC).
    b. herpes simplex keratoconjunctivitis.
    c. trachoma.
    d. adult inclusion conjunctivitis.

14. The differential diagnosis for chronic follicular conjunctivitis includes all of the following except
    a. EKC.
    b. medicamentosa.
    c. Parinaud's oculoglandular syndrome.
    d. trachoma.

15. Infectious etiologies of pseudomembranous or membranous conjunctivitis include all of the following except
    a. *Gonococcus*.
    b. herpes simplex.
    c. adult inclusion conjunctivitis.
    d. *Candida*.

9

16. Immunologic etiologies of a pseudomembranous or membranous conjunctivitis include all of the following except
    a. ocular cicatricial pemphigoid (OCP).
    b. vernal keratoconjunctivitis.
    c. ligneous keratoconjunctivitis.
    d. atopic keratoconjunctivitis.

17. Superficial opacification of the cornea in a horizontal fashion between the eyelid margins is best referred to as
    a. superficial punctate keratitis.
    b. micropannus.
    c. band keratopathy.
    d. gross corneal pannus.

18. The predominant cell forms seen in "mutton-fat" KPs are
    a. lymphocytes.
    b. epithelioid histiocytes.
    c. PMNs.
    d. red blood cells.

19. Which of the following is an advantage of PRK when compared to LASIK?
    a. reduced incidence of stromal haze.
    b. more rapid epithelial healing.
    c. reduced incidence of postoperative endophthalmitis.
    d. reduced postoperative pain.

20. A corneal ulcer recalcitrant to routine treatment is rescraped for special staining and cultures. The Gram stain is reported as growing moderate diphtheroids. Which special stain is most likely to be of value in determining the actual diagnosis?
    a. Ziehl-Neelsen stain.
    b. Warthin-Starry stain.
    c. Giemsa stain.
    d. periodic acid-Schiff (PAS) stain.

21. The most common agent involved in mycotic ocular infections in the northern half of the United States is
    a. *Aspergillus.*
    b. *Fusarium.*
    c. *Penicillium.*
    d. *Candida.*

22. The most common agent involved in mycotic ocular infections in the southern half of the United States is
    a. *Aspergillus.*
    b. *Fusarium.*
    c. *Penicillium.*
    d. *Candida.*

23. The most basic difference between *Candida* and *Fusarium* is
    a. *Fusarium* is a mold, and *Candida* is dimorphic.
    b. *Fusarium* is dimorphic, and *Candida* is a mold.
    c. *Fusarium* is a mold, and *Candida* is a yeast.
    d. *Fusarium* as a yeast has pseudohyphae, whereas *Candida* has true hyphae.

24. The most common ocular manifestation of cryptococcal infection is
    a. membranous conjunctivitis.
    b. orbital cellulitis.
    c. endogenous endophthalmitis.
    d. ulcerative keratitis.

25. Factors that increase the difficulty of laboratory identification of fungal pathogens include all of the following except
    a. inclusion of cycloheximide in various media.
    b. fastidiousness of the fungal agents.
    c. discarding of plates before full identification of fungal species.
    d. confusion of pathogenic fungal species as contaminants.

26. Which of the following Epstein-Barr virus (EBV) antibodies does not peak in serum level within the first 6 to 12 weeks of infection?
    a. viral capsid antigen IgM (VCA-IgM).
    b. VCA-IgG.
    c. early antigen-diffuse (EA-D).
    d. Epstein-Barr nuclear antigen (EBNA).

9

27. Which of the following is NOT true regarding laser-assisted subepithelial keratomileusis (LASEK)?
    a. There is no stromal flap created.
    b. The procedure may offer increased comfort for the patient when compared to LASIK.
    c. 20% ethanol can be used to trephine the epithelium.
    d. The procedure has less haze associated with it than LASIK.

28. Biologic features of chlamydiae that render them closer to bacterial than viral life forms include all of the following except
    a. nucleic acid content.
    b. mechanism of replication.
    c. cell wall properties.
    d. full complement of organelles.

29. At what point do most flap folds occur after LASIK?
    a. within 1 week.
    b. after 2 weeks.
    c. after 1 month.
    d. after 1 year.

30. Which one of the following regarding louse infections of the eye is false?
    a. *Pediculus capitis* and *Phthirus pubis* are the only organisms that infect the periocular structures.
    b. Ocular irritation is due to injection of toxic louse saliva into lid tissue.
    c. Sexual contact is felt to be the significant mode of transmission.
    d. Eradication of organisms depends on suffocation, either by bland ointments or paralytic medications such as eserine.

31. The method of choice for documenting intracytoplasmic inclusion bodies is
    a. Giemsa stain.
    b. blood agar with *Staphylococcus aureus* cultures.
    c. Sabouraud's agar.
    d. Ziehl-Neelsen stain.

32. Which of the following antivirals has in vivo activity against herpes simplex virus (HSV)?
    a. idoxuridine.
    b. vidarabine.
    c. trifluridine.
    d. acyclovir.

33. Which of the following is false regarding radial corneal incisions?
    a. Radial incisions cause a local flattening of the cornea.
    b. Radial incisions cause flattening 90° away from the meridian of the incision.
    c. Radial incisions have a greater effect as they move further away from the visual axis.
    d. Radial incisions have a greater effect the larger they are (up to 11 mm).

34. All of the following have been described as signs of antiviral toxicity except
    a. follicular conjunctivitis.
    b. anterior uveitis.
    c. indolent corneal ulceration.
    d. preauricular lymphadenopathy.

35. The drug of choice for presumed filamentous keratomycosis is
    a. topical amphotericin.
    b. oral ketoconazole.
    c. topical clotrimazole.
    d. topical natamycin.

36. The drug of choice for *Aspergillus* keratitis is
    a. clotrimazole.
    b. flucytosine.
    c. natamycin.
    d. amphotericin.

37. Which of the following organ systems is most likely to be the target of toxicity from the polyene class of antifungal agents?
    a. central nervous system (CNS).
    b. hepatic.
    c. renal.
    d. hematopoietic.

9

38. Which of the following organ systems is most likely to be the target of the imidazole class of antifungal agents?
    a. central nervous system (CNS).
    b. hepatic.
    c. renal.
    d. hematopoietic.

39. The cellular element generally responsible for inflammatory corneal damage is the
    a. macrophage.
    b. lymphocyte.
    c. polymorphonuclear leukocyte (PMN).
    d. eosinophil.

40. Which of the following statements regarding intracorneal rings (ICRs) is false?
    a. One advantage of ICR implantation is the reversible nature of the procedure.
    b. Decreased corneal sensation can be a postoperative complication.
    c. The most common complication, corneal perforation, can lead to severe visual loss.
    d. More than 90% of patients have <1 D change in refraction at 1-year postoperative follow-up.

41. The topical steroid preparation with the greatest antiinflammatory activity within the cornea is
    a. prednisolone phosphate 1.0%.
    b. dexamethasone phosphate 1.0% ointment.
    c. prednisolone acetate 1.0%.
    d. dexamethasone alcohol 0.1% suspension.

42. A patient presents 6 hours after receiving a prescription for topical antibiotic for a suspected bacterial blepharoconjunctivitis. The patient complains of itching and tearing, and an examination documents severe chemosis and mild hyperemia. The most likely diagnosis is
    a. anaphylactoid reaction.
    b. toxic follicular conjunctivitis.
    c. toxic papillary conjunctivitis.
    d. contact allergic reaction.

43. A patient presents approximately 6 days after daily use of antibiotic ointment following cataract surgery. The patient describes a gradual onset of scaling and itching of the skin and increasing redness of the eye. The hypersensitivity pattern most likely at play is
    a. type I.
    b. type II.
    c. type III.
    d. type IV.

44. The two organisms most frequently involved in phlyctenulosis are
    a. *Coccidioides immitis* and *Mycobacterium tuberculosis*.
    b. *Coccidioides* and *Staphylococcus*.
    c. *Chlamydia trachomatis* and *Staphylococcus*.
    d. *Mycobacterium tuberculosis* and *Staphylococcus*.

45. The most common cause of hyperacute purulent conjunctivitis is
    a. *Haemophilus influenzae*.
    b. *Neisseria meningitidis*.
    c. *Streptococcus pneumoniae*.
    d. *Neisseria gonorrhoeae*.

46. The only bacterial conjunctivitis that routinely leads to preauricular lymphadenopathy is
    a. *Haemophilus influenzae*.
    b. *Neisseria meningitidis*.
    c. *Streptococcus pneumoniae*.
    d. *Neisseria gonorrhoeae*.

47. Which of the following would be the most appropriate treatment of culture-proven gonococcal conjunctivitis?
    a. ceftriaxone 1 g intramuscularly daily for 5 days and doxycycline orally twice daily for 3 weeks.
    b. topical penicillin G four times daily with doxycycline 100 mg orally twice daily for 1 week.
    c. topical penicillin G four times daily and topical tetracycline four times daily for 1 week.
    d. ceftriaxone 1 g intramuscularly daily for 5 days.

9

48. A child presents with the findings below and associated inferior follicular conjunctivitis. The most likely diagnosis is
    a. phlyctenulosis.
    b. staphylococcal blepharoconjunctivitis.
    c. molluscum contagiosum.
    d. primary herpes simplex dermatitis.

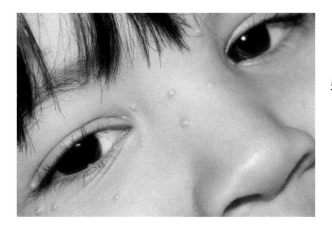

49. Classic epidemic keratoconjunctivitis (EKC) is typically caused by
    a. enterovirus type 70.
    b. adenovirus types 3 and 7.
    c. coxsackievirus A24.
    d. adenovirus types 8 and 19.

50. The most important element in the management of a patient with EKC is
    a. fastidious hygiene.
    b. topical trifluridine drops.
    c. topical bacitracin.
    d. topical prednisolone.

51. Successful long-term management of adult inclusion conjunctivitis includes
    a. recurrent oral tetracycline therapy.
    b. chronic daily use of a mild topical steroid preparation.
    c. conjunctival transplantation.
    d. examination with treatment, if necessary, of personal contacts.

52. Important differences between neonatal inclusion conjunctivitis and adult inclusion conjunctivitis include all of the following except
    a. more prominent follicular response in neonates.
    b. more discharge in neonates.
    c. more prominent cytoplasmic inclusion bodies in neonates.
    d. better response to topical therapy in neonates.

53. Which of the following disorders is most likely to respond quickly to topical antihistamine therapy?
    a. season allergic conjunctivitis.
    b. phlyctenulosis.
    c. atopic keratoconjunctivitis.
    d. giant papillary conjunctivitis (GPC).

54. For which disorder is chronic use of systemic antihistamine most important?
    a. season allergic conjunctivitis.
    b. phlyctenulosis.
    c. atopic keratoconjunctivitis.
    d. giant papillary conjunctivitis (GPC).

55. Features distinguishing atopic keratoconjunctivitis from vernal keratoconjunctivitis include all of the following except
    a. age range of typically affected patient.
    b. seasonal variations of incidence.
    c. presence of extensive conjunctival and corneal scarring.
    d. presence of eosinophils in conjunctival scrapings.

56. To secure the diagnosis of atopic keratoconjunctivitis, it is critical to inquire about a previous or active history of
    a. asthma.
    b. sinusitis.
    c. vesicular rash consistent with HSV.
    d. eczema.

9

215

57. An obese 35-year-old man presents to an ophthalmologist complaining of increasing redness and irritation of his left eye (pictured below), progressive over the previous 4 to 6 months. Examination discloses mildly edematous and erythematous left eyelids with mild conjunctival injection and scant mucus discharge. The conjunctival findings are much more prominent superiorly. The right eye appears normal. With this patient, the critical historical feature to inquire about is
   a. use of over-the-counter eye medications.
   b. any history of previous sexually transmitted diseases.
   c. which side of his body he generally chooses to sleep on.
   d. any previous history of allergic disorders.

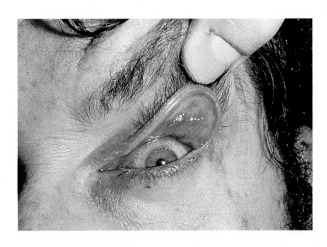

58. The two leading causes of corneal blindness in the United States are
   a. trachoma and trauma.
   b. trachoma and herpes simplex.
   c. trauma and herpes simplex.
   d. trachoma and onchocerciasis.

59. Latent type 1 HSV (responsible for recurrent orofacial infection) generally resides in the
   a. oculomotor nucleus.
   b. gasserian ganglion.
   c. sphenopalatine ganglion.
   d. superior cervical ganglion.

60. Clinical features differentiating primary from recurrent HSV infection include all of the following except
   a. prominent follicular membranous conjunctivitis.
   b. preauricular lymphadenopathy.
   c. duration and size of corneal dendrites.
   d. vesicular blepharitis.

61. Potential outcomes of overtreatment with topical antivirals for HSV keratitis include all of the following except
   a. sterile corneal ulceration.
   b. pseudodendrites.
   c. punctate keratitis with photophobia.
   d. bacterial superinfection.

62. Two weeks after initial diagnosis and topical therapy of HSV epithelial keratitis, a patient returns with a 4 mm, oval, central epithelial defect with smooth rolled edges. Factors that may be important in the pathogenesis of this finding include all of the following except
   a. active intraepithelial virus replication.
   b. underlying stromal inflammation.
   c. overuse of prescribed topical antivirals.
   d. impaired corneal sensation.

63. Which of the following is not seen as part of the spectrum of HSV disciform keratitis?
   a. Descemet's folds.
   b. peripheral anterior synechiae.
   c. mild anterior uveitis with KP.
   d. glaucoma.

64. A circular, superficial distribution of neutrophils around an area of corneal edema or inflammation is called
   a. Wessely ring.
   b. disciform keratitis.
   c. metaherpetic ulcer.
   d. ring ulcer.

9

65. All of the following features of corneal dendrites favor the diagnosis of herpes zoster ophthalmicus except
    a. a large, frequently branching dendrite.
    b. a dendrite with no terminal bulb.
    c. coarse, ropy dendrites with blunt ends.
    d. a dendrite with dull fluorescein and no rose-bengal staining.

66. Which of the following is not a systemic risk factor for the development of bacterial keratitis?
    a. drug abuse.
    b. diabetes mellitus.
    c. vitamin deficiency.
    d. hypertension.

67. Which of the following is not considered an independent risk factor for the development of fungal keratitis?
    a. prolonged use of topical corticosteroids.
    b. previous history of herpetic keratitis.
    c. prolonged use of broad-spectrum topical antibiotics.
    d. corneal trauma.

68. Leading causes of interstitial keratitis (IK) in the United States include all of the following except
    a. sarcoidosis.
    b. lepromatous leprosy.
    c. herpes zoster virus (HZV).
    d. syphilis.

69. Cogan's syndrome is frequently associated with which systemic disorder?
    a. polyarteritis nodosa.
    b. Wegener's granulomatosis.
    c. rheumatoid arthritis.
    d. systemic lupus erythematosus.

70. Which one of the following regarding Thygeson's superficial punctate keratitis is false?
    a. The presenting symptom is typically photophobia or tearing.
    b. There is usually an associated follicular conjunctivitis.

c. The corneal deposits may resemble those of EKC.
    d. Topical steroids have been used for symptomatic relief but may prolong the natural history of the disorder.

71. There is a definite association of superior limbic keratoconjunctivitis (SLK) with
    a. valvular heart disease.
    b. thyroid disease.
    c. inflammatory bowel disease.
    d. systemic lupus erythematosus.

72. Which class of chemicals constitutes the greatest threat for ocular injury?
    a. solvents.
    b. petroleum products.
    c. acids.
    d. alkali.

73. After thorough and copious irrigation of the conjunctival fornices, the next most important step in initial management of a patient with a chemical burn is
    a. topical steroid agents.
    b. topical antibiotic agents.
    c. debridement of any foreign bodies.
    d. topical ascorbate.

74. The primary goal in intermediate therapy of chemical burns is
    a. normalization of intraocular pressure.
    b. reestablishment of limbal blood flow.
    c. control of intraocular inflammation.
    d. reepithelialization of the corneal surface.

75. Which one of the following regarding episcleritis is false?
    a. Both nodular and diffuse forms have been described.
    b. The majority of cases are sectoral.
    c. The majority of cases will be recurrent.
    d. The condition may lead to scleritis if not promptly treated.

9

76. The most benign form of scleritis is
    a. diffuse anterior scleritis.
    b. nodular anterior scleritis.
    c. necrotizing scleritis with inflammation.
    d. scleromalacia perforans.

77. The scleritis associated with the gravest systemic prognosis is
    a. diffuse anterior scleritis.
    b. nodular anterior scleritis.
    c. necrotizing scleritis with inflammation.
    d. scleromalacia perforans.

78. The scleritis most likely to be associated with rheumatoid arthritis is
    a. diffuse anterior scleritis.
    b. nodular anterior scleritis.
    c. necrotizing scleritis with inflammation.
    d. scleromalacia perforans.

79. Infectious scleritis may be seen due to all of the following except
    a. *Chlamydia*.
    b. syphilis.
    c. tuberculosis.
    d. herpes zoster.

80. Agents helpful in the medical management of autoinflammatory sclerokeratitis include all of the following except
    a. topical indomethacin.
    b. oral prednisone.
    c. subtenon's injection of corticosteroid.
    d. cyclosporine A.

81. The most common cause of acute, painful enlargement of the lacrimal gland is
    a. sarcoidosis.
    b. Sjögren's syndrome.
    c. bacterial dacryoadenitis.
    d. herpes zoster virus.

82. The most common cause of painless, bilateral enlargement of lacrimal glands is
    a. sarcoidosis.
    b. Sjögren's syndrome.
    c. bacterial dacryoadenitis.
    e. herpes zoster virus (HZV).

83. Mikulicz's syndrome refers to the combination of chronic dacryoadenitis with
    a. rheumatoid arthritis.
    b. enlargement and inflammation of the parotid glands.
    c. keratoconjunctivitis sicca.
    d. dacryocele.

84. The treatment of choice for the most common cause of chronic canaliculitis is
    a. topical tetracycline for 2 weeks.
    b. oral tetracycline for 3 weeks.
    c. surgical evacuation of the canaliculus.
    d. topical corticosteroids.

85. A patient presents with a tender mass below the medial canthal tendon and mucopurulent discharge from the inferior canaliculus. One week of oral antibiotic treatment and warm compresses leads to an increase in size and fluctuance of the mass. The next step in treatment should be
    a. change in antibiotic agents.
    b. increasing the frequency of dosage of the antibiotic agent.
    c. probing and irrigation of the nasolacrimal system.
    d. incision and drainage of the fluctuant mass.

86. A 2-month-old infant with unilateral epiphora in the left eye is brought to the ophthalmologist by her parents. Gentle compression of the lacrimal sac produces reflux of mucus from the canaliculi, but only on the left. There is obviously increased tear flow on the left as well. The next step should probably be
    a. reassurance with once daily antibiotic ointment and gentle medial canthal massage.
    b. probing and irrigation of the nasolacrimal system on the left.
    c. incision and drainage of the lacrimal sac.
    d. oral antibiotics.

87. A 13-month-old infant with chronic epiphora and discharge in the left eye is brought to the ophthalmologist by his parents. Gentle massage of the medial canthal area produces a reflux of mucus from the left canaliculi. The next step in management should be
    a. reassurance with once daily antibiotic ointment and gentle medial canthal massage.
    b. probing and irrigation of the nasolacrimal system on the left.
    c. incision and drainage of the lacrimal sac.
    d. oral antibiotics.

88. Which of the following with regard to wavefront analysis and wavefront aberrations is true?
    a. Wavefront analysis is only used to describe reference spheres and cannot be used in patients with irregular astigmatism.
    b. A penetrating keratoplasty using eight interrupted sutures will produce a four-leaf clover.
    c. Spherical aberration occurs when central rays focus more in front of peripheral rays, leading to night myopia in some postoperative LASIK patients.
    d. An eye with no astigmatism will have no wavefront aberration.

89. In which of the following conditions would lamellar keratoplasty be least efficacious?
    a. Terrien's marginal degeneration.
    b. pellucid marginal degeneration.
    c. Salzmann nodular degeneration.
    d. Fuchs endothelial dystrophy.

90. Which of the following statements accurately represents Munnerlyn's formula?
    a. The ablation depth (in microns) is equal to the (diopters of myopia divided by 3) multiplied by the square of the optical zone (in millimeters).
    b. The ablation depth (in microns) is equal to the (diopters of myopia multiplied by 3) divided by the square of the optical zone (in millimeters).
    c. The ablation depth (in microns) is equal to the (diopters of myopia divided by 5) multiplied by the cube of the optical zone (in millimeters).
    d. The ablation depth (in microns) is equal to the (diopters of myopia multiplied by 3) divided by the cube of the optical zone (in millimeters).

91. Which of the following is not a common feature of a conjunctival papilloma?
    a. hyperkeratosis.
    b. acanthosis.
    c. parakeratosis.
    d. anaplasia.

92. A 33-year-old man presents to an ophthalmologist complaining of a "growth" on his eyelid. He maintains that the lesion developed over the preceding 4 weeks and is nontender. He produces a driver's license photo from 4 months earlier, which shows normal eyelids. Examination discloses a 3.5-cm round elevated lesion of the right lower eyelid with a central depressed area and debris within. There is no pigmentation. The most likely diagnosis is
    a. seborrheic keratosis.
    b. actinic keratosis.
    c. keratoacanthoma.
    d. basal cell carcinoma.

93. Which one of the following regarding seborrheic keratosis is false?
    a. It is a lesion most commonly seen in elderly people.
    b. The lesion must be carefully distinguished from actinic keratosis.
    c. Texturally, the lesion appears dry and scaly.
    d. Histopathologically, there is prominent dyskeratosis and hyperpigmentation in a papillary growth pattern.

9

94. With regard to the photograph below, which one of the following true?
    a. Growth is typically explosively rapid.
    b. In 25%, the conjunctiva is primarily involved with secondary skin involvement.
    c. The upper eyelid is affected more frequently than the lower eyelid.
    d. Nuclei at the periphery of tumor cell nests retain polarity with palisading.

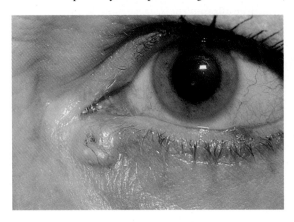

95. Which of the following growth patterns of basal cell carcinoma carries the worst prognosis?
    a. fibrosing.
    b. cystic.
    c. adenocystic.
    d. nodular.

96. Which location of basal cell carcinoma carries the poorest prognosis?
    a. lateral lower lid.
    b. lateral canthus.
    c. upper lid.
    d. medial canthus.

97. Basal cell carcinoma causes the most significant systemic morbidity and mortality via
    a. hematogenous metastasis to the brain.
    b. local invasion of skull and central nervous system (CNS).
    c. lymphatic metastasis.
    d. hematogenous metastasis to liver.

98. Which one of the following regarding squamous cell carcinoma of the eyelid is false?
    a. Growth pattern is usually rapid.
    b. Chronic actinic exposure plays a role in its development.

c. The upper eyelid is more frequently involved than the lower eyelid.
d. Metastatic potential is greater than for basal cell carcinoma.

99. A 68-year-old woman complains to her ophthalmologist that her stye just will not go away, despite 3 months of warm compresses and two surgical drainages. She undergoes full-thickness biopsy of her lower lid; a light microscopic section is shown below. Which of the following is true regarding her situation?
    a. The disorder typically affects middle-aged or elderly people.
    b. Prompt drainage of the initial chalazion would have been curative.
    c. The lesion is likely derived from Moll's glands.
    d. Mohs' micrographic techniques can be curative at this stage.

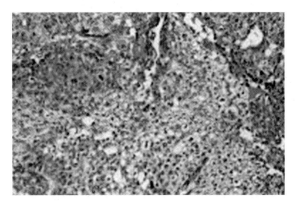

100. The biopsy specimen from the patient in question 99 should also have undergone which one of the following histopathologic techniques?
    a. electron microscopy.
    b. cell surface marker studies.
    c. cellular adhesion studies.
    d. frozen section processing.

101. Adnexal tumors of hair follicle origin include all of the following except
    a. syringoma.
    b. trichoepithelioma.
    c. trichilemmoma.
    d. pilomatrixoma.

102. Which of the following tumors is most likely to calcify?
    a. syringoma.
    b. trichoepithelioma.
    c. trichilemmoma.
    d. pilomatrixoma.

103. Which one of the following regarding nevi is false?
    a. Pigmentation and growth generally increase around the onset of puberty.
    b. With time, nevi tend to advance superficially, toward the surface epithelium.
    c. Junctional activity carries the greatest potential for malignant transformation.
    d. Subepithelial or dermal activity carries the least potential for malignant transformation.

104. Which one of the following regarding Kaposi's sarcoma is false?
    a. The disorder is generally more aggressive and lethal in the immunocompromised individual.
    b. The disorder is endemic in Central Africa.
    c. In the setting of normal immune regulation, the disease typically affects the lower extremities of older men.
    d. Radiation currently plays no role in the management of ocular Kaposi's sarcoma.

105. Potential etiologies for multiple discrete eyelid nodules include all of the following except
    a. juvenile xanthogranuloma.
    b. Hand-Schüller-Christian disease.
    c. xanthelasma.
    d. syringoma

106. A 32-year-old man from North Carolina presents to an ophthalmologist for routine examination. The ophthalmologist notes bilateral bulbar leukoplakia at the nasal and temporal limbus. On further questioning, the patient reports that these lesions have been present for many years and that several of his siblings have similar findings. Examination of which of the following is most likely to confirm the probable diagnosis?

    a. the patient's fundus.
    b. history of sunlight exposure.
    c. intertriginous areas of the patient's body.
    d. the patient's mouth.

107. Epithelial neoplasms of the conjunctiva and cornea bear striking pathologic similarities to neoplasms of the
    a. stomach.
    b. ovary.
    c. cervix.
    d. urinary bladder.

108. Which one of the following is not a risk of clear lens exchange as a corrective treatment for high myopia?
    a. endophthalmitis.
    b. stromal flap dehiscence.
    c. IOL dislocation or decentration.
    d. retinal detachment.

109. The most common location of origin for corneal intraepithelial neoplasia is
    a. the inferior fornix.
    b. the superior fornix.
    c. the limbus.
    d. the bulbar conjunctiva.

110. The key structure preventing local invasion of squamous cell carcinoma of the cornea is
    a. corneal stroma.
    b. Bowman's layer.
    c. endothelium.
    d. Descemet's membrane.

9

111. Which one of the following regarding conjunctival nevi is false?
    a. Because of the absence of a dermal layer, conjunctival nevi are of the junctional variety only.
    b. Conjunctival nevi are frequently cystic.
    c. Due to sudden enlargement, mucus secretion within nevi can lead to the false impression of malignant transformation.
    d. Conjunctival nevi are more frequently amelanotic or lightly pigmented than skin nevi.

112. With regard to the diagnosis associated with the photograph below, which of the following statements is accurate?
    a. This entity is equally common among Caucasians, African Americans, and Asians.
    b. This entity is more common in Caucasians, but malignant transformation to melanoma is more common in African Americans and Asians.
    c. This entity is more common in Asians and African Americans, in whom malignant transformation is more common.
    d. This entity is more common in Asians and African Americans, but malignant transformation is more common in Caucasians.

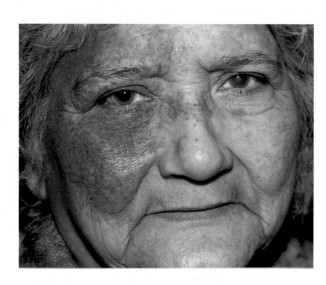

113. Which of the following regarding primary acquired melanosis of the conjunctiva is not true?
    a. The pigmented lesions represent proliferation of intraepithelial melanocytes.
    b. It is primarily a disorder of the middle-aged and elderly.
    c. The most troublesome sign (indicating potential malignant transformation) is nodular thickening.
    d. The most frequently involved region is the palpebral conjunctiva.

114. The anterior segment dysgeneses reflect developmental abnormalities related to what cell line?
    a. surface ectoderm.
    b. neuroectoderm.
    c. neural crest.
    d. mesoderm.

115. An abnormally prominent Schwalbe's line is referred to as
    a. posterior embryotoxon.
    b. Rieger's anomaly.
    c. Peters' anomaly.
    d. Axenfeld's anomaly.

116. A patient presents with bilateral glaucoma. Gonioscopy reveals an anteriorly displaced, prominent Schwalbe's line with attached iris processes and slit lamp exam is significant for iris stromal hypoplasia and polycoria. There are no other obvious systemic abnormalities noted. This patient's clinical condition would be most correctly termed
    a. posterior embryotoxon.
    b. Axenfeld-Rieger syndrome.
    c. Peters anomaly.
    d. ICE syndrome.

117. All cases of Peters' anomaly share which of the following features?
    a. Central absence of Descemet's membrane and endothelium.
    b. cataract or ectopia lentis.
    c. posterior embryotoxon.
    d. polycoria.

118. Which of the following regarding corneal birth trauma is true?
    a. There are no means of distinguishing the findings from those of congenital glaucoma.
    b. The presenting finding is typically corneal stromal edema in the first postnatal week and may recur later in life.
    d. If corneal edema clears, there are no permanent physical findings.
    c. If corneal edema clears, there are no visual consequences.

9

119. Which one of the following regarding pingueculae is false?
    a. The agent most frequently implicated in the pathogenesis is ultraviolet light.
    b. Histologically, accumulation of abnormal elastin material can be observed.
    c. The nasal limbus is more frequently involved than the temporal limbus.
    d. Surgical excision is generally not pursued unless there are cosmetic or comfort issues.

120. Which of the following regarding pterygia is/are true?
    a. Epidemiologically and histologically, pterygia are clearly extensions of pingueculae.
    b. Corneal invasion is limited in depth by the epithelial basement membrane.
    c. Mild inflammation and copper lines at the leading edge are typically seen.
    d. Like pingueculae, surgical intervention is usually mandated for comfort.

121. Methods to diminish the recurrence rate of pterygia following excision include all of the following except
    a. conjunctival autotransplantation.
    b. beta-irradiation.
    c. topical mitomycin C.
    d. 5-fluorouracil.

122. The stain of choice for suspected amyloid deposits of the external eye is
    a. hematoxylin and eosin (H&E).
    b. congo red.
    c. periodic acid-Schiff (PAS).
    d. alcian blue.

123. A conjunctival deposit of amyloid is examined via biopsy and stained with Congo red. As a polarizing filter between the illuminating light and the specimen is rotated 90°, the amyloid deposits seem to change from cherry red to apple green. This phenomenon is known as
    a. birefringence.
    b. autofluorescence.
    c. metachromasia.
    d. dichroism.

124. The most common form of conjunctival amyloidosis is
    a. primary localized.
    b. primary systemic.
    c. secondary localized.
    d. secondary systemic.

125. The most common type of eyelid amyloidosis is
    a. primary localized.
    b. primary systemic.
    c. secondary localized.
    d. secondary systemic.

126. Corneal forms of amyloidosis include all of the following except
    a. limbal girdle of Vogt.
    b. primary gelatinous droplike dystrophy.
    c. lattice dystrophy type I.
    d. Meretoja's syndrome.

127. Which one of the following regarding corneal arcus is false?
    a. The deposits generally begin in the interpalpebral fissure and spread superiorly and inferiorly with time.
    b. Incidence approaches 100% in patients over the age of 80.
    c. There is generally a lucent zone between the limbus and the peripheral edge of the arcus.
    d. Unilateral corneal arcus may be seen in the setting of contralateral high-grade carotid stenosis.

128. A 65-year-old woman is examined as part of a routine annual checkup. On retroillumination of the cornea, fleck-like deposits in the deep corneal stroma are detectable centrally. Visual acuity is normal, and there are no other ocular findings. The most likely diagnosis is
    a. Hassall-Henle bodies.
    b. cornea guttae.
    c. cornea farinata.
    d. central cloudy dystrophy.

9

129. Clinically and histopathologically, the earliest calcium deposits in band keratopathy are located in the
    a. horizontal peripheral cornea, Descemet's membrane.
    b. vertical peripheral cornea, Descemet's membrane.
    c. vertical peripheral cornea, Bowman's layer.
    d. horizontal peripheral cornea, Bowman's layer.

130. The two most commonly encountered chemical compositions of band keratopathy are
    a. urate and cholesterol.
    b. cholesterol and calcium.
    c. urate and calcium.
    d. cholesterol and amyloid.

131. Which of the following corneal degenerations is generally seen only in association with corneal neovascularization?
    a. Salzmann's nodular degeneration.
    b. spheroidal degeneration.
    c. Coats' white ring.
    d. lipid keratopathy.

132. A 63-year-old woman presents with a red, painful right eye (photographed below). Examination discloses an ulcerative, circumferential marginal keratitis with a leading, undermined edge and early neovascularization. Which one of the following regarding the condition is false?
    a. There is dysregulation in both cellular and humoral immunity.
    b. A milder, less painful variant may be seen in young African American men.
    c. Medical management might include oral prednisone, cyclophosphamide or methotrexate.
    d. An evaluation for connective tissue disease is mandatory.

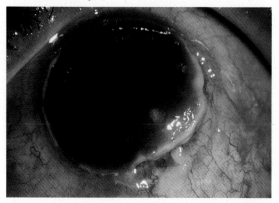

133. The most common anterior corneal dystrophy is
    a. Meesman dystrophy.
    b. map-dot-fingerprint dystrophy.
    c. central cloudy dystrophy.
    d. Reis-Bückler dystrophy.

134. Which one of the following regarding anterior membrane dystrophy is false?
    a. Examination of family members may disclose a familial pattern.
    b. Abnormalities in basement membrane production are manifest as map and fingerprint lines.
    c. Dots represent calcification of epithelial debris.
    d. Symptoms are generally related to defective epithelial adherence.

135. Treatment modalities useful in symptomatic anterior membrane dystrophy include all of the following except
    a. copious lubrication.
    b. hypertonic saline ointments.
    c. stromal puncture.
    d. penetrating keratoplasty (PK).

136. A 28-year-old patient presents to an ophthalmologist complaining of irritation and episodic blurry vision bilaterally. Slit-lamp examination reveals intraepithelial bubbles that are too numerous to count and that are visible only on retroillumination (photographed below). These bubbles appear entirely transparent. A lamellar keratoplasty specimen should reveal
    a. areas of reduplicated basement membrane and trapped epithelial cells.
    b. PAS staining of epithelially contained "peculiar substance."
    c. focal areas of absence of basement membrane and fibrocellular invasion of Bowman's zone.
    d. hyaline deposits in the anterior stroma.

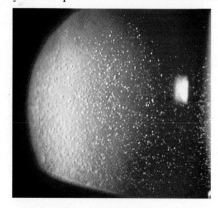

9

137. Which of the following corneal dystrophies is the most disabling visually?
   a. anterior membrane dystrophy.
   b. Reis-Bückler dystrophy.
   c. Meesman dystrophy.
   d. central cloudy dystrophy.

138. A 29-year-old woman undergoes a routine ophthalmic examination. Visual acuity is normal. Slit-lamp examination discloses numerous crumblike deposits in the anterior corneal stroma as shown in the photograph below, which are bilaterally symmetric, densest centrally. Intervening stroma is clear. Which one of the following is likely to be false?
   a. Careful history may elicit a history of recurrent corneal erosions.
   b. Examination of family members will disclose similar findings.
   c. Visual acuity generally remains normal throughout life.
   d. Histopathologic review will reveal hyaline deposits on the Masson trichrome stain.

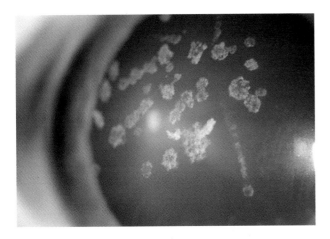

139. A 38-year-old man presents to the ophthalmologist complaining of gradual diminution in vision bilaterally. Visual acuity is 20/100 in both eyes. Slit-lamp examination reveals focal gray deposits in the stroma, densest centrally but extending to the limbus. Intervening areas of stroma have an ill-defined haze as photographed at the right column. Which one of the following regarding this condition is likely to be false?

   a. The patient's siblings may be affected, but his offspring are unlikely to be.
   b. It is the stromal dystrophy most likely to be associated with recurrent erosions.
   c. It is the least common of the stromal dystrophies.
   d. A blood test may aid in the diagnosis.

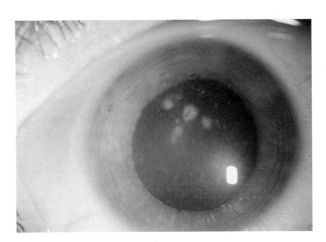

140. A 59-year-old woman presents to the ophthalmologist complaining of gradual loss of vision in each eye over the previous 5 years. Visual acuity is 20/80 in both eyes. Slit-lamp examination reveals the findings represented in the photograph shown at the top of the next page. The peripheral corneal is clear. Both eyes are symmetrically involved. Which one of the following statements is likely to be false?
   a. Each of the patient's children has a 50% chance of being affected with the same disorder.
   b. Recurrence in donor corneas following penetrating keratoplasty is more likely with this disorder than any other related disorder.
   c. The patient, on further questioning, will probably complain of a history of double vision or facial droop.
   d. With polarizing filters on both sides of the specimen, light microscopic evaluation of the patient's corneal button following keratoplasty will reveal birefringence of the abnormal deposits.

9

225

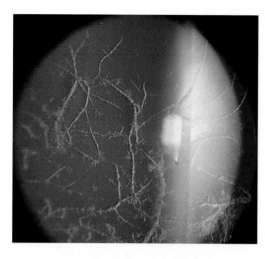

141. Which of the stromal dystrophies is photographed below and may be associated with systemic hyperlipidemia?
    a. granular dystrophy.
    b. central crystalline dystrophy.
    c. fleck dystrophy.
    d. central cloudy dystrophy of Francois.

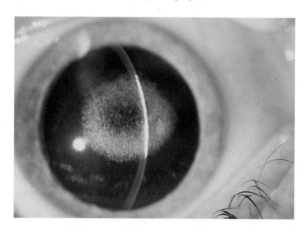

142. Which one of the stromal dystrophies may be associated with keratoconus, atopy, or pseudoxanthoma elasticum?
    a. granular dystrophy.
    b. central crystalline dystrophy.
    c. fleck dystrophy.
    d. central cloudy dystrophy of Francois.

143. Which one of the following stromal dystrophies is least likely to be associated with poor vision?
    a. granular dystrophy.
    b. lattice dystrophy.
    c. macular dystrophy.
    d. central cloudy dystrophy of Francois.

144. Which one of the following regarding Fuchs' endothelial dystrophy is false?
    a. At one end of the spectrum are corneal guttata; at the other are epithelial bullae.
    b. Symptoms usually consist of blurry vision and pain, worse in the evening.
    c. Typically, stromal edema develops before epithelial abnormalities are noted.
    d. Penetrating keratoplasty (PK) may need to be undertaken at the time of cataract surgery, even though corneal symptoms are minimal or nonexistent.

145. An infant is born with bilaterally thickened, hazy corneas with epithelial edema as demonstrated in the photograph below. Corneal diameters are normal. There is associated nystagmus. Which one of the following regarding this condition is false?
    a. Intraocular pressure (IOP) is likely to be elevated.
    b. Another variant of the disorder exists in which there is no nystagmus and the onset is later.
    c. Features distinguishing this disorder from congenital hereditary stromal dystrophy include corneal thickening and epithelial edema.
    d. Descemet's membrane may be thickened but there are no guttata.

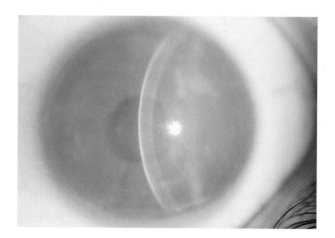

9

146. A 28-year-old man presents claiming "someone said my eyes look funny." Visual acuity is normal bilaterally. Slit-lamp examination reveals multiple abnormalities on the posterior corneal surface, including groups of blisterlike deposits, scalloped banding, and irregular maplike grayish deposits on the endothelium with focal stromal edema. These findings are bilateral, as is corectopia, with the pupil drawn temporally. Careful questioning fails to reveal any family history of eye disorders. Which one of the following regarding this condition is probably false?
    a. Careful examination of a sibling may reveal milder but similar findings.
    b. The most likely diagnosis is iridocorneal endothelial syndrome (ICE).
    c. Gonioscopy may reveal anteriorly placed peripheral anterior synechiae.
    d. Histopathologic findings of the eye, if reviewed, would reveal an abnormally proliferative corneal endothelium with desmosomes and microvilli.

147. The most common finding in the contralateral eye of a patient with unilateral keratoconus is
    a. Vogt's striae.
    b. horizontal breaks in Descemet's membrane.
    c. fleck dystrophy.
    d. myopia with high astigmatism.

148. The time of greatest progression of keratoconus is during the
    a. first decade.
    b. second decade.
    c. third decade.
    d. The condition is generally static.

149. A patient with known keratoconus presents to the ophthalmologist with a sudden decrease in vision and tearing from the right eye. Which one of the following regarding this situation is probably false?
    a. The "tearing" represents spontaneous perforation and demands immediate surgery.
    b. The corneal findings at the slit lamp may slowly resolve with time.

c. There may be considerable associated pain.
    d. Typically, the condition is painless.

150. A patient presents to the ophthalmologist unhappy with his latest refraction. Examination discloses vision of 20/50 with each eye through his new pair of spectacles. This improves to 20/25+ with a pinhole over either lens. Keratometry reveals 45.5 D at 180° and 53.5 D at 90° in each eye. The next logical intervention should be
    a. photorefractive keratectomy.
    b. toric soft contact lens fitting.
    c. rigid gas permeable contact lens fitting.
    d. penetrating keratoplasty.

151. Contact lens fitting is usually most challenging for patients with
    a. keratoconus.
    b. keratoglobus.
    c. pellucid marginal degeneration.
    d. posterior keratoconus.

152. At what point does diffuse lamellar keratitis post-LASIK surgery typically manifest?
    a. 6 to 12 hours postoperatively.
    b. 24 to 48 hours postoperatively.
    c. Within the first week postoperatively.
    d. Within the first month after LASIK.

153. Which one of the following regarding tear deficiency states is false?
    a. Classic signs include ropy mucus discharge, corneal filaments, and punctate rose bengal staining in the exposure zone.
    b. Pathophysiologically, the problem is a loss of adequate tear volume.
    c. Patients may complain of epiphora.
    d. Tests to be considered in the evaluation of potential tear deficiency include Schirmer's tests, rose bengal stain, and observation of tear breakup time.

9

154. A patient presents with complaints typical for dry eye syndrome. Schirmer's testing with and without anesthesia is normal. A hypothesis of tear deficiency state due to inadequate tear lipid or mucus layer would be best confirmed by
    a. tear breakup time testing.
    b. tear osmolarity testing.
    c. rose bengal staining.
    d. tear lysozyme testing.

155. Classic Sjögren's syndrome consists of keratoconjunctivitis sicca, xerostomia, and
    a. eczema.
    b. arthritis.
    c. Raynaud's phenomenon.
    d. SS-A and SS-B autoantibodies.

156. Patients with primary Sjögren's syndrome are not at increased risk for subsequent development of
    a. autoimmune thyroiditis.
    b. Waldenström's macroglobulinemia.
    c. lymphoma.
    d. adenoid cystic carcinoma of the lacrimal gland.

157. A patient with established dry eye syndrome is suffering persistent discomfort and blurry vision despite hourly topical artificial tears. The next most appropriate intervention might be
    a. warm compresses to both eyes twice a day.
    b. lateral tarsorrhaphy.
    c. a trial of temporary inferior punctal occlusion with collagen plugs.
    d. permanent thermal punctal occlusion for all four puncta.

158. A patient with a history of previous severe herpes zoster keratitis presents with Bell's palsy and decreased corneal sensation. Appropriate intervention at this point should include
    a. hourly artificial tears.
    b. bandage contact lens.
    c. lateral tarsorrhaphy.
    d. conjunctival flap.

159. Which one of the following regarding rosacea is false?
    a. It is more common in fair-skinned races.
    b. Facial lesions include telangiectasis, papules, pustules, and comedones.
    c. Nasal skin thickening (rhinophyma) is a late sign.
    d. Alcohol consumption can aggravate the disorder.

160. A 42-year-old man of Irish descent presents to the ophthalmologist complaining that his eyes have been red for several months. Examination discloses multiple brow and cheek telangiectasias with small papillary rash at the tip of the nose. All four eyelids are thickened with telangiectasias crossing the lid margin. There is focal meibomian gland loss. Both eyes have moderate conjunctival injection, and the right eye has a marginal infiltrate under intact epithelium at the inferior temporal limbus. An effective treatment strategy might include all of the following except
    a. topical bacitracin ointment to the eyelids twice a day.
    b. topical prednisolone 1.0% to the right eye every 2 to 4 hours.
    c. topical metronidazole for the skin findings.
    d. long-term oral doxycycline.

161. The mucous membrane most frequently involved in cicatricial pemphigoid is
    a. oral.
    b. conjunctival.
    c. pharyngeal.
    d. genitourinary.

162. Which one of the following regarding the clinical features of ocular cicatricial pemphigoid (OCP) is false?
    a. Women are more commonly affected than men.
    b. The disease most typically presents as insidious, bilaterally asymmetric chronic conjunctivitis.
    c. Chronic use of topical ocular medications may induce a clinically identical picture.
    d. The most sensitive region of the eye to examine for early findings is the superior tarsus.

163. The classic histologic finding in ocular cicatricial pemphigoid (OCP) is
    a. complement and immunoglobulin bound to epithelial basement membrane.
    b. intraepithelial immunoglobulin and intraepithelial bullae.
    c. granulomatous destruction of epithelial basement membrane.
    d. mast cells and eosinophils in the epithelium and subepithelial stroma.

164. Ocular findings consistent with vitamin A deficiency include all of the following except
    a. keratinization and bacterial superinfection of bulbar conjunctiva.
    b. tear deficiency state.
    c. deep white lesions of the peripheral retina.
    d. focal corneal necrosis with ulceration.

165. Bilateral corneal ulceration should be presumed to be due to vitamin A deficiency until proved otherwise all of the following patients except
    a. patients with cystic fibrosis.
    b. patients with history of gastric bypass surgery.
    c. patients with cirrhosis.
    d. patients with normal nutrition and a history of heavy smoking.

166. A 32-year-old woman presents to the ophthalmologist complaining of recurrent pain and tearing of her right eye over the previous 1 to 2 months. Closer questioning discloses that her symptoms are virtually always present upon awakening and disappear after 2 or 3 hours. She denies any history of contact lens use. Which of the following statements is least likely to be true?
    a. Careful questioning may reveal a history of corneal abrasion or trauma in the right eye.
    b. Careful examination of the right eye may disclose a focal abnormality in tear breakup.
    c. Careful examination of the left eye may reveal map or fingerprint abnormalities.
    d. This syndrome may be seen more frequently in patients with hypertension.

167. Modalities accepted for treatment of recurrent erosion syndrome include all of the following except
    a. pressure patching.
    b. 5% sodium chloride ointment at bedtime for 2 to 4 weeks.
    c. bandage contact lens.
    d. anterior stromal puncture with a 27-gauge needle.

168. Which of the following concerning the mucopolysaccharidoses (MPS) is false?
    a. Lysosomal enzyme defects lead to accumulation of metabolites within keratocytes.
    b. The MPS least likely to demonstrate corneal clouding is type III (Sanfilippo's syndrome).
    c. Metabolites that accumulate include keratan sulfate, dermatan sulfate, and heparan sulfate.
    d. These disorders are all inherited on an autosomal-recessive basis.

169. The typical corneal finding in a patient with Fabry's disease is
    a. corneal clouding.
    b. anterior membrane dystrophy.
    c. vortex keratopathy.
    d. corneal neovascularization.

170. A 26-year-old woman presents for a routine ophthalmic examination. Slit-lamp examination discloses a vortex keratopathy bilaterally with telangiectatic conjunctival vessels. Her mother and father are both healthy. Which one of the following is false?
    a. A careful drug history should be taken.
    b. The patient should be warned of potentially lethal renal failure.
    c. Fundus findings might include telangiectatic retinal vessels.
    d. Half of the patient's brothers will be seriously affected by the same disorder.

9

229

171. A patient presents with photophobia and blurry vision. Examination discloses crystalline deposits throughout the entire stroma, most dense peripherally. Findings important in determining the correct diagnosis include all of the following except
    a. family history of eye findings.
    b. previous history of kidney transplant.
    c. history of peptic ulcer disease (PUD).
    d. presence of pigmentary retinopathy in each eye.

172. The corneal findings in tyrosinemia most closely resemble those of
    a. anterior membrane dystrophy.
    b. herpes simplex keratitis.
    c. Wilson's disease.
    d. ochronosis.

173. Which one of the following regarding vortex keratopathy is false?
    a. Drugs associated with the finding include amiodarone, indomethacin, chloroquine, and chlorpromazine.
    b. The findings in drug-induced vortex keratopathy are identical to those of Fabry's disease.
    c. The drug-induced varieties are accompanied by a pigmentary retinopathy.
    d. Cessation of drug therapy will usually lead to resolution of vortex keratopathy.

174. A patient is sent to an ophthalmologist by a gastroenterologist to "rule out Wilson's disease." The key part of the ophthalmologist's examination should be
    a. visual acuity measurement.
    b. slit-lamp examination.
    c. gonioscopy.
    d. dilated funduscopy.

175. The most accurate characterization of donor endothelial cell counts following penetrating keratoplasty is
    a. no significant change.
    b. slow, steady increase in endothelial cell count over 10 to 15 years.

    c. rapid loss of endothelial cells over the first postoperative year, slow loss of endothelial cells over the next 10 to 15 years, with stable cell counts after 15 years.
    d. slow, progressive loss of endothelial cells over 10 to 15 years with stabilization thereafter.

176. Currently, the most frequent indication for penetrating keratoplasty in the United States is
    a. keratoconus.
    b. bullous keratopathy following cataract extraction.
    c. Fuchs' dystrophy.
    d. herpes simplex keratitis.

177. Which of the following is considered a favorable prognostic factor for penetrating keratoplasty?
    a. relatively young age.
    b. glaucoma.
    c. large graft size (>8.5 mm).
    d. no previous history of graft rejection.

178. The primary cause of poor vision following penetrating keratoplasty (PK) for aphakic bullous keratopathy is
    a. glaucoma.
    b. endophthalmitis.
    c. cystoid macular edema.
    d. graft rejection.

179. The condition in which same-size or smaller-than-host-bed donor buttons often used is
    a. keratoconus.
    b. Fuchs' dystrophy.
    c. bullous keratopathy after cataract surgery.
    d. corneal stromal dystrophies.

180. Which method of closure of penetrating keratoplasty (PK) causes the greatest amount of irregular astigmatism (prior to suture removal)?
    a. interrupted.
    b. single running.
    c. double running.
    d. combined interrupted plus single running.

9

181. A patient returns for follow-up 8 weeks after penetrating keratoplasty (PK). The central cornea is clear but too irregular to permit accurate keratometry. Vision is 20/400, pinholing to 20/30. What is the most reliable and effective method of visual rehabilitation?
    a. random removal of sutures, one per week.
    b. removal of sutures that appear tightest at the slit lamp.
    c. use of keratoscope to guide suture removal.
    d. contact lens refraction and correction.

182. A 62-year-old woman presents complaining of slow loss of vision in each eye. She denies any previous ocular history. Visual acuities are 20/400 in the right eye and 20/100 in the left eye. Slit-lamp examination reveals corneal guttata in both eyes with central stromal thickening more prominent on the right. The corneal epithelium is normal bilaterally. There is dense nuclear sclerosis on the right and moderate nuclear sclerosis on the left. The view of the fundus is consistent with the patient's vision. The next appropriate step for visual rehabilitation in this patient might be
    a. cataract extraction only in the right eye.
    b. cataract extraction with posterior chamber intraocular lens (PCIOL) in the right eye.
    c. penetrating keratoplasty (PK) alone in the right eye.
    d. PK, cataract extraction, and PCIOL in the right eye.

183. Mucous membrane grafting in anticipation of penetrating keratoplasty is most hazardous in patients with
    a. Stevens-Johnson syndrome.
    b. ocular cicatricial pemphigoid (OCP).
    c. trachoma.
    d. keratoconjunctivitis sicca.

184. Persistent epithelial defects of the donor cornea following PK are likely to be seen in all of the following except
    a. ocular cicatricial pemphigoid (OCP).
    b. alkali burns.

    c. keratoconus.
    d. herpes zoster ophthalmicus.

185. Recurrence of the original disease process has been reported following penetrating keratoplasty for each of the following conditions except
    a. lattice dystrophy.
    b. herpes simplex keratitis.
    c. Reis-Bückler dystrophy.
    d. Fuchs' dystrophy.

186. The most common postoperative complication seen after penetrating keratoplasty is
    a. infectious keratitis.
    b. recurrence of the original disease process.
    c. high astigmatism.
    d. wound leak.

187. A patient presents to the ophthalmologist 12 weeks following penetrating keratoplasty. Complaints consist of increasing redness and discomfort in the operated eye. Visual acuity is the same as the previous office visit 2 weeks earlier. Examination discloses a white, crystalline infiltrate at the donor/host interface between sutures. The infiltrate has indistinct borders, and the stroma appears thickened by it. There is overlying epithelial irregularity but no confluent epithelial defect. Gram's stain of a corneal scraping reveals gram-positive cocci in chains. Cultures on blood agar grow multiple colonies with alpha hemolysis. Which one of the following statements regarding this condition is false?
    a. The causative organism, as with cases originally described, is *Streptococcus viridans*.
    b. This infection is generally slowly progressive.
    c. This condition is generally quite responsive to topical antibiotics.
    d. Historical factors most significant in the development of the lesion include topical steroid use and keratoplasty.

9

28. **d.** Like bacteria (and unlike viruses), chlamydiae have both DNA and RNA, replicate via binary fission, have lipopolysaccharide cell walls, and respond to certain antibiotics. Unlike bacteria, chlamydiae do not possess all organelles and require a host cell for replication.

29. **a.** More than 50% of flap folds occur within the first day, and more than 90% of flap folds occur within the first week postoperatively. Not all folds need to be repaired, but visually significant folds should be repaired within 24 hours.

30. **a.** Only *Phthirus pubis* (crab) has been associated with lash infestation. *Pediculus capitis* (head louse) resides only in the scalp. Therefore, ocular "pediculosis" is a misnomer (the better term is "phthiriasis").

31. **a.** This is useful for suspected chlamydial disease.

32. **d.** Topical acyclovir is available in Europe for HSV keratitis.

33. **c.** Radial incisions have a greater effect as they move closer to the visual axis. These incisions can sometimes be used to correct postoperative astigmatism.

34. **b.** The hypersensitivity reaction to idoxuridine is so strong that it may induce lymphadenopathy.

35. **d.** Topical natamycin is the drug of choice for presumed filamentous keratomycosis.

36. **a.** Clotrimazole is the drug of choice for *Aspergillus* keratitis.

37. **c.** Polyenes are insoluble in water and have systemic toxicity via binding to renal tubular cells and erythrocytes.

38. **b.** Liver enzymes should be monitored during long-term ketoconazole therapy.

39. **c.** PMNs release hydrolytic enzymes that denature protein and cause tissue necrosis.

40. **c.** Intracorneal rings are currently being used for the treatment of low myopia. They are also being studied as a potential treatment for keratoconus. Corneal perforation is a potential complication of the procedure, but occurs less frequently than decreased corneal sensation.

41. **c.** Although drug levels in the cornea do not necessarily correlate with antiinflammatory activity, studies involving rabbit corneas indicate that prednisolone acetate has the greatest antiinflammatory activity.

42. **a.** An anaphylactoid reaction is rapid in onset with itching, conjunctival erythema, and chemosis and is usually caused by penicillin, bacitracin, sulfacetamide, or anesthetics.

43. **d.** Allergic contact reactions (type IV) are slow and gradual in onset and characterized by itching with eczematoid dermatitis and conjunctival injection.

44. **d.** The most common cause of phlyctenulosis is *Staphylococcus*, followed by active or latent tuberculosis.

45. **d.** It is important to recognize and treat hyperacute purulent conjunctivitis; untreated, it can rapidly progress to corneal ulceration and perforation.

46. **d.** This is the only bacterial conjunctivitis that routinely causes preauricular adenopathy.

47. **a.** Doxycycline (or tetracycline) is added to treat potential chlamydial infection (sexually transmitted diseases tend to run together).

48. **c.** Removal of the lesions is curative.

49. **d.** Pharyngoconjunctival fever is typically caused by adenovirus types 3 and 7.

50. **a.** Adenoviral conjunctivitis is highly contagious, and infection can be transferred by fomites several weeks after onset. Epidemic keratoconjunctivitis may produce a hemorrhagic or membranous conjunctivitis.

51. **d.** Personal contacts must be examined and treated because of the venereal nature of the disease.

52. **a.** The follicular response of inclusion conjunctivitis is rarely seen in the neonatal form. Although neonatal inclusion conjunctivitis usually responds to topical therapy, systemic erythromycin is recommended because of associated chlamydial infections, such as otitis media and pneumonitis.

53. **a.** Seasonal allergic conjunctivitis is ideally treated with topical antihistamines.

54. **c.** Topical antihistamines do not work well in atopic keratoconjunctivitis; systemic antihistamines are critical for its control.

55. **d.** Although conjunctival scraping in atopic disease usually reveals fewer eosinophils than in vernal keratoconjunctivitis, their mere presence is not a useful differentiating factor.

56. **d.** By definition, atopic keratoconjunctivitis is an IgE-mediated process that occurs in patients who have atopic dermatitis (eczema).

57. **c.** This history is classic for the floppy eyelid syndrome. Spontaneous eyelid eversion occurs during sleep with minimal pillow (or bedsheet) contact. The condition is treated by mechanically protecting the involved eye (taping, shield). If these conservative measures fail, horizontal lid tightening procedures may be attempted.

58. **c.** Trachoma is the most common cause of irreversible blindness in the world, but not in the United States.

59. **b.** Type 2 herpes usually resides latently in spinal ganglia. The gasserian (or trigeminal) ganglion,

located in Meckel's cave, contains the cell bodies of the trigeminal nerve.

60. **d.** Vesicular blepharitis may occur in either primary or recurrent HSV infection. Dendrites are fleeting in primary infection. Lymphadenopathy is rare in secondary disease.

61. **d.** Overtreatment with topical antivirals is common and should be avoided. Bacterial superinfection is not a complication of overtreatment.

62. **a.** This ulcer is typical of a "metaherpetic" lesion and does not reflect epitheliitis. Corneal epithelial healing is impaired by decreased sensation, stromal inflammation, and antiviral toxicity.

63. **b.** Peripheral anterior synechiae occur commonly following anterior uveitis due to HSV but are not usually seen with disciform keratitis.

64. **a.** The phenomenon is identical to the immunoprecipitate formed in the Ouchterlony gel.

65. **a.** Herpes zoster "dendrites" (pseudodendrites) are typically smaller and less branching than their simplex counterparts.

66. **d.** Drug abuse, particularly crack cocaine smoking, is associated with contamination and damage of corneal epithelium. Diabetes mellitus is associated with defective epithelial adherence, as is aging (which also comes with relative hypesthesia).

67. **b.** Fortunately, herpetic keratitis does not appear to increase the risk of subsequent fungal keratitis.

68. **b.** Leprosy is a cause of IK worldwide, but is uncommon in the United States.

69. **a.** Patients are also at risk of aortitis with dissecting aneurysms.

70. **b.** The conjunctiva is usually normal in Thygeson's disease.

9

71. **b.** About one-half of patients with SLK have some form of thyroid disease. Treatment of the thyroid disorder, however, has little effect on the SLK. A recent study suggests that orbital decompression for thyroid optic neuropathy is required more frequently in patients with thyroid-associated SLK.

72. **d.** Alkali injury has the potential to cause the most long-term damage as these agents have the potential to significantly penetrate ocular tissue. Alkaline substances saponify cell membranes. For any chemical burn, the ocular surface must be irrigated until pH is normal (6.8 to 7.2). Corneal epithelial loss, clarity, and limbal ischemia (whitening) are critical early prognostic factors.

73. **c.** Retained foreign bodies represent a hazardous depot of alkaline material. These must be removed immediately upon detection.

74. **d.** Epithelial continuity is essential for the prevention of infections, inflammation, and scarring. Unfortunately, severe chemical injuries retard healing. Avoiding drugs that are toxic to the epithelium (e.g., neomycin, tobramycin, gentamicin) is very important, as these agents will inhibit corneal epithelial healing. If corticosteroids are to be used, they should be restricted to the first 5 to 10 days. They are useful in reducing corneal and intraocular inflammation and helpful in combating the formation of symblepharon. However, corticosteroids may enhance collagenase-induced corneal melting, which often begins 1 to 2 weeks after the injury.

75. **d.** Episcleritis is a recurrent, transient, self-limited, and usually nonspecific disease of young adults. Simple episcleritis is sectoral in 70% and generalized in 30% of cases. Pingueculae may show a distinct form of episcleritis with local superficial inflammation similar to nodular episcleritis. Episcleritis rarely progresses to scleritis; however, episcleritis nearly always accompanies scleritis. Two-thirds of patients with episcleritis have recurrences, and the condition is usually self-limited without treatment. The condition can be treated with topical steroids and/or oral nonsteroidal agents.

76. **a.** Diffuse anterior scleritis is the most benign form of scleritis and is associated with the least severe systemic conditions.

77. **c.** Necrotizing scleritis with inflammation is the most destructive form of scleritis. Sixty percent of affected patients develop complications (in addition to scleral thinning), and 40% suffer visual loss. These patients are at risk for mortality, secondary to associated autoimmune disease.

78. **d.** Patients with scleromalacia perforans (necrotizing scleritis without signs of inflammation) often have long-standing rheumatoid arthritis.

79. **a.** Scleritis can occur in association with various systemic infectious diseases, including leprosy, tuberculosis, herpes zoster, and syphilis. Metabolic diseases such as gout also may be associated with scleritis. Approximately one-half of patients with scleritis have an associated systemic disease. Scleritis is frequently associated with autoimmune connective tissue diseases such as systemic lupus erythematosus, rheumatoid arthritis, polyarteritis nodosa, or Wegener's granulomatosis. Inflammatory bowel disease also has been reported in conjunction with peripheral ulcerative keratitis.

80. **c.** Subtenon's injections of corticosteroids are relatively contraindicated in patients with auto-inflammatory sclerokeratitis because these drugs may result in scleral thinning and increased potential for perforation.

81. **c.** Acute dacryoadenitis is most often caused by ascending staphylococcal infection, often in patients who suffer from dehydration, and is associated with a purulent conjunctival discharge. Viral dacryoadenitis is frequently painless.

82. **a.** Chronic dacryoadenitis is usually associated with systemic disease such as lymphoma, sarcoidosis, syphilis, or tuberculosis. Sarcoidosis is the most common cause of painless bilateral enlargement of the lacrimal gland.

83. **b.** Chronic dacryoadenitis is sometimes accompanied by inflammation and swelling of the salivary glands, which is referred to as Mikulicz's syndrome. Biopsy may be required for diagnosis.

84. **c.** *Actinomyces israelii* is usually found with expression or curettage of the canaliculus. *A. israelii* is a gram-positive, branching, filamentous bacterium. Canaliculitis occurs more frequently in females.

85. **d.** A lacrimal sac abscess has formed and is not responsive to oral antibiotics. It should be drained.

86. **a.** Congenital obstruction of the nasolacrimal system usually produces epiphora. The lumen of the nasolacrimal duct is blocked near the lower ostium (valve of Hasner) by epithelial debris or a mucosal membrane. The ostium will open spontaneously in 90% during the first 9 months of life. Gentle probing and irrigation of the nasolacrimal system are performed by 6 to 9 months of age, if the system does not open spontaneously. If probing is unsuccessful, silicone tube intubation should be considered.

87. **b.** Because of the patient's age, probing and irrigation should be performed; few blocked ducts will open spontaneously after 12 months of age.

88. **d.** Eyes without any astigmatism will not have any wavefront aberration. Wavefront analysis is used to analyze irregular astigmatism. An eight-leaf clover will be produced with a PKP using eight interrupted sutures (and a four-leaf clover will be produced using four interrupted sutures). Spherical aberration occurs when peripheral rays focus in front of central rays, leading to night myopia in postoperative LASIK patients.

89. **d.** Lamellar keratoplasty does not effectively treat conditions with damaged corneal endothelium.

90. **a.** Munnerlyn's formula estimates the ablation depth needed centrally to perform photorefractive keratectomy. It is most useful with low amounts of correction (<7 D). Note that the amount of ablation needed is directly proportional to the square of the optical zone, so a larger optical zone requires more ablation.

91. **d.** These benign tumors demonstrate hyperkeratosis, parakeratosis, and epidermidalization, in addition to lobular acanthosis surrounding vascular cores. Papillomas of the eyelid in young people are often caused by the human papillomavirus.

92. **c.** Keratoacanthoma is a reactive tumor that develops rapidly over 4 to 8 weeks. It is a large, elevated, and round cutaneous tumor that contains a central core of keratin. Although acanthosis, hyperkeratosis, and dyskeratosis may be extreme, dysplasia is often absent. Inflammation is prominent because keratoacanthoma is a type of pseudoepitheliomatous hyperplasia. Keratoacanthoma is likely a low-grade squamous cell carcinoma. The other lesions listed in the question are primarily disorders of the elderly.

93. **c.** Seborrheic keratoses are usually verrucoid and "greasy" looking.

94. **d.** This is an example of basal cell carcinoma, a slowly growing tumor of the skin. Conjunctival involvement is rare, and lesions are most commonly found on the lower lid.

95. **a.** The fibrotic type is also known as morpheaform. This pattern features strands of tumor cells infiltrating out from the central, clinically apparent lesion. Thus, it is much more difficult to define the margins of the lesion. They are also less responsive to radiation therapy. The other forms listed tend to be more localized.

9

96. **d.** Tumors here tend to be more deeply invasive, and the involved structures are more difficult to free of tumor.

97. **b.** Distant metastases of any kind are very rare for this tumor. Its invasive, burrowing nature is reflected in its historical pseudonym, "rodent ulcer."

98. **a.** These lesions tend to be slow growing.

99. **a.** The histopathology indicates a sebaceous cell carcinoma of the eyelid, a disorder of later life. Only prompt recognition of the diagnostic possibility with prompt resection offers hope for complete cure. All too often, chalazia are repeatedly drained, with no pathologic review to exclude this critical diagnosis. Because of this tumor's tendency to produce "skip" lesions (discontinuous areas of diseased tissue), Mohs' techniques may leave residual tumor behind. Map biopsies are generally necessary. Potential sites of origin of sebaceous cell carcinoma are glands of Zeis, glands of the caruncle, and meibomian glands: all sebaceous type glands. Moll's glands are apocrine sweat glands.

100. **d.** Frozen section techniques allow for preservation of tissue lipid, staining for which (oil-red O stain) plays a role in diagnosing sebaceous cell carcinoma.

101. **a.** The syringoma is derived from sweat gland tissue.

102. **d.** An alternate name for pilomatrixoma is the "calcifying epithelioma of Malherbe."

103. **b.** The opposite is true. They tend to move deeper into the subepithelial space, migrating into the dermis (or conjunctival substantia propria).

104. **d.** Radiation therapy is a very important and effective modality for treating these lesions.

105. **c.** Xanthelasma tend to be flat, plaquelike lesions, as opposed to nodules.

106. **d.** Oral mucosal leukoplakic lesions are the other common finding in benign hereditary intraepithelial dyskeratosis—an obscure, dominantly inherited condition found in a paucity of North Carolinians.

107. **c.** The grading of epithelial dysplasia is identical, as is the acronym (CIN: conjunctival, corneal, or cervical intraepithelial neoplasia).

108. **b.** Clear lens exchange is the same procedure as phacoemulsification with posterior chamber lens implantation. However, patients with high myopia are already at risk for retinal detachment, and intraocular surgery can increase this risk further. Also, if posterior capsular opacification develops, an Nd:YAG capsulotomy will also increase the risk of retinal detachment. Ptosis is also a risk of cataract surgery. Flap dehiscence does not occur with clear lens exchange, because unlike LASIK, there is no stromal flap created.

109. **c.** The same is true for conjunctival neoplasms.

110. **b.** By definition, the neoplasia of the corneal epithelium is not invasive until it has begun to penetrate Bowman's layer.

111. **a.** Although the conjunctiva does not have a dermal layer, subepithelial conjunctival nevi occur and are equivalent to dermal nevi of the skin. The nevus cells, with time, migrate down into the substantia propria.

112. **d.** Ocular melanocytosis is a congenital blue nevus of the episclera and is most common in Caucasians. When ocular melanocytosis occurs in combination with periocular cutaneous melanosis (nevus of Ota), it is termed oculodermal melanocytosis. This is more common in African Americans and Asians and is nearly always unilateral. Malignant transformation is rare, but it seems to occur almost exclusively in Caucasians.

113. **d.** Primary acquired melanosis is most frequently found on the bulbar conjunctiva or in the fornices. Nodular thickening is an indication for excisional biopsy.

114. c. Although the anterior segment dysgenesis anomalies were once felt to be a result of mesodermal dysgenesis, it is now believed that the affected tissues are of neural crest origin.

115. a. Posterior embryotoxon is a centrally displaced Schwalbe's line that is visible without gonioscopy.

116. b. Axenfeld-Rieger syndrome is a spectrum of anterior segment defects characterized by an anteriorly displaced Schwalbe's line. Patients may have glaucoma, developmental defects of facial bones and teeth. It is most commonly inherited in an autosomal dominant pattern. In the past, "Rieger's anomaly" was defined as the components of "Axenfeld's anomaly" plus atrophy of the iris stroma. "Rieger's syndrome" was defined as "Rieger's anomaly" with additional findings of skeletal, dental, or craniofacial abnormalities. However, the term Axenfeld-Rieger syndrome is now more appropriate given the high incidence of overlapping findings, rather than rigidly defining each syndrome/anomaly.

117. a. An anterior cataract or dislocated lens may be present but is not necessary for the diagnosis. Peters anomaly is bilateral in two-thirds of cases.

118. b. Congenital glaucoma can be distinguished from birth trauma by the presence of increased intraocular pressure and horizontal (as opposed to vertical) breaks in Descemet's membrane. In corneal birth trauma, residual hypertrophic ridges in Descemet's membrane are often visible even after the corneal edema clears.

119. b. The actinic damage seen in pingueculae results in changes in the subepithelial collagen. Although these fibers stain with some elastin stains, the fibers are not true elastin and will not be degraded by elastase. This finding is known as "elastosis."

120. a. Pterygia invade the cornea down to Bowman's layer, producing fibrovascular ingrowth at this layer. Because excised pterygia can recur with vigor, surgery is indicated only when the visual axis has been obscured or if there is extreme irritation. Pterygia are assicated with iron lines, often referred to as Stocker's lines.

121. d. Mitomycin C, beta-irradiation with strontium 90, and conjunctival autotransplantation all have been shown to reduce the recurrence rate of pterygia.

122. b. Amyloid exhibits dichroism and birefringence when stained with Congo red.

123. d. Note that only one polarizing filter is required to elicit dichroism.

124. a. Primary localized amyloidosis consists of conjunctival amyloid plaques, which occur without systemic involvement and without a local cause.

125. b. Primary systemic amyloidosis produces ecchymotic, waxy eyelid papules. Other ocular structures also may be infiltrated, including vitreous and uveal tract.

126. a. The white limbal girdle of Vogt consists of white flecklike deposits at the nasal and temporal limbus. It consists of subepithelial elastotic degeneration and is sometimes accompanied by calcium deposition. Meretoja's syndrome is a form of systemic amyloidosis combined with corneal lattice dystrophy.

127. a. The lipid deposition in arcus senilis tends to occur at the superior and inferior poles (where the local temperature is highest) and then spreads into the palpebral fissure. In the setting of high-grade carotid stenosis, the ipsilateral eye is protected from lipid deposition. There is an increased incidence of arcus in African Americans.

9

128. c. Cornea farinata is a condition that is characterized by asymptomatic tiny deep stromal opacities that are best viewed by retroillumination. Corneal guttae are at the level of the corneal endothelium. Hassall-Henle bodies are normal aging changes found in the peripheral cornea.

129. d. Band keratopathy starts at the horizontal periphery. It may spread centrally to form a horizontal band. Occasionally, it starts paracentrally. It is always in Bowman's layer.

130. c. The urate form is much less common and may be associated with gout or hyperuricemia.

131. d. Salzmann's nodular degeneration, spheroidal degeneration, and Coats' white ring are corneal degenerations that typically do not involve neovascularization. (However, if located peripherally, each of the three may have surface neovascularization.)

132. b. The variety of Mooren's ulcer that occurs in young men of African anscestry is usually more aggressive and responds poorly to medical or surgical management. Perforation is more common in this group. It is felt that some patients in this group may have developed the corneal ulceration as a result of antigen–antibody reactions to helminthic toxins. The toxins may get deposited during the blood-borne phase of certain parasitic infections.

133. b. Both congenital and acquired (degenerative) forms of map-dot-fingerprint dystrophy may be seen. The latter may develop in the setting of recurrent erosions associated with trauma, contact lens use, or chronic blepharoconjunctivitis. Reis-Bückler dystrophy involves Bowman's zone, whereas lattice and central cloudy dystrophies are stromal dystrophies.

134. c. Dots seen in anterior membrane dystrophy are clumps of degenerated epithelial cells and basement membrane material within the epithelium. They are also known as microcysts.

Cogan's microcystic edema is the eponym for the pure "dot" form of this disorder.

135. d. Successful treatment is generally targeted toward stimulating production of new, healthier basement membrane material via epithelial removal or stimulation (debridement or puncture), occlusion therapy (patching, contact lenses, lubrication), and/or epithelial dehydration (for recurrent erosions).

136. b. Epithelial cysts are seen in both map-dot-fingerprint and Meesman dystrophies. The cysts in the former are translucent or opaque and represent degenerated epithelial cells and basement membrane. Those of Meesman dystrophy are transparent and are filled with PAS-positive material known as "peculiar substance." Fibrocellular invasion of Bowman's zone (pannus) is typical of Reis-Bückler dystrophy; hyaline stromal deposits are seen in granular dystrophy. Congophilic stromal deposits are the hallmark of lattice dystrophies.

137. b. Recurrent erosions and anterior corneal scarring lead to visual loss in Reis-Bückler dystrophy sooner and to a greater degree than in the others. Pre-Descemet's dystrophy is usually clinically silent, like central cloudy dystrophy.

138. c. In granular dystrophy, recurrent erosions are seen, but much less commonly than for the anterior dystrophies or lattice dystrophy. Transmission is autosomal dominant. Visual acuity is generally affected, but not until later in life (fifth decade or later). Stromal deposits of hyaline are diagnostic and may be associated with amyloid deposits in certain subtypes (Avellino variant).

139. b. Macular dystrophy may have focal stromal deposits but differs from granular dystrophy in several ways. First, the intervening stroma is cloudy. Second, the peripheral cornea is involved much earlier in macular dystrophy. Third, macular dystrophy is inherited recessively,

so that parents or offspring are unlikely to be involved, whereas siblings are likely to be involved. Patients with macular dystrophy have a deficiency in enzymatic synthesis of keratan sulfate, and serum levels are typically depressed. The mnemonic for stromal dystrophies (dystrophy, deposit, stain) is *Marilyn Monroe Always Gets Her Man in Los Angeles County*. Marilyn Monroe Always (Macular/Mucopolysaccharide/Alcian blue) Gets Her Man (Granular/Hyaline/Masson trichrome) in Los Angeles County (Lattice/Amyloid/Congo red).

140. **c.** Lattice dystrophy also may have granular deposits but also features linear, branching (lattice) deposits. Both types of deposits are amyloid and will demonstrate birefringence and dichroism when stained with Congo red. In type I, as in this patient, the deposits are randomly distributed, greater centrally. This form is localized. In type II, the deposits are along the course of the corneal nerves, so they are denser peripherally. Type II is seen only in familial amyloidotic polyneuropathy type IV (Meretoja's syndrome) and is associated with cranial nerve palsies and dry, redundant skin. Like granular dystrophy, lattice dystrophies are inherited dominantly. This is the stromal dystrophy most likely to be associated with recurrent erosions.

141. **b.** Central crystalline dystrophy of Schnyder represents intrastromal accumulation of cholesterol crystals. Like xanthelasma and corneal arcus, a minority of patients have systemic hyperlipidemia.

142. **c.** This disorder may be highly asymmetric or unilateral and associated with a wide range of ocular or systemic disorders. Tiny flecks are visible in corneal stroma. Vision is not affected.

143. **d.** Central cloudy dystrophy is nearly always clinically silent.

144. **b.** Symptoms of Fuchs' dystrophy are typically worse in the morning, when the corneal epithelium is more hydrated. Mild corneal stromal edema may be silent in the setting of visually significant cataract, so that triple procedures (penetrating keratoplasty, cataract extraction, intraocular lens placement) may be indicated despite asymptomatic corneal changes (with preexistent corneal edema, further decompensation is almost certain). If there are no signs (as opposed to symptoms) of corneal decompensation (stromal or epithelial edema), then cataract extraction and intraocular lens implantation may be undertaken alone.

145. **a.** In the setting of normal corneal diameters, glaucoma is less likely. Congenital hereditary endothelial dystrophy presents like congenital glaucoma, except the corneal diameters and IOP are normal. In congenital hereditary stromal dystrophy, the clinical appearance is similar, except the stroma has normal thickness (but diffusely hazy), and the epithelium is spared. This disorder reflects an abnormality in neural crest cell migration or differentiation.

146. **b.** This bilateral disorder presenting in a young man is less likely to be ICE than posterior polymorphous dystrophy (PPMD). Transmission is autosomal dominant, but expression is highly variable and asymmetric. Clinical findings may be similar to those of ICE. Histopathologically, the disorder may simulate epithelial downgrowth, but the cell of origin is the corneal endothelial cell.

147. **d.** The earliest stage of keratoconus is progressive myopia with high astigmatism. Exactly when an eye may be declared to have keratoconus is a matter of opinion.

148. **b.** Corneal thinning, myopia, and astigmatism are most likely to progress significantly during adolescence, although progression can occur at any time.

149. **a.** Acute hydrops reflects sudden stromal edema associated with an acute break in Descemet's

9

membrane. Pain may be severe, but frequently the only symptom is blurry vision. Once the break in Descemet's membrane spontaneously seals (in 6–10 weeks), the stromal edema clears. Residual scarring may or may not require penetrating keratoplasty.

150. c. Rigid gas permeable (RGP) contact lenses are the optical correction of choice in keratoconus because these lenses are the most successful at eradicating irregular astigmatism.

151. c. Higher corneal protrusion above the area of corneal thinning makes fitting very difficult in pellucid degeneration. Scleral contact lenses have been tried with some success.

152. c. Diffuse lamellar keratitis, also known as "Sands of the Sahara," typically manifests itself within the first week after LASIK surgery. If it is diagnosed early, topical steroid treatment usually provides for an excellent prognosis. However, later stages (clumping of white blood cells in the central visual axis) usually require flap lifting, irrigation, intense topical steroids, and occasionally systemic steroids.

153. b. Typically, tear volume is deficient in dry eye syndrome (inadequate aqueous phase), but an important subset of patients have problems with surface wetting due to deficiencies of the other phases (mucus problems in keratinizing disorders, lipid problems in blepharitis). Schirmer's testing in these cases may be normal or supranormal despite a history and examination suggestive of dry eye. Tear breakup time is frequently the important clue.

154. a. Schirmer's testing in these cases may be normal or supranormal despite a history and examination suggestive of dry eye. Tear breakup time is frequently the important clue.

155. b. The most frequent association is classic rheumatoid arthritis.

156. d. A variety of autoimmune diseases have been reported to develop following chronic primary Sjögren's syndrome. There is no known association with epithelial lacrimal gland neoplasms.

157. c. Punctal occlusion is safe and effective therapy for severe dry eye syndrome. Epiphora is the most likely adverse effect, so a graded, stepwise approach is generally taken. Temporary occlusion of inferior puncta allows assessment of response prior to permanent occlusion.

158. c. The combination of corneal hypesthesia and exposure/lagophthalmos is nearly always disastrous for the corneal surface. Lateral tarsorrhaphy is advisable before irreversible, destructive changes can commence.

159. b. Comedones are not a feature of rosacea dermatitis. This differentiates acne rosacea from acne vulgaris. Demodex folliculorum may play an adjuvant role in what is primarily a type IV hypersensitivity reaction to unknown stimuli.

160. b. Potent steroids may precipitate melting in eyes with rosacea keratitis. Any steroid preparation should probably be avoided in the setting of frank corneal ulceration. Once epithelial continuity has been restored and secondary infection adequately treated (hygiene, antibiotic ointments, oral tetracycline), mild steroid preparations are probably safe but must be used with adequate surveillance.

161. b. Oral and conjunctival epithelia are the most frequently involved, with a slight preponderance of the latter.

162. d. The inferior fornix is generally the most rewarding area of the eye to examine in OCP. Here, subepithelial fibrosis and fornix foreshortening may be seen to precede symblepharon formation. The superior tarsus may show subconjunctival scarring. For treatment, dapsone is an acceptable first choice in mild to moderate cases in patients with no evidence of

glucose-6-phosphate dehydrogenase deficiency (in whom dapsone can cause a fatal hemolytic anemia). The most reliable prognostic indicator for long-term outcome in OCP is the severity and rapidity of active inflammation. Thus, severe cases should be treated with more potent immunosuppressive agents from the outset, such as cyclophosphamide.

163. **a.** This is in distinction to pemphigus, in which epithelial acantholysis and intraepithelial bullae are characteristic features.

164. **d.** Areas of metaplastic keratinization of the conjunctiva within the exposure zone are known as Bitot's spots. Secondary infection by xerosis bacilli (Corynebacterium xerosis) is common. A peripheral retinopathy of minimal functional significance also has been described. Keratomalacia, *diffuse* corneal necrosis and melting, is the most disastrous of manifestations.

165. **d.** Any deficiency of fat absorption may lead to hypovitaminosis A. Chronic alcoholics with very poor nutrition should be suspected of relative hypovitaminosis A and undergo serum vitamin A level testing in the setting of bilateral dry eye or corneal ulceration.

166. **d.** The history is most compatible with recurrent erosion syndrome. Predisposing factors are numerous and include previous corneal abrasion, particularly recalcitrant ones; contact lens use; anterior corneal dystrophies (map-dot-fingerprint, Reis-Bückler); and diabetes mellitus (defective basal epithelial adherence).

167. **b.** Hypertonic saline may be useful in maintaining epithelial deturgescence and enhancing adherence but must be used for several (4–6) months if it is to have long-term effect.

168. **d.** Type III (Sanfilippo's syndrome) is virtually never associated with corneal clouding. Type II (Hunter's syndrome) is rarely associated with corneal clouding (only adults with the milder variety). Type II is inherited on an X-linked–recessive basis.

169. **c.** The findings are indistinguishable from medication-induced vortex keratopathy.

170. **b.** Fabry's disease is an X-linked recessive disorder featuring accumulation of cerebrosides in the cardiovascular system and kidneys. Affected male patients develop renal failure, but female carriers do not.

171. **c.** Three forms of cystinosis are recognized. The infantile form is the most severe, followed by the juvenile or adolescent form. Renal failure is expected in both. The adult form is mild (renal failure is unusual). Monoclonal gammopathies may be associated with corneal crystals, with immunoglobulin deposits in the peripheral cornea. PUD is not associated with cystinosis or myeloma. Bietti's crystalline dystrophy features crystalline keratopathy and a pigmentary retinopathy.

172. **b.** In tyrosinemia, elevated serum tyrosine levels lead to lysosomal instability with dermal and ocular inflammation, as well as mental retardation. Nonstaining pseudodendrites may recur and be misdiagnosed as HSV.

173. **c.** Of the agents known to cause vortex keratopathy, only chlorpromazine is associated with pigmentary retinopathy. The two are generally independent. (Chloroquine can cause a bull's-eye maculopathy as well.)

174. **c.** The earliest sign of copper deposition in Descemet's membrane (Kayser-Fleischer ring) is detectable only at the far periphery with gonioscopy. Slit-lamp examination alone is insufficient.

175. **c.** After corneal transplant, there is often rapid loss of endothelial cells over the first postoperative year, slow loss of endothelial cells over the next 10 to 15 years, with stable cell counts after 15 years.

9

176. **b.** Bullous keratopathy following cataract extraction is the most frequent indication for corneal transplant.

177. **d.** Other favorable factors include lack of neovascularization, lack of inflammation, and no history of previous graft failure. Unfavorable factors include stromal vascularization, tear deficiency state, corneal hypesthesia, youth, larger grafts, and glaucoma.

178. **c.** Most IOLs capable of causing corneal decompensation also can cause chronic intraocular inflammation and secondary cystoid macular edema.

179. **a.** Smaller-than-host donor buttons tend to be flatter and thus more hyperopic than the larger-than-host buttons. This effect helps to neutralize part of the high myopia seen in eyes with keratoconus.

180. **a.** Interrupted sutures, without a running suture, induce the greatest amount of irregular astigmatism.

181. **c.** Keratoscopy gives qualitative information regarding corneal topography when the surface is too irregular to permit quantification with keratometry.

182. **d.** In the setting of corneal edema and cataract, the triple procedure is probably advisable. Guttae alone are not a sufficient indication for this procedure. There should be stromal or epithelial edema before it is undertaken.

183. **b.** Ocular surgery may precipitate increased disease activity in OCP. Once the other disorders have become quiescent, they typically remain so.

184. **c.** Preexistent epithelial and/or surface disorders predispose the graft to chronic epithelial defects. Keratoconus has an excellent prognosis after PK.

185. **d.** Unless the donor endothelium is unhealthy or damaged at the time of transplantation (primary graft failure), the findings of Fuchs' dystrophy do not recur. Primary failure is different than true recurrence, which has been reported numerous times for each of the other disorders.

186. **c.** This complication can frequently be controlled with selective suture removal, but in some cases refractive surgery is necessary.

187. **c.** Frequently, prolonged topical and systemic antibiotic therapy is necessary, with or without surgical therapy (lamellar or penetrating excision). This infectious crystalline keratopathy (IKC) is closely associated with keratoplasty and topical steroid use.

188. **d.** Immunologic graft failure never presents within 24 hours of transplantation.

189. **b.** Epithelial rejection is typically mild and of no long-term significance because host epithelium quickly populates the donor surface. Endothelial rejection is of far greater visual significance and may be precipitated by seemingly innocuous events, all of which stimulate ocular inflammation. Endothelial graft rejection should be treated as an emergency with intensive topical and systemic steroids.

190. **c.** Lattice dystrophy typically involves the deeper stroma, so lamellar surgery is not definitive.

191. **c.** The absence of significant heat release makes adhesives safer and more reliable.

192. **a.** A conjunctival flap will not provide an adequate seal over an underlying fistula or perforation. The "hole" must be closed with a tectonic graft (full-thickness or lamellar, with sclera or cornea) before a flap may be advanced.

193. **d.** The Herpetic Eye Disease Study has answered several questions regarding the utility

of topical steroids in herpes simplex stromal keratitis. Topical steroids reduced persistence or progression of stromal keratitis compared with placebo. Delayed initiation of steroid therapy slowed resolution but did not affect long-term (6 months) visual outcome. Recurrences following steroid taper responded well to a more gradual taper. Topical trifluridine was used in both treatment arms of the study to help lower the incidence of epithelial keratitis. A large proportion of patients treated with trifluridine and placebo suffered significant progression of herpetic inflammation, implying that trifluridine alone does not exert a significant beneficial effect for stromal keratitis.

194. **c.** Azithromycin and clarithromycin are among the class of bacterial ribosomal inhibitors known as azalides. They are related chemically to erythromycin but are much more rapidly distributed to tissues with better absorption, bioavailability, and higher intracellular penetration. Azithromycin's tissue half-life is also quite long, 2 to 4 days, rendering it useful as a single-dose agent. This enhances compliance relative to the traditional prolonged topical treatment and also offers the advantage of treating extraocular reservoirs of chlamydia.

195. **c.** Following incisional keratotomy, radial corneal wounds regain up to 50% of unincised corneal tensile strength.

196. **b.** Keratoconus is not considered a risk factor for the development of bacterial keratitis.

197. **d.** Diabetes is not associated with keratoconus.

198. **b.** These are probably due to precipitation of drug, which requires low pH for solubility. Ofloxacin may not be subject to this complication.

199. **b.** This patient has contact lens associated bacterial keratitis. In order to better direct antibiotic therapy, appropriate laboratory analysis should be performed including gram staining, culture, and sensitivity of the organism. PK is indicated if there is significant corneal perforation. Vitreous tap and inject is utilized if endophthalmitis is suspected (unlikely if there is no vitreous cell). This patient's cultures demonstrated *Pseudomonas* resistant to beta-lactams.

200. **c.** With a large, purulent ulcer, topical fortified antibiotics every hour should be the initial management of choice. Topical moxifloxacin is easier to obtain but should be reserved for smaller, noncentral ulcers. Steroids should be avoided as initial management but may play a role in minimizing corneal scarring later in the treatment regimen. Topical chlorhexidine is used in corneal ulcers from acanthamoeba and would not be used initially in this clinical scenario.

9

CHAPTER 10

Pediatric Ophthalmology and Strabismus

Questions

1. At birth, the length of the average infant human eye is
   a. 8 to 9 mm.
   b. 12 to 13 mm.
   c. 16 to 17 mm.
   d. 20 to 21 mm.

2. The factor primarily responsible for the shallow anterior chamber in a normal infant eye is:
   a. The infant cornea is flatter than the adult cornea.
   b. The infant iris is relatively thicker than the adult iris.
   c. The infant lens is relatively thicker than the adult lens.
   d. There is more positive vitreous pressure in the infant eye than in the adult eye.

3. The reason for relatively miotic pupils in infancy include
   a. relative delay in sympathetic innervation of the eye.
   b. excessive supranuclear input to the Edinger-Westphal nucleus.
   c. increased sensitivity of the light-induced miosis reflex.
   d. immaturity of the dilator pupillae muscle.

4. Which of the following gives the least amount of information in regard to estimating visual acuity in the preverbal child?
   a. optokinetic nystagmus testing (OKN).
   b. preferential looking testing (PLT).
   c. visual evoked potentials (VEP).
   d. electroretinography (ERG).

5. Congenital colobomas of the eyelids are associated with which systemic syndrome?
   a. Goldenhar's syndrome.
   b. Pierre Robin's syndrome.
   c. Hallermann-Streiff syndromc.
   d. Stickler's syndrome.

6. Which of the following is true?
   a. Both congenital ectropion and entropion involve the upper lid more frequently than the lower lid.
   b. Like congenital entropion, distichiasis generally does not cause significant keratopathy.
   c. There are three varieties of epicanthus: palpebralis, tarsalis, and inversus.
   d. Telecanthus is synonymous with hypertelorism.

7. Which of the following is not part of the syndrome depicted in the photograph below?
   a. simple epicanthus (palpebralis).
   b. ptosis.
   c. telecanthus.
   d. lid phimosis.

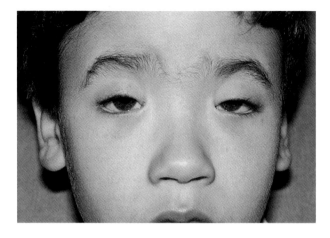

8. Which of the following concerning congenital toxoplasmosis is true?
   a. Fetal infection earlier in gestation generally results in less severe involvement.
   b. The incidence of congenital toxoplasmosis, both symptomatic and asymptomatic, is approximately 1 in 10,000 live births.
   c. A majority of pregnant women are seronegative (i.e., susceptible to infection).
   d. When placental transfer occurs, the infant nearly always develops some obvious manifestation of the infection.

9. Which of the following is not a sign or symptom typical of congenital toxoplasmosis?
   a. hepatosplenomegaly.
   b. seizures with intracranial calcifications.
   c. vomiting and diarrhea.
   d. diffuse pigmentary retinopathy.

10. Which of the following medications is not important in the control of ocular toxoplasmosis?
    a. folic acid.
    b. pyrimethamine.
    c. sulfadiazine.
    d. prednisone.

11. Which of the following concerning the epidemiology of congenital rubella infection is true?
    a. The majority of pregnant women are seronegative (susceptible to rubella infection).
    b. Seroconversion of a mother from negative to positive nearly guarantees infection of the fetus.
    c. Symptomatic fetal defects are uncommon, even with viremia.
    d. Maternal infection during the third trimester rarely leads to fetal infection.

12. The most common clinical finding in infants with congenital rubella syndrome is
    a. pigmentary retinopathy.
    b. sensorineural hearing loss.
    c. mental retardation.
    d. cataract.

13. Which two signs of congenital rubella infection are unlikely to be found simultaneously?
    a. microphthalmia and congenital cataract.
    b. pigmentary retinopathy and congenital cataract.
    c. congenital cataract and glaucoma.
    d. congenital cataract and a poorly dilating iris.

14. The postoperative course following extraction of infantile cataract associated with the congenital rubella syndrome is distinguished by
    a. a higher incidence of retinal detachment.
    b. a higher incidence of glaucoma.
    c. difficulty tolerating aphakic contact lenses.
    d. severe inflammation.

15. The most common congenital infection in humans is
    a. toxoplasmosis.
    b. rubella.
    c. cytomegalovirus (CMV).
    d. herpes simplex virus (HSV).

16. The most common ocular manifestation of congenital CMV infection is
    a. cataract.
    b. microphthalmia.
    c. retinochoroiditis.
    d. strabismus.

10

17. Which of the following in regard to pediatric viral infections is true?
    a. Most cases of congenital herpes simplex (HSV) infection are due to maternal viremia during gestation.
    b. Most cases of congenital CMV infection are due to maternal viremia during gestation.
    c. Like congenital CMV infection, congenital HSV infection is frequently asymptomatic.
    d. The ocular manifestations of congenital HSV infection resemble those of acquired infections in adolescence and adulthood.

18. Which of the following microorganisms is generally transmitted through an infected birth canal as opposed to a transplacental route?
    a. *Toxoplasma*.
    b. CMV.
    c. *Treponema pallidum*.
    d. herpes simplex.

19. Hutchinson's triad, considered diagnostic of congenital syphilis infection, includes
    a. peg-shaped teeth, eighth nerve deafness, and interstitial keratitis.
    b. rhagades, interstitial keratitis, and hepatosplenomegaly.
    c. pseudoretinitis pigmentosa, interstitial keratitis, and peg-shaped teeth.
    d. pseudoretinitis pigmentosa, eighth nerve deafness, and interstitial keratitis.

20. Each of the following is a valid conclusion of the Multicenter Trial of Cryotherapy for Retinopathy of Prematurity except:
    a. Treatment of threshold disease reduces the incidence of retinal detachment relative to no treatment.
    b. Treatment of threshold disease reduces the incidence of blindness relative to no treatment.
    c. Treatment of threshold disease results in better long-term Snellen acuity relative to no treatment.
    d. Treatment benefit is independent of birth weight, race, and number of sectors of stage 3 involvement.

21. Which of the following is not considered a common etiologic agent for conjunctivitis in children?
    a. *Streptococcus pneumoniae*.
    b. *Hemophilus influenzae*.
    c. *Staphylococcus aureus*.
    d. *Streptococcus pyogenes*.

22. Which of the following viral infections is not associated with a pronounced keratitis?
    a. herpes simplex (HSV).
    b. adenovirus type 3.
    c. adenovirus type 8.
    d. herpes zoster.

23. Which of the following concerning Parinaud's oculoglandular syndrome is not true?
    a. Histopathology reveals nongranulomatous inflammation.
    b. Common etiologic agents include the cat-scratch fever organism, rickettsiae, Treponema pallidum, and mycobacterial species.
    c. Clinically, follicles are prominent with a moderate discharge.
    d. Historical features may include contact with animals.

24. The agent most commonly responsible for preseptal cellulitis in children is
    a. *Staphylococcus aureus*.
    b. *Pseudomonas aeruginosa*.
    c. *Streptococcus pyogenes*.
    d. *Haemophilus influenzae*.

25. The agent most frequently associated with orbital cellulitis following bacterial conjunctivitis is
    a. *Staphylococcus aureus*.
    b. *Pseudomonas aeruginosa*.
    c. *Streptococcus pyogenes*.
    d. *Haemophilus influenzae*.

26. The focus of primary infection in most cases of orbital cellulitis is
    a. maxillary sinus.
    b. ethmoid sinus.
    c. frontal sinus.
    d. orbital foreign body.

27. Sudden deterioration in ocular motility without a dramatic increase in proptosis suggests which complication of orbital cellulitis?
    a. panophthalmitis.
    b. meningitis.
    c. cavernous sinus thrombosis.
    d. subperiosteal abscess.

28. Which of the following concerning vernal conjunctivitis is true?
    a. It is primarily a disease of the elderly.
    b. It affects girls more frequently than boys.
    c. Prominent symptoms include photophobia and itching.
    d. The palpebral form of the disease is typically more severe inferiorly.

29. Which of the following is not a corneal manifestation of vernal disease?
    a. deep stromal vascularization.
    b. superficial punctate keratitis.
    c. superior corneal pannus.
    d. transverse oval sterile ulceration in the superior cornea.

30. In regard to vernal keratoconjunctivitis and trachoma, which of the following is true?
    a. The limbal nodules of vernal keratoconjunctivitis are actually follicles.
    b. Horner-Trantas dots and Herbert's pits are histopathologically indistinguishable.
    c. The presence of superior corneal pannus favors the diagnosis of trachoma over vernal conjunctivitis.
    d. The shield ulcers of vernal keratoconjunctivitis are primarily due to mechanical abrasion by tarsal papillae.

31. Which of the following is not a diagnostic criterion for Kawasaki's disease?
    a. bilateral uveitis.
    b. mucous membrane injection with fissures.
    c. strawberry tongue.
    d. desquamating rash of the palms and/or soles.

32. Systemic mortality due to Kawasaki's disease is most frequently due to
    a. stroke.
    b. respiratory failure.
    c. myocardial infarction.
    d. acute renal failure.

33. Which one of the following concerning the anatomy of the nasolacrimal system is false?
    a. The canaliculi normally run vertically for 1 or 2 mm before running medially toward the nasolacrimal sac.
    b. The medial palpebral ligament straddles the lower one-third of the nasolacrimal sac.
    c. The nasolacrimal canal extends downward, posteriorly, and laterally through the lateral nasal wall.
    d. The lining of the canaliculi is a stratified squamous epithelium, whereas that of the nasolacrimal sac and canal is a bilayered columnar epithelium.

34. Which one of the following concerning congenital impatency of nasolacrimal system is false?
    a. It may mimic a medial canthal hemangioma.
    b. Acute dacryocystitis is uncommon.
    c. The defect in canalization is within the intraosseous portion of the nasolacrimal duct.
    d. Common symptoms include epiphora and mucus discharge.

35. An infant presents with bilateral findings as demonstrated in the photograph shown at the top of the next page. The intraocular pressure is normal. There is no increase in corneal diameter. What is the most likely diagnosis?
    a. congenital glaucoma.
    b. congenital hereditary endothelial dystrophy (CHED).
    c. bacterial keratitis.
    d. sclerocornea.

10

52. Which one of the following concerning ocular histoplasmosis is false?
    a. Symptoms consistent with histoplasmosis include a flulike syndrome and malaise.
    b. There is a geographic, but not a seasonal, predilection for the development of systemic or ocular histoplasmosis.
    c. The vitritis that may accompany the ocular infection may lead to decreased visual acuity.
    d. Although skin testing may support the diagnosis, it may lead to worsening of the macular disease.

53. Which of the following concerning toxocariasis is not true?
    a. The infectious cycle in humans generally starts with the consumption of fecally contaminated soil.
    b. The condition may present as a peripheral granuloma in an otherwise quiet eye.
    c. There may be an associated peripheral eosinophilia.
    d. The associated uveitis is due to a hypersensitivity reaction to living organism.

54. Which of the following concerning idiopathic pars planitis is not true?
    a. It may have a mild course, with floaters as the only symptom.
    b. Peripheral retinal periphlebitis is frequently associated.
    c. Infectious etiologies are usually not found.
    d. It is usually unilateral.

55. Findings in a patient with known JRA and uveitis that should prompt an increase in topical steroid administration include
    a. aqueous cells.
    b. worsening cataract.
    c. flare.
    d. band keratopathy.

56. Which one of the following concerning persistent hyperplastic primary vitreous (PHPV) is false?
    a. The presence of dense leukocoria in an eye that is abnormally small suggests the diagnosis of retinoblastoma rather than PHPV.

    b. In severe cases, fibrovascular overgrowth within the primary vitreous may invade the lens substance itself.
    c. A common complication is glaucoma, either secondary to vitreous hemorrhage or secondary angle closure.
    d. The condition is typically unilateral.

57. The incidence of retinopathy of prematurity of any stage in premature children weighing <1,250 g at birth is approximately
    a. 5%.
    b. 25%.
    c. 50%.
    d. 65%.

58. Which one of the following concerning Coats' disease is false?
    a. True Coats' disease is a disorder of childhood, more often affecting boys.
    b. The condition is more commonly bilateral than unilateral.
    c. Diagnosis of Coats' disease may not be made in the setting of subretinal exudate without obvious abnormal retinal vessels.
    d. In up to one-half of untreated cases, the condition may be nonprogressive.

59. Children of diabetic mothers are at increased risk for the development of
    a. Coats' disease.
    b. pigmentary glaucoma.
    c. pseudotumor cerebri.
    d. optic nerve hypoplasia.

60. The most common fundus finding in a patient with acute leukemic oculopathy is
    a. choroidal infiltration (creamy elevated subretinal patches).
    b. nerve fiber layer hemorrhages.
    c. cotton-wool spots.
    d. Roth's spots.

61. Which of the following concerning the gangliosidoses is/are true?
    a. The most common is Sandhoff's disease.
    b. Inheritance is generally on an X-linked recessive basis.
    c. Prominent cherry-red spots are typically seen in Tay-Sachs and Sandhoff's diseases.
    d. Patients generally succumb to neurologic deterioration in their late teens or early twenties.

62. Which one of the following concerning the oculorenal syndromes is false?
    a. Lowe's syndrome is inherited on an X-linked recessive basis.
    b. Female carriers of Lowe's syndrome may be detected by punctate cortical opacities of the lens.
    c. The most common ocular disorder in Lowe's syndrome is glaucoma.
    d. The most common ocular finding in Alport's syndrome is anterior lenticonus and/or anterior polar cataract.

63. Which of the following is true in regard to pediatric vitreoretinal disease?
    a. In albinism, more ganglion cell fibers decussate at the chiasm than in normal visual pathways.
    b. The tyrosinase-negative type of albinism generally has more severe clinical findings than the tyrosinase-positive type.
    c. The vitreous is normal in juvenile retinoschisis.
    d. Most cases of sector retinitis pigmentosa ultimately progress to macular involvement with a poor visual prognosis.

64. The most common underlying disorder in a patient with a "bull's-eye" maculopathy is
    a. Stargardt's disease.
    b. cone dystrophy.
    c. chloroquine retinopathy.
    d. Best's disease.

65. Which one of the following regarding the various forms of congenital stationary night blindness (CSNB) is false?
    a. Retinitis punctata albescens is associated with dots deep in the retina.
    b. Fundus albipunctatus reveals normalization of the scotopic ERG after prolonged dark adaptation (after 3 to 12 hours).
    c. One variety may have a normal scotopic A-wave with no apparent B-wave.
    d. Oguchi's disease displays the Mizuo phenomenon: a golden sheen of the retina returning to normal after several hours of dark adaptation.

66. Which of the following findings is not associated with Leber's congenital amaurosis?
    a. oculodigital sign.
    b. keratoconus.
    c. high myopia.
    d. sensorineural hearing loss.

67. Which of the following is not true?
    a. Visual acuity, although usually better in blue cone monochromatism than rod monochromatism, is not reliable for distinguishing between the two.
    b. In most cases designated as Stargardt's disease, the presenting symptom is night blindness.
    c. Visual function in the pattern dystrophies of the retinal pigment epithelium (RPE) is usually good.
    d. Colobomata involving the optic nerve may be associated with nonrhegmatogenous retinal detachment.

68. All of the following are features of Aicardi's syndrome except
    a. X-linked recessive inheritance.
    b. agenesis of the corpus callosum.
    c. lacunar chorioretinal degeneration.
    d. severe mental retardation.

69. Which of the following findings is not consistent with the tilted disc syndrome?
    a. prominence of the superior portion of the disc.
    b. an inferior or inferonasal scleral crescent.
    c. situs inversus.
    d. binasal field defects.

10

70. Which of the following concerning optic nerve hypoplasia is not true?
    a. The condition may be unilateral or bilateral.
    b. Visual acuity may vary from normal to no light perception.
    c. A classic finding is the double ring sign.
    d. The association of optic nerve hypoplasia, absence of the septum pellucidum, midline central nervous system (CNS) anomalies, and hypothalamic–pituitary abnormalities is stronger for unilateral than for bilateral optic nerve hypoplasia.

71. The most common location for optic disc pits is
    a. superonasal.
    b. superotemporal.
    c. inferotemporal.
    d. inferonasal.

72. Aids in distinguishing pseudopapilledema with buried drusen from true papilledema include
    a. red free photographs.
    b. magnetic resonance imaging (MRI).
    c. visual fields.
    d. ultrasonography.

73. Which one of the following concerning the fibroosseous disorders of the orbit is false?
    a. The distinction between fibrous dysplasia and ossifying fibroma is generally made radiologically.
    b. Generally, fibrous dysplasia stabilizes after skeletal maturity is attained.
    c. The polyostotic variety of fibrous dysplasia may be accompanied by sexual precocity and hyperpigmented skin macules.
    d. The most significant visual implication of fibroosseous orbital lesions is optic nerve compression.

74. Which one of the following is false in regard to the lesion depicted in the photograph shown at the top of the next column?
    a. They are more common in girls than in boys.
    b. They characteristically blanch with pressure.
    c. Phlebolith formation is common.
    d. Indications for treatment include occlusion amblyopia and/or significant astigmatism.

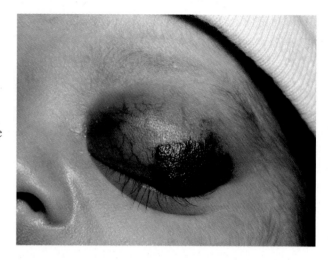

75. Which of the following concerning lymphangiomas is not true?
    a. They are primarily a disorder of the pediatric age range.
    b. Superficial lesions may have a bluish or violaceous hue.
    c. Classic presenting symptoms include proptosis with crying and following upper respiratory infections, and spontaneous ecchymosis.
    d. Surgical intervention is indicated early in the course of the disorder in order to remove the tumor while it is small.

76. Which of the following concerning the epidemiology of rhabdomyosarcoma is not true?
    a. It is one of the most common soft-tissue malignancies in children.
    b. It is the most common solid malignant tumor of the orbit in children.
    c. A common presentation is an orbital cellulitis-like picture.
    d. The average age at diagnosis is 2 years.

77. Which of the following regarding the histopathology of rhabdomyosarcoma is true?
    a. The embryonal type is the least common.
    b. The embryonal type has the best prognosis.
    c. The alveolar type has the worst prognosis.
    d. The differentiated (pleomorphic) type is the second most common.

10

78. Which of the following concerning the neurilem-moma (schwannoma) is true?
    a. The majority of patients with neurofibromato-sis will develop at least one.
    b. The lesion can be exquisitely tender or painful.
    c. Malignant degeneration is common.
    d. There are three classic histopathologic patterns.

79. Which of the following concerning neurofibroma is true?
    a. The nodular neurofibroma is the most specific for neurofibromatosis.
    b. Like schwannomas, neurofibromas grow in close relation to peripheral nerves.
    c. Neurofibromas are generally osteosclerotic.
    d. The association of neurofibroma with con-genital glaucoma is strongest with lesions of the upper eyelid.

80. Which of the following regarding the epidemiol-ogy of neuroblastoma is not true?
    a. This tumor presents as metastases in over half of the cases.
    b. In some pediatric series, the incidence is greater than that of rhabdomyosarcoma.
    c. The second most common site of origin is the retroperitoneal sympathetic chain.
    d. The site of origin is the adrenal gland in at least half of the cases.

81. Common presentations for neuroblastoma meta-static to the orbit include all of the following except
    a. rapidly developing proptosis.
    b. enophthalmos.
    c. spontaneous ecchymoses.
    d. orbital cellulitis.

82. All of the following are features of the histopa-thology of metastatic neuroblastoma except
    a. sheets of indistinct round cells with scanty cytoplasm.
    b. areas of tumor necrosis.

    c. Homer-Wright rosettes.
    d. bony invasion.

83. Which of the following is considered an ominous prognostic factor for metastatic neuroblastoma?
    a. bone metastases.
    b. liver metastases.
    c. age more than 1 year.
    d. bone marrow metastases.

84. The paraneoplastic syndrome most commonly associated with metastatic neuroblastoma is
    a. photoreceptor degeneration.
    b. optic neuropathy.
    c. opsoclonus.
    d. facial myokymia.

85. Which of the following concerning Ewing's sar-coma is true?
    a. Like neuroblastoma, this tumor may present with an orbital cellulitis-like picture.
    b. Invasion of the globe is common.
    c. The age at onset is younger than for neuroblastoma.
    d. Unlike neuroblastoma, there is no role for radiotherapy.

86. Which one of the following concerning ocular adnexal dermoid cysts is false?
    a. The most common location is the superonasal orbital rim.
    b. Generally, they do not enlarge after the first year of life.
    c. Rupture may lead to an orbital cellulitis-like picture.
    d. Radiography of orbital lesions generally dem-onstrates bony excavation.

87. The epibulbar lesion most commonly seen in children under the age of 15 years is
    a. dermoid.
    b. dermolipoma.
    c. nevus.
    d. epithelial inclusion cyst.

10

257

124. A vertical slit pattern is projected onto the fovea of the right eye, whereas a horizontal slit pattern is projected onto the fovea of the left eye. The subject perceives rapidly alternating images of each pattern—first one then the other, never simultaneously. This perception is an example of
    a. fusion.
    b. stereopsis.
    c. suppression.
    d. retinal rivalry.

125. Which of the following regarding amblyopia is true?
    a. The incidence in the general population is approximately 0.2%.
    b. The presence of an afferent pupillary defect clearly establishes an organic etiology for visual loss, rather than amblyopia.
    c. Patients with amblyopia will frequently perform better with single-symbol acuity test targets than with line targets (crowded stimuli).
    d. A neutral density filter placed over an amblyopic eye will generally cause a greater decrement in visual acuity than the same filter placed over an eye with maculopathy.

126. In which of the following types of strabismus is amblyopia least frequently seen?
    a. infantile esotropia.
    b. esotropia with high accommodative convergence to accommodation ratio (AC/A).
    c. alternating esotropia.
    d. esotropia associated with Duane's syndrome.

127. A 7-year-old patient presents to a pediatric ophthalmologist after failing his school vision test. Visual acuity is 20/20 in the right eye and 20/50 in the left eye, tested with patching and Snellen targets. Motility is full, and there is no apparent tropia on cover–uncover testing. The child has stereoacuity with targets disparate by no <60 seconds of arc. Distance Worth four-dot testing reveals fusion. Convergence and divergence amplitudes are normal at distance. The most likely diagnosis is
    a. cyclic esotropia.
    b. monofixation syndrome.

c. central fixation with anomalous retinal correspondence.
    d. factitious visual loss.

128. The patient in question 127 has no history of previous eye surgery. The remainder of his examination is most likely to disclose
    a. high axial myopia bilaterally.
    b. retraction of the globe on adduction.
    c. anisometropia > 2D.
    d. esotropia developing sometime within the next 24 hours.

129. The most practical and valuable test to perform next on the patient above would be
    a. Lancaster red-green test.
    b. afterimage testing.
    c. Bagolini glass testing.
    d. four-prism-diopter base-out test.

130. A 42-year-old patient presents to the emergency room with a manifest right esotropia. A red glass is placed over the left eye and the patient is asked to fixate at a distant point-light target. In the absence of suppression, and with normal retinal correspondence, the patient should perceive the red light
    a. above the white light.
    b. below the white light.
    c. to the right of the white light.
    d. to the left of the white light.

131. Which of the following regarding the afterimage test for retinal correspondence is true?
    a. It is best to flash the vertical line into the fixating eye.
    b. Regardless of fixation behavior, in the setting of normal retinal correspondence, the patient will perceive a cross with a single central gap.
    c. A patient with a right exotropia, central fixation, and harmonious anomalous retinal correspondence will perceive the vertical line flashed into his right eye as being to the left of the horizontal image placed into his fixating left eye (crossed diplopia).
    d. To appropriately interpret this test, the patient's fixation behavior must be determined.

110

78. Which of the following concerning the neurilemmoma (schwannoma) is true?
    a. The majority of patients with neurofibromatosis will develop at least one.
    b. The lesion can be exquisitely tender or painful.
    c. Malignant degeneration is common.
    d. There are three classic histopathologic patterns.

79. Which of the following concerning neurofibroma is true?
    a. The nodular neurofibroma is the most specific for neurofibromatosis.
    b. Like schwannomas, neurofibromas grow in close relation to peripheral nerves.
    c. Neurofibromas are generally osteosclerotic.
    d. The association of neurofibroma with congenital glaucoma is strongest with lesions of the upper eyelid.

80. Which of the following regarding the epidemiology of neuroblastoma is not true?
    a. This tumor presents as metastases in over half of the cases.
    b. In some pediatric series, the incidence is greater than that of rhabdomyosarcoma.
    c. The second most common site of origin is the retroperitoneal sympathetic chain.
    d. The site of origin is the adrenal gland in at least half of the cases.

81. Common presentations for neuroblastoma metastatic to the orbit include all of the following except
    a. rapidly developing proptosis.
    b. enophthalmos.
    c. spontaneous ecchymoses.
    d. orbital cellulitis.

82. All of the following are features of the histopathology of metastatic neuroblastoma except
    a. sheets of indistinct round cells with scanty cytoplasm.
    b. areas of tumor necrosis.
    c. Homer-Wright rosettes.
    d. bony invasion.

83. Which of the following is considered an ominous prognostic factor for metastatic neuroblastoma?
    a. bone metastases.
    b. liver metastases.
    c. age more than 1 year.
    d. bone marrow metastases.

84. The paraneoplastic syndrome most commonly associated with metastatic neuroblastoma is
    a. photoreceptor degeneration.
    b. optic neuropathy.
    c. opsoclonus.
    d. facial myokymia.

85. Which of the following concerning Ewing's sarcoma is true?
    a. Like neuroblastoma, this tumor may present with an orbital cellulitis-like picture.
    b. Invasion of the globe is common.
    c. The age at onset is younger than for neuroblastoma.
    d. Unlike neuroblastoma, there is no role for radiotherapy.

86. Which one of the following concerning ocular adnexal dermoid cysts is false?
    a. The most common location is the superonasal orbital rim.
    b. Generally, they do not enlarge after the first year of life.
    c. Rupture may lead to an orbital cellulitis-like picture.
    d. Radiography of orbital lesions generally demonstrates bony excavation.

87. The epibulbar lesion most commonly seen in children under the age of 15 years is
    a. dermoid.
    b. dermolipoma.
    c. nevus.
    d. epithelial inclusion cyst.

10

88. Which of the following concerning the incidence of retinoblastoma is not true?
    a. The most frequent age at diagnosis is 18 months.
    b. Ninety percent of cases are diagnosed by the age of 3 years.
    c. Almost 95% of newly diagnosed cases will have no family history of retinoblastoma.
    d. The most reliable clue to the presence of a new germline mutation is unilateral involvement.

89. A couple gives birth to a child who, at the age of 9 months, is diagnosed with bilateral retinoblastoma. There is no previous family history of the disorder. Which one of the following statements regarding this situation is incorrect?
    a. The child most likely carries one abnormal copy of chromosome 13 in each of his cells.
    b. The chance of this child having an affected brother or sister is approximately 6%.
    c. Either the mother or the father must carry an abnormal copy of chromosome 13 in their germ cells.
    d. The child's life expectancy is less than normal.

90. Two years later, the same couple gives birth to another child who, at the age of 15 months, is diagnosed with bilateral retinoblastoma. When the parents inquire about the probability of their next child developing retinoblastoma, they should be told that the probability is approximately
    a. <1%.
    b. 6%.
    c. 25%.
    d. 40%.

91. Patients who have received radiation therapy for bilateral retinoblastoma are at increased risk for the development of all of the following except
    a. choroidal osteoma.
    b. osteogenic sarcoma of the long bones.
    c. osteogenic sarcoma of the orbital bones.
    d. leiomyosarcomas of the eye or orbit.

92. Which of the following is the most common presentation for retinoblastoma?
    a. decreased vision.
    b. strabismus.
    c. incidental finding.
    d. leukocoria.

93. Which of the following statements pertaining to retinoblastoma is true?
    a. Retinoblastoma that grows into the vitreous in a mushroom or spherical shape is termed "exophytic."
    b. An interesting light microscopic characteristic of retinoblastoma is zonal necrosis of tumor surrounding blood vessels.
    c. The genetic implications of retinoma (retinocytoma) are identical to those of retinoblastoma.
    d. Case reports of pineal gland neoplasms associated with retinoblastoma probably represent central nervous system metastasis.

94. The blood vessels in a retinoblastoma may absorb released nucleic acids from the necrotic cells and take on what appearance microscopically?
    a. eosinophilia.
    b. basophilia.
    c. fibrinoid necrosis.
    d. xanthomatization.

95. Which of the following is the most common site of retinoblastoma spread outside the eye?
    a. skull bones.
    b. liver.
    c. lymph nodes.
    d. central nervous system (CNS).

96. Which one of the following regarding the treatment of retinoblastoma is false?
    a. For large tumors, treatment generally includes enucleation.
    b. In advanced or metastatic cases, chemotherapy is used.
    c. Cryotherapy is avoided because it typically leads to dissemination of viable tumor cells within the eye.
    d. Cobalt plaque therapy has been used in eyes that have incompletely responded to external beam irradiation.

10

97. Which one of the following regarding medullo-epithelioma (diktyoma) is false?
   a. The cell of origin is probably nonpigmented ciliary epithelium.
   b. Like hemangiopericytoma, tumors with benign histopathologic features have a significant metastatic potential.
   c. A teratoid variant exists that may contain cartilage, muscle, or neural tissue.
   d. Leukocoria may be the presenting finding.

98. A 17-year-old girl undergoes dilated funduscopic examination after being fit for contact lenses. A creamy orange, geographic placoid elevation deep to the retina is noted (photograph below). Ultrasonography reveals a very highly reflective thickening of choroid in the same region. Computed tomography (CT) reveals calcification. The most likely diagnosis is
   a. amelanotic melanoma.
   b. choroidal hemangioma.
   c. choroidal osteoma.
   d. choroidal metastasis from an ovarian primary.

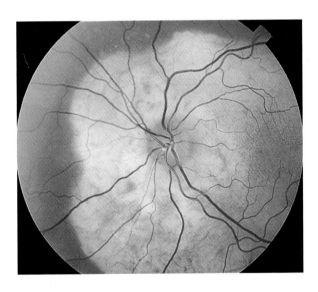

99. Which of the following tests is most likely to be normal in severe unilateral optic nerve hypoplasia?
   a. visual acuity test.
   b. swinging flashlight test.
   c. electroretinography.
   d. visual evoked responses.

100. Seizures, mental retardation, and facial angiofibroma (as depicted in the photograph below) form the classic triad for
   a. neurofibromatosis.
   b. tuberous sclerosis.
   c. von Hippel-Lindau disease.
   d. ataxia–telangiectasia.

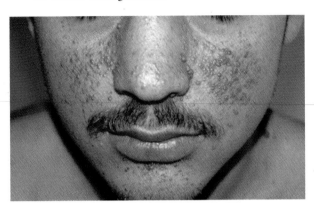

101. Which of the following is true in regard to Sturge-Weber syndrome?
   a. The complete Sturge-Weber syndrome includes facial hemangioma, ipsilateral glaucoma, and ipsilateral epilepsy.
   b. The classic fundus finding in a patient with Sturge-Weber syndrome is the focal choroidal hemangioma.
   c. The glaucoma seen ipsilateral to facial hemangioma in Sturge-Weber syndrome is due entirely to elevated episcleral venous pressure (EVP).
   d. In Sturge-Weber syndrome, iris neovascularization may complicate the course of retinal angiomatosis.

102. What percentage of patients with capillary hemangiomas of the retina will develop hemangioblastomas of the cerebellum?
   a. 5%.
   b. 20%.
   c. 50%.
   d. 75%.

103. Which of the following disorders is inherited on an autosomal-recessive basis?
   a. tuberous sclerosis.
   b. Sturge-Weber syndrome.
   c. von Hippel-Lindau disease.
   d. ataxia–telangiectasia.

10

104. Potential ocular manifestations of the craniosyn-ostoses include all of the following except
    a. optic nerve hypoplasia.
    b. papilledema.
    c. exposure keratitis.
    d. tortuous retinal vasculature.

105. The strabismus most frequently associated with the craniosynostoses is
    a. double elevator palsy.
    b. Duane's syndrome.
    c. V-pattern exotropia.
    d. A-pattern esotropia.

106. Which of the following is not a feature of the Pierre Robin sequence?
    a. cleft palate.
    b. bird face.
    c. glossoptosis.
    d. micrognathia.

107. Lower lid colobomas, pronounced antimongol-oid slant (downward displacement of the lateral canthus), and orbital rim defects are typical of
    a. Hallermann-Streiff syndrome.
    b. Treacher Collins' syndrome.
    c. Goldenhar's syndrome.
    d. Waardenburg's syndrome.

108. Ocular findings in the patient photographed below least likely include
    a. optic nerve hypoplasia.
    b. hypertelorism.
    c. anterior segment dysgeneses.
    d. tortuous retinal vessels.

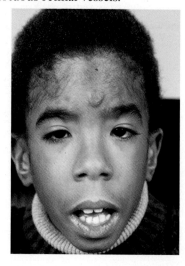

109. Which of the following arises from the annulus of Zinn?
    a. superior oblique.
    b. levator palpebrae superioris.
    c. superior rectus.
    d. inferior oblique.

110. The action(s) of the medial rectus muscle with the eye in primary position is/are
    a. adduction, elevation, intorsion.
    b. adduction, depression, intorsion.
    c. adduction and intorsion.
    d. adduction.

111. To maximize the elevation generated by the superior rectus, how must the eye be rotated from primary position?
    a. adducted 51°.
    b. abducted 51°.
    c. adducted 23°.
    d. abducted 23°.

112. To maximize the depression generated by the superior oblique, how must the eye be rotated?
    a. adducted 51°.
    b. abducted 51°.
    c. adducted 23°.
    d. abducted 23°.

113. Which of the following in regard to extraocular muscles is true?
    a. Both oblique muscles are characterized by a physical distinction between the anatomic origin and the mechanical origin.
    b. The superior oblique tendon passes between the superior rectus muscle and the globe on the way to its insertion.
    c. The inferior oblique muscle passes between the inferior rectus muscle and the globe on the way to its insertion.
    d. The superior oblique muscle becomes tendinous after turning through the trochlea.

114. The primary intorter of the globe in primary position is the
    a. superior oblique.
    b. superior rectus.
    c. inferior oblique.
    d. inferior rectus.

115. The extraocular muscle with the shortest length of active muscle belly is the
    a. superior rectus.
    b. inferior rectus.
    c. superior oblique.
    d. inferior oblique.

116. Which of the following changes in lid position are consistent with the muscle surgery described?
    a. narrowing of palpebral fissure with superior rectus recession.
    b. narrowing of palpebral fissure with inferior rectus recession.
    c. narrowing of the palpebral fissure with inferior rectus resection.
    d. narrowing of the palpebral fissure with superior oblique tenotomy.

117. Each of the following is a correct match of muscular synergist and antagonist except
    a. lateral rectus: synergist, superior oblique; antagonist, medial rectus.
    b. superior rectus: synergist, superior oblique; antagonist, inferior rectus.
    c. inferior rectus: synergist, superior oblique; antagonist, superior rectus.
    d. inferior oblique: synergist, superior rectus; antagonist, superior oblique.

118. Which one of the following constitutes a violation of Hering's law?
    a. cyclic esotropia.
    b. dissociated vertical deviation (DVD).
    c. Brown's syndrome.
    d. Duane's syndrome.

119. Which one of the following constitutes a violation of Sherrington's law?
    a. cyclic esotropia.
    b. dissociated vertical deviation (DVD).

    c. Brown's syndrome.
    d. Duane's syndrome.

120. The site of origin of neural impulses leading to a rightward saccade is the
    a. right frontal lobe.
    b. left frontal lobe.
    c. right parietooccipital lobe.
    d. left parietooccipital lobe.

121. The site of origin of neural impulses leading to a leftward pursuit movement is the
    a. right frontal lobe.
    b. left frontal lobe.
    c. right parietooccipital lobe.
    d. left parietooccipital lobe.

122. Which of the following is true?
    a. Physiologically, any point not lying on the empirical horopter will be perceived doubly by the human visual system.
    b. If simultaneous stimulation of retinal areas in two eyes leads to the perception of one image, normal retinal correspondence is said to exist.
    c. For fusion to exist, there must be simultaneous stimulation of corresponding retinal areas with normal retinal correspondence.
    d. For fusion to exist, the two retinal images must be similar in size and shape.

123. Which one of the following statements concerning motor fusion is false?
    a. Motor fusion is the act by which similar retinal images are made to fall on corresponding retinal areas.
    b. A normal convergence amplitude at distance is 14 prism diopters and at near is 38 prism diopters.
    c. A normal divergence amplitude at distance is 14 D and at near is 16 D.
    d. Normal vertical fusional amplitude varies from 2 to 4 prism diopters and is independent of fixation distance.

10

124. A vertical slit pattern is projected onto the fovea of the right eye, whereas a horizontal slit pattern is projected onto the fovea of the left eye. The subject perceives rapidly alternating images of each pattern—first one then the other, never simultaneously. This perception is an example of
    a. fusion.
    b. stereopsis.
    c. suppression.
    d. retinal rivalry.

125. Which of the following regarding amblyopia is true?
    a. The incidence in the general population is approximately 0.2%.
    b. The presence of an afferent pupillary defect clearly establishes an organic etiology for visual loss, rather than amblyopia.
    c. Patients with amblyopia will frequently perform better with single-symbol acuity test targets than with line targets (crowded stimuli).
    d. A neutral density filter placed over an amblyopic eye will generally cause a greater decrement in visual acuity than the same filter placed over an eye with maculopathy.

126. In which of the following types of strabismus is amblyopia least frequently seen?
    a. infantile esotropia.
    b. esotropia with high accommodative convergence to accommodation ratio (AC/A).
    c. alternating esotropia.
    d. esotropia associated with Duane's syndrome.

127. A 7-year-old patient presents to a pediatric ophthalmologist after failing his school vision test. Visual acuity is 20/20 in the right eye and 20/50 in the left eye, tested with patching and Snellen targets. Motility is full, and there is no apparent tropia on cover–uncover testing. The child has stereoacuity with targets disparate by no <60 seconds of arc. Distance Worth four-dot testing reveals fusion. Convergence and divergence amplitudes are normal at distance. The most likely diagnosis is
    a. cyclic esotropia.
    b. monofixation syndrome.

c. central fixation with anomalous retinal correspondence.
    d. factitious visual loss.

128. The patient in question 127 has no history of previous eye surgery. The remainder of his examination is most likely to disclose
    a. high axial myopia bilaterally.
    b. retraction of the globe on adduction.
    c. anisometropia > 2D.
    d. esotropia developing sometime within the next 24 hours.

129. The most practical and valuable test to perform next on the patient above would be
    a. Lancaster red-green test.
    b. afterimage testing.
    c. Bagolini glass testing.
    d. four-prism-diopter base-out test.

130. A 42-year-old patient presents to the emergency room with a manifest right esotropia. A red glass is placed over the left eye and the patient is asked to fixate at a distant point-light target. In the absence of suppression, and with normal retinal correspondence, the patient should perceive the red light
    a. above the white light.
    b. below the white light.
    c. to the right of the white light.
    d. to the left of the white light.

131. Which of the following regarding the afterimage test for retinal correspondence is true?
    a. It is best to flash the vertical line into the fixating eye.
    b. Regardless of fixation behavior, in the setting of normal retinal correspondence, the patient will perceive a cross with a single central gap.
    c. A patient with a right exotropia, central fixation, and harmonious anomalous retinal correspondence will perceive the vertical line flashed into his right eye as being to the left of the horizontal image placed into his fixating left eye (crossed diplopia).
    d. To appropriately interpret this test, the patient's fixation behavior must be determined.

10

132. During routine examination, an alternate-cover test reveals outward fixation shifts of each eye as the cover is moved. The cover–uncover test reveals no shift of either eye as the cover is placed over either eye. The correct description of the patient's motility status would be
 a. orthophoric, esotropic.
 b. orthotropic, esophoric.
 c. orthotropic, exophoric.
 d. This set of findings is not possible.

133. During a routine examination, the cover–uncover test reveals an outward fixation shift of either eye as the cover is placed over the contralateral eye. The alternate-cover test reveals no shift as the cover is moved back and forth. The correct description of this patient's motility status would be
 a. orthophoric, esotropic.
 b. orthotropic, esophoric.
 c. orthotropic, exophoric.
 d. This set of findings is not possible.

134. Which of the following ocular alignment tests does not require foveal fixation in the deviated eye for quantification of the angle of strabismus?
 a. the cover–uncover test with prisms.
 b. the alternate-cover test with prisms.
 c. the simultaneous prism-cover test.
 d. the Krimsky test.

135. A patient with strabismus is asked to fixate a penlight held by the examiner. The examiner notes that the corneal reflex in the right eye is central, whereas that in the left eye is displaced approximately 3 mm temporal to the center of the pupil. Using Hirschberg's method for estimating the angle of strabismus, the examiner concludes that the patient has a
 a. 45-degree esotropia.
 b. 45-prism-diopter esotropia.
 c. 45-degree exotropia.
 d. 45-prism-diopter exotropia.

136. When used with prisms, which of the following is best suited for quantification of a tropia only, with no contribution from a phoria?
 a. cover–uncover test.
 b. alternate-cover test.
 c. Maddox rod testing.
 d. simultaneous prism-cover test.

137. When tested with a Maddox rod held over the affected eye with its cylinders running horizontally, a patient with new-onset excyclotropia will perceive
 a. a horizontal line.
 b. a vertical line.
 c. an oblique line running superotemporal to inferonasal.
 d. an oblique line running superonasal to inferotemporal.

138. An adult with a right esotropia due to an acquired right abducens paresis is tested with the Lancaster red-green test. He wears the goggles with the red glass over his right eye and the green glass over his left. An examiner holds the green light central on the chart and gives the patient the red light. The patient is then instructed to superimpose his red light on the examiner's green light. To the examiner
 a. the red light will appear to the left of the green light.
 b. the red light will appear above the green light.
 c. the red light will appear to the right of the green light.
 d. the lights will be superimposed.

139. To the patient described above in question 138:
 a. the red light will appear to the left of the green light
 b. the red light will appear above the green light.
 c. the red light will appear to the right of the green light.
 d. the lights will be superimposed.

140. The same patient described in question 139 is retested with the goggles reversed, that is, the green lens over the right eye and the red lens over the left eye. The examiner holds the green light as a fixation target centrally, and patient moves the red light. This time, the examiner will observe
   a. the red light to the left of the green light at the same distance between the two as before.
   b. the red light to the left of the green light at a larger distance between the two than before.
   c. the red light to the right of the green light with the same distance between the two as before.
   d. the red light to the right of the green light at a larger distance than before.

141. Broad nasal bridges with abnormally large angle kappa may lead to an error in the diagnosis of strabismus with which of the following methods?
   a. alternate-cover tests.
   b Maddox rod testing.
   c. cover–uncover testing.
   d. Hirschberg testing.

142. To accurately quantify an esodeviation, prism is most appropriately placed over either eye
   a. base up.
   b. base out.
   c. base down.
   d. base in.

143. A 31-year-old man with moderate hyperopia presents for routine examination. There is a 10-prism-diopter alternating esotropia at distance. While reading through his distance correction at 20 cm, there is a 35-prism-diopter esotropia. Eye movements are full, and he denies any history of prior surgery. You conclude that
   a. He must have amblyopia in one eye.
   b. He probably has restrictive strabismus.
   c. He probably will note double vision if questioned appropriately.
   d. He has a high AC/A ratio.

144. In regard to question 143, the examiner elects to calculate the patient's AC/A ratio. His interpupillary distance is 60 mm, and his near deviation increases to 50 prism diopters when he views an acuity target through a 1.00 D sphere over each eye. By the gradient method, his AC/A ratio measures
   a. 5:1.
   b. 11:1.
   c. 15:1.
   d. 25:1.

145. For the patient above, using the heterophoria method the AC/A ratio measures
   a. 5:1.
   b. 11:1.
   c. 15:1.
   d. 25:1.

146. In the patient shown below, what is the most likely diagnosis?
   a. right superior oblique palsy.
   b. left superior oblique palsy.
   c. right superior rectus palsy.
   d. left superior rectus palsy.

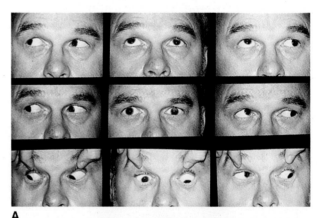

A

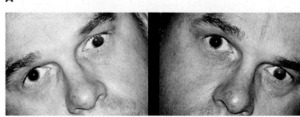

B

147. A patient undergoes left orbital exploration for biopsy of a suspicious infiltrate on computed tomography (CT) scanning. Postoperatively, the patient is noted to have a widely dilated pupil and poor vision at near in the left eye. He also complains of binocular diplopia. You note an inability to elevate the eye when it is adducted. What findings would you expect on the three-step test?
   a. a right hypertropia worse in right gaze and left head tilt.
   b. a left hypertropia worse in left gaze and right head tilt.
   c. a right hypertropia worse in right gaze and right head tilt.
   d. a left hypertropia worse in right gaze and left head tilt.

148. Atropine is relatively contraindicated in all of the following groups except
   a. albinos.
   b. neonates.
   c. patients with Down's syndrome.
   d. patients with heart block.

149. Systemic manifestations of cycloplegic intoxication include all of the following except
   a. flushing.
   b. agitation.
   c. bradycardia.
   d. somnolence.

150. Which of the following concerning the patient represented in the photograph at the top of the right column is most likely true?
   a. Although it is typically seen in isolation, these findings may be associated with neurologic abnormalities.
   b. Amblyopia will likely develop as the child cross-fixates.
   c. Characteristically, the esotropia is small (<25 prism diopters).
   d. There is never an accommodative component found in this clinical scenario.

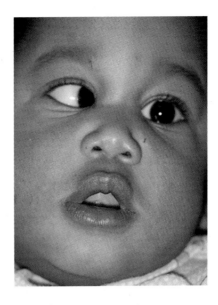

151. Findings commonly associated with infantile esotropia on examination include all of the following except
   a. latent nystagmus.
   b. high AC/A ratio.
   c. overaction of the inferior obliques.
   d. disassociated vertical divergence (DVD).

152. Appropriate options for initial surgical intervention in infantile esotropia include all of the following except
   a. bimedial recession.
   b. bilateral resection.
   c. ipsilateral medial rectus recession and lateral rectus resection.
   d. bimedial resection.

153. Parents bring their 3-year-old boy for examination after they note the development of "cross-eyes." Upon closer review, the parents report that they originally noted the deviation to be present throughout the day at age 2. A brief "glance" at the child makes a constant moderate-angle esotropia obvious. Which of the following is most likely true?
   a. Amblyopia is highly unlikely.
   b. With further careful questioning, it may be possible to document that the deviation was originally intermittent.
   c. The child should be able to perceive the wings of the Titmus fly in three dimensions.
   d. It would be surprising to find a family history of a similar disorder.

10

265

154. As part of the comprehensive examination of the patient in question 153, a cycloplegic refraction is performed and reveals +8.50 D in both eyes. Which of the following is/are true?
    a. There may be unilateral amblyopia.
    b. The deviation will certainly be greater at near than at distance.
    c. +3.00 D lenses are likely to have little effect on the distance deviation.
    d. The deviation at distance is likely to measure >50 prism diopters.

155. The initial step in management of the patient above must be
    a. penalization with atropine bilaterally.
    b. full correction of the cycloplegic refractive error.
    c. bifocals.
    d. bimedial recession.

156. Parents bring their child to the ophthalmologist after noting "cross-eyes." On further questioning, they report that they noted the deviation to be present throughout the day since approximately age 2. A quick glance at the child reveals an obvious intermittent moderate-angle esotropia. It seems to be larger when the child plays with an object in his hands. Cycloplegic refraction reveals +1.50 D in both eyes. Which of the following is likely false?
    a. The deviation at distance is not likely to be large.
    b. The deviation at near is likely to be moderate (20 to 30 prism diopters).
    c. The deviation at near is likely to be lessened with +3.00 D lenses over each eye.
    d. The AC/A ratio is likely to be <5.

157. Which of the following regarding the treatment of esotropia is true?
    a. Accommodative esotropia is more likely to require surgical intervention than infantile esotropia.
    b. Bifocals are most helpful in the management of patients with refractive accommodative esotropia.
    c. If refractive correction fails to solve the problem, the only solution is surgical.
    d. Accommodative esotropia may progress over the first 5 to 7 years of life and should be monitored carefully.

158. Clinical features of esotropia that are predictive of the need for future surgical intervention include all of the following except
    a. presence of overaction of the inferior obliques.
    b. large-angle esotropia (>50 prism diopters).
    c. age of onset between 2 and 3 years.
    d. low hyperopia or myopia.

159. Which of the following regarding the treatment of accommodative esotropia is true?
    a. No improvement of esotropia with miotic therapy rules out the possibility of an accommodative component.
    b. Delay in refractive correction of an accommodative esotropia increases the probability of a permanent residual esotropia after full correction is given.
    c. It is important to attempt surgical realignment before prolonged occlusion therapy.
    d. Surgical realignment resulting in a residual esotropia of <20 prism diopters may permit the development of peripheral fusion.

160. In intermittent accommodative esotropia, some ophthalmologists do not prescribe full hyperopic correction because
    a. Distance vision will be blurred.
    b. The greater deviation at near will not be fully compensated.
    c. The patient may be converted to a constant esotropia without glasses.
    d. The patient may become exotropic with full hyperopic correction.

161. Divergence insufficiency resembles lateral rectus palsy except
    a. There is typically an esodeviation.
    b. The deviation is generally worse at distance.
    c. There are commonly no associated neurologic abnormalities.
    d. The deviation is comitant.

162. Findings that favor the diagnosis of spasm of the near reflex rather than accommodative esotropia include
    a. new hyperopia.
    b. esotropia worse at near than at distance.
    c. miosis on attempted lateral gaze.
    d. no vertical component.

163. The feature least consistent with acquired abducens paresis include all of the following except
    a. esotropia.
    b. deviation greater at distance than near.
    c. amblyopia.
    d. head turn toward the side of the paretic muscle.

164. An exodeviation that is greater at distance than at near is known as
    a. basic exotropia.
    b. divergence excess exotropia.
    c. basic exophoria.
    e. convergence insufficiency exotropia.

165. To distinguish true divergence excess exotropia from "simulated divergence excess" exotropia,
    a. The deviations are remeasured after cycloplegia.
    b. The AC/A ratio is calculated by the hetero-phoria method.
    c. The AC/A ratio is calculated by the gradient method.
    d. The deviations are remeasured after pro-longed (30–45 minutes) monocular occlusion.

166. The most common etiology for constant exotro-pia is
    a. decompensated intermittent exotropia.
    b. sensory exotropia.
    c. third nerve palsy.
    d. Duane's syndrome type II.

167. Clinical features frequently associated with intermittent exotropia include all of the follow-ing except
    a. variable angle of deviation.
    b. high AC/A ratio.
    c. reflex closure of one eye in bright light.
    d. amblyopia.

168. Useful treatment modalities for intermittent exotropia include
    a. plus lenses.
    b. phospholine iodide.
    c. base-in prism.
    d. bilateral rectus resections.

169. Clinical features of convergence insufficiency include all of the following except
    a. asthenopia.
    b. blurry reading vision.
    c. diplopia while reading.
    d. exophoria at near.

170. A patient presents for evaluation of "wandering eyes." On alternate-cover testing, with the left eye covered, the right eye fixes a distance target. As the cover is shifted to the right eye, the left eye moves down to pick up fixation. As the cover is moved back over the left eye, the right eye moves upward to reassume fixation. This set of findings is consistent with
    a. right hyperdeviation.
    b. left hyperdeviation.
    c. overaction of the inferior obliques.
    d. dissociated vertical deviation (DVD).

171. A patient presents for evaluation of "wandering eyes." On alternate-cover testing, with the left eye covered, the right eye fixes a distance target. As the cover is shifted to the right eye, the left eye moves down to pick up fixation. As the cover is shifted back over the left eye, the right does not move in order to reassume fixation. This set of findings is most consistent with
    a. right hyperdeviation.
    b. left hyperdeviation.
    c. overaction of the inferior obliques.
    d. dissociated vertical deviation (DVD).

172. A 4-year-old child with a moderate-angle eso-tropia is noted to have a left hypertropia on right gaze and a right hypertropia on left gaze. When fixing with the left eye in right gaze, there is a right hypotropia, and when fixing with the right eye in left gaze, there is a left hypotropia. The most likely clinical diagnosis is
    a. right hypotropia.
    b. left hypotropia.
    c. esotropia associated with overaction of the inferior oblique muscles.
    d. esotropia with DVD.

10

267

173. Which of the following features argue for a bilateral rather than a unilateral superior oblique paresis?
    a. head tilt.
    b. symptomatic excyclotorsion.
    c. a pattern esotropia.
    d. aggravation of diplopia with right or left head tilt.

174. Surgical strategies for the management of a right superior oblique paresis with symptomatic diplopia include all of the following except
    a. right inferior oblique myectomy.
    b. right superior oblique tuck.
    c. right inferior rectus recession.
    d. left superior oblique tenectomy.

175. The surgical procedure of choice in a superior oblique paresis with excyclotorsion only (no vertical diplopia) is the
    a. ipsilateral superior oblique tuck.
    b. ipsilateral inferior oblique myectomy.
    c. recession of the ipsilateral superior rectus muscle.
    d. lateral transposition of the superior oblique tendon.

176. In young healthy eyes, anterior segment ischemia becomes a concern after surgery on how many rectus muscles?
    a. 1.
    b. 2.
    c. 3.
    d. 4.

177. Of the following acuity tests, which is least likely to lead to an overestimation of actual recognition acuity?
    a. single Snellen letters.
    b. illiterate E.
    c. optotype cards.
    d. Allen cards.

178. All of the following are features consistent with double elevator palsy except
    a. ptosis.
    b. forced ductions indicating inferior rectus restriction.

    c. chin-down head position.
    d. poor Bell's phenomenon on the side of the palsy.

179. Which one of the following regarding Brown's syndrome is false?
    a. Both congenital and acquired forms exist.
    b. A common manifestation is hypotropia of the involved eye in adduction.
    c. Duction and version testing mimic weakness of the ipsilateral superior oblique muscle.
    d. Forced duction testing is necessary to confirm the diagnosis.

180. Late clinical findings consistent with an inferior blowout fracture of the orbit include all of the following except
    a. proptosis.
    b. paresthesia or hypesthesia of the infraorbital region.
    c. ipsilateral hypotropia on upgaze.
    d. ipsilateral hypertropia on downgaze.

181. Which of the following regarding A and V patterns of horizontal strabismus is true?
    a. A patterns must measure at least 15 prism diopters difference between upgaze and downgaze to be considered significant.
    b. V patterns must measure at least 10 prism diopters between upgaze and downgaze to be considered significant.
    c. These forms of noncomitance are seen in fewer than 5% of horizontal strabismus.
    d. All the extraocular muscles (in varying combinations) have been implicated as responsible for these patterns.

182. A patient presents with an exotropia measuring 15 prism diopters in primary position. In downgaze, it diminishes to <5 prism diopters, and in upgaze it increases to >30 prism diopters. There is no significant oblique muscle dysfunction noted. Appropriate surgical intervention might include all of the following except
    a. recession of the ipsilateral lateral rectus.
    b. resection of the ipsilateral medial rectus.
    c. upward transposition of the lateral rectus and downward transposition of the medial rectus.
    d. inferior oblique myectomy.

183. A patient presents with a 20-prism-diopter eso-tropia in primary gaze that increases to 35 prism diopters in downgaze and diminishes to 15 prism diopters in upgaze. There is overaction of the inferior obliques bilaterally. Appropriate surgical intervention might include all of the following except

    a. upward transposition of the lateral rectus and downward transposition of the medial rectus muscles ipsilaterally.
    b. recession of ipsilateral medial rectus muscle.
    c. resection of the ipsilateral lateral rectus muscle.
    d. bilateral inferior oblique myectomies.

184. The most common cause of third nerve palsy in the pediatric population is

    a. congenital.
    b. traumatic.
    c. inflammatory.
    d. tumor.

185. In adults, the most common cause of third nerve palsy is

    a. microvascular.
    b. traumatic.
    c. aneurysm.
    d. tumor.

186. Strabismus surgery for patients with Graves' ophthalmopathy generally is performed before

    a. orbital decompression.
    b. orbital radiation.
    c. tarsorrhaphy.
    d. eyelid surgery.

187. A child's nystagmus is noted to have equal velocity in all directions and to be symmetric in direction, amplitude, and frequency in each eye. The nystagmus would most appropriately be described as

    a. pendular, conjugate.
    b. jerk, conjugate.
    c. pendular, disconjugate.
    d. jerk, disconjugate.

188. Characteristics considered classic for spasmus nutans include all of the following except

    a. head nodding.
    b. a small-amplitude, disconjugate nystagmus.
    c. torticollis.
    d. hypertonia.

189. The entity in the differential diagnosis with spasmus nutans that must be ruled out is

    a. optic nerve meningioma.
    b. parasellar glioma.
    c. pontine glioma.
    d. cerebellar astrocytoma.

190. Treatment for a patient with congenital nystagmus whose null zone is in right gaze and who has adopted an extreme left head turn might include

    a. prism base down in both eyes.
    b. prism base in both eyes.
    c. prism base in the right eye and base out in the left eye.
    d. prism base out in the right eye and base in the left eye.

191. A 3-year-old child presents to the ophthalmologist with parents complaining of "cross-eyes" for approximately 1 year. Examination discloses visual acuity of 20/30 in the right eye and 20/100 in the left eye with Allen cards. There is a 35-prism-diopter esotropia at distance increasing to 45 prism diopters at near. Refraction reveals +3.50 D in both eyes. Initial steps in managing this patient should include

    a. bimedial recessions.
    b. bilateral resections.
    c. prescription of +3.50 in both eyes with add +3.50 in both eyes (bifocals).
    d. prescription of +3.50 D in both eyes and patching of the right eye.

10

269

192. A 7-year-old boy presents with an exotropia. His deviation measures 30 prism diopters in primary position, 20 prism diopters in right gaze, and 40 prism diopters in left gaze. Near deviation is 15 prism diopters in all directions. Fixation appears to alternate, and visual acuity is 20/20 in both eyes. The patient's parents strongly desire some form of correction. You recommend
    a. addition of −2.00 D to his current distance refraction.
    b. bilateral rectus recessions, equal on each side.
    c. bilateral rectus recessions with a greater distance of recession on the left.
    d. bilateral rectus recessions with a greater distance of recession on the right.

193. A patient presents with symptomatic vertical diplopia from a right hypertropia that is greatest in left eye: left upgaze and left downgaze. Appropriate surgical intervention could include all of the following except
    a. right superior oblique tuck.
    b. left superior oblique tenotomy.
    c. right inferior oblique myectomy.
    d. right superior rectus resection.

194. A 1-year-old child is brought to the ophthalmologist by his parents who have noted that "cross-eyes" developed over the previous 6 months. Your examination reveals an approximatcly 40-prism-diopter esotropia at near that does not seem to diminish significantly when the child fixes at longer distances. The child can maintain fixation with either eye easily. Cycloplegic refraction reveals +1.50 D in both eyes. An appropriate step in the management of this patient might next be
    a. prescription of +1.50 D glasses in both eyes.
    b. prescription of +1.50 D in both eyes with +3.50 add in both eyes.
    c. alternate patching throughout the day.
    d. bilateral rectus recession of 8 mm in both eyes.

195. After treating a child with mixed mechanism esotropia for 8 months with full hyperopic correction and occlusion therapy, surgery is

undertaken to realign his eyes. Visual acuity measures 20/50 in the right eye and 20/25 in the left eye with HOTV cards. There is an esotropia of 30 prism diopters in all directions of gaze. Appropriate surgical intervention would consist of
    a. bimedial rectus recession of 4.5 mm in both eyes.
    b. bilateral rectus resection of 7 mm in both eyes.
    c. bimedial rectus recession of 7 mm in both eyes.
    d. recession of the right medial rectus 4.5 mm and resection of the right lateral rectus 7 mm.

196. A 6-year-old patient presents to an ophthalmologist for the first time after failing a school eye examination. Complete ophthalmic examination discloses a visual acuity of 20/20 in the right eye and 20/100 in the left eye. There is a comitant left exotropia measuring 30 prism diopters. Cycloplegic refraction reveals +0.50 D in both eyes. A year of occlusion therapy of the right eye is undertaken, with little improvement in acuity in the left eye. The next step in the management of this patient might be
    a. prescription of −1.50 D in both eyes.
    b. base-in prism.
    c. bilateral rectus recession of 7 mm.
    d. recession of the left lateral rectus 7 mm and resection of the left medial rectus 6 mm.

197. Which of the following regarding diplopia after surgery for esotropia is true?
    a. Children with acquired strabismus are more likely to suffer from symptoms than adults.
    b. Postoperative diplopia is most likely to develop in undercorrection of intermittent exotropia.
    c. A trial of preoperative prisms may be helpful in predicting who is likely to suffer from this complication.
    d. The complication, if persistent, must be managed with a second surgical procedure.

198. A 2-year-old child undergoes bimedial recession for infantile esotropia. On the first post-operative day, the deviation is measured as <10 prism diopters of residual esotropia, with fairly good versions. At the 1-week visit, there is a prominent right exotropia, which increases in left gaze. Duction testing reveals an inability to adduct the right eye past the midline. The most likely diagnosis is
a. surgical undercorrection.
b. consecutive exotropia due to surgical overcorrection.
c. postoperative third nerve palsy.
d. lost or slipped right medial rectus.

199. Early signs in the development of malignant hyperthermia include all of the following except
a. tachycardia/arrhythmia.
b. elevated body temperature.
c. darkening of the blood in the operative field.
d. trismus.

200. The most common complication of botulinum injections is
a. vertical strabismus.
b. Adie's pupil.
c. ptosis.
d. perforation of the globe.

10

144. **c.** By the gradient method, AC/A ratio equals the difference in the deviation induced by a lens divided by the specific accommodative gradient (of an extra lens over the distance correction). Minus lenses stimulate accommodation, whereas plus lenses blunt it. Here, 50−35 divided by 1 = 15:1.

145. **b.** By the heterophoria method, the AC/A ratio equals the near deviation minus the distance deviation divided by the accommodative demand at near, plus the pupillary distance (PD) in centimeters. Here, this is
35 − 10 = 25,
divided by 5 (reading at 20 cm) = 5
plus 6 (PD in cm) = 11:1.

146. **a.** This patient presents with right hypertropia in primary gaze. Three step testing is presented here. The right hypertropia is worse on left gaze and worse on right head tilt. This maps to a right superior oblique palsy. In straight upgaze, there is a small exotropia or V pattern from the secondary abducting action of the overacting inferior oblique. In gazing down and to the patient's right, the left eye is slightly lower, reflecting the slight overaction of the normal left *superior oblique* muscle. This may be caused by a contracted or tight right superior rectus muscle from the chronic, longstanding higher right eye. The overaction of the opposite *superior oblique* is a common finding in these patients.

147. **c.** The clinical findings of mydriasis and accommodative paresis indicate damage to the parasympathetic supply to the globe. These nerves travel with the nerve to the inferior oblique before forming the short root of the ciliary ganglion. The motility findings in this case indicate a probable inferior oblique palsy (inability to elevate the adducted eye). The three-step test should show a left hypotropia (right hypertropia) worsened in right gaze and right head tilt.

148. **d.** Exaggerated sensitivity to cholinergic blockade has been reported in albinos and patients with Down's syndrome. Infants are also particularly sensitive. Atropine is a treatment for heart block (acutely) and should not cause arrhythmias in patients with this disorder.

149. **c.** Atropine's central nervous system side effects include both alerting/agitation and somnolence. Flushing and tachycardia are particularly common in infants.

150. **a.** This is a classic example of infantile esotropia. With cross-fixation, amblyopia is less likely to develop because the youngster will use each eye at different times. An accommodative component may be discovered in many cases of infantile esotropia. There is usually a large esotropia measuring more than 30 prism diopters as seen in this clinical photograph.

151. **b.** Latent nystagmus, overacting inferior obliques, and DVD are such common concomitants that they should be specifically sought in the examination of a child with infantile esotropia. A high AC/A ratio may be seen but is not typical.

152. **d.** Surgery for esotropia must provide either weakening of the medial rectus muscles (recession) or strengthening of the lateral rectus muscles (resection). Recession always has a greater effect than a resection of the same amount. Thus, bimedial recession is generally performed before bilateral resection. In some cases, however, bilateral resection may be the first procedure (for instance, in esotropia that is greater at distance). Combined medial and lateral resection is an equally effective alternative.

153. **b.** Amblyopia is certainly possible given the constant esotropia. A large-angle turn might provide cross-fixation, but amblyopia must be ruled out. Given the age of onset, an accommodative component is likely, so an originally intermittent turn is also possible. No patient with manifest strabismus has any stereopsis whatsoever. Certainly, a family history of esotropia of any mechanism is possible.

154. c. This patient probably has refractive accommodative esotropia. Amblyopia is possible bilaterally, given the high ametropia in both eyes. The deviation may be greater at near than distance, but this is not highly likely because patients with refractive accommodative esotropia typically have normal AC/A ratios. In this type of esotropia, the turn is usually moderate (20 to 40 prism diopters), although it may be greater. +3.00 lenses may lessen *non*refractive accommodative esotropia but typically have little effect on this type (with +3.00 lenses, there would still be a residual 5 D of hyperopia).

155. b. In all cases of accommodative esotropia, full hyperopic correction is warranted immediately. Penalization with atropine may be useful in cases of noncompliance with spectacles and/or patching therapy. Bifocals may be of value with high AC/A ratio with a residual turn at near after full correction.

156. d. This is probably a case of nonrefractive accommodative amblyopia (intermittent turn, worse at near, with normal refractive error and high AC/A ratio). +3.00 D lenses for near work will relieve the accommodative demand and prevent accommodative convergence from causing an esotropia.

157. d. Surgery is necessary in virtually all cases of infantile esotropia, whereas many cases of pure accommodative esotropia will resolve with time and refractive correction. Bifocals are generally most helpful in nonrefractive accommodative esotropia, where high AC/A ratios make the esotropia worse at near. If full refractive correction is not the solution, some experts advocate atropine penalization with full correction or pilocarpine treatment to provide accommodation without convergence. These steps frequently fail, however, and are controversial.

158. c. Age of onset between 2 and 3 years makes an accommodative mechanism more likely, with better prognosis for refractive correction. The other findings are consistent with a large-angle, congenital esotropia.

159. b. Persistent esotropia on pilocarpine treatment may be seen in accommodative esotropia, so spectacle correction must always be attempted. Surgical results are much more stable and predictable in the setting of maximal visual acuity (after occlusion therapy). Surgical realignment resulting in a residual esotropia of <10 prism diopters may permit the development of peripheral fusion.

160. c. Correction with full hyperopic prescription may weaken the patient's fusional divergence, which is the force keeping accommodative esotropia intermittent at its outset. Then, the esotropia may become constant without the "crutch" of the spectacles.

161. d. Divergence insufficiency is indistinguishable from sixth nerve palsy, except it is typically comitant. Sixth nerve palsy is more likely to have an esotropia at near as well.

162. c. New myopia favors the diagnosis of spasm of the near reflex; the myopia may be hard to establish if the spasm is intermittent, but the miosis is detectable and is the diagnostic "clincher." Also, the angle of turn is highly variable and unpredictable.

163. c. Unless the palsy is acquired early in childhood, goes untreated (with occlusion), and/or does not resolve, amblyopia is highly unlikely. Some children will develop a permanent esotropia after abducens palsy, probably representing a decompensated esophoria. Thus, all cases must be followed to resolution. Although many experts will obtain timely neuroimaging tests (CT/MRI), abducens palsy in a child is a common postviral syndrome and typically resolves uneventfully. The second most common etiology is increased intracranial pressure (central nervous system mass lesions, pseudotumor cerebri).

164. b. Exotropia that is equal at distance and near is basic. If the deviation is greater at near, then it

10

5. Systemic findings in a patient with the retinal pathology in the image below may include all of the following except
   a. Café-au-lait spots.
   b. Pancreatic and renal cysts.
   c. Hemangioblastomas of the brainstem.
   d. Pheochromocytoma.

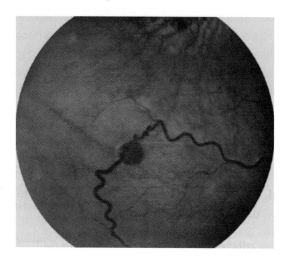

6. Which one of the following concerning aphakic or pseudophakic cystoid macular edema (CME) is false?
   a. The incidence of CME is lower with extracapsular surgery compared with intracapsular surgery.
   b. Intraocular lens implantation decreases the incidence of CME following cataract surgery.
   c. More than 75% of mild cases demonstrate regression within 6 months.
   d. Topical nonsteroidal anti-inflammatory medications have been shown to reduce the incidence as well as to improve vision in CME following cataract surgery.

7. Which of the following statements regarding Eales' disease is true?
   a. It is primarily a disease of childhood and young adulthood, more commonly affecting girls.
   b. It can be associated with tuberculosis, epistaxis, and cerebral vasculitis.
   c. It is generally bilateral.
   d. It generally affects males from the Middle East.

8. Which of the following statements regarding optical coherence tomography (OCT) is false?
   a. Obtaining retinal OCT images is generally not possible in eyes with dense vitreous hemorrhage because the light is unable to penetrate through the hemorrhage.
   b. Current OCT machines offer much better resolution than ultrasound.
   c. Fourier-domain OCT offers the ability for registration in order to measure changes in macular volume in the same patient during subsequent patient visits.
   d. Fourier-domain OCT offers better resolution images although they generally take longer to obtain than time-domain OCT.

9. Which of the following molecules is generally defective in Stargardt's disease?
   a. All-trans retinol.
   b. ATP-binding cassette transporter of the retina.
   c. 11-trans-retinaldehyde.
   d. Rhodopsin.

10. The pathology demonstrated in the image below anatomically represent breaks within
    a. The RPE.
    b. Bruch's membrane.
    c. Retinal photoreceptors.
    d. Outer plexiform layer.

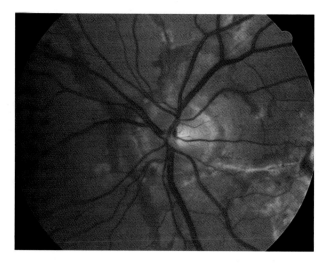

11. All of the following statements are true, except
    a. Nanophthalmos typically is characterized by thickened sclera that can impede outflow leading to uveal effusion syndrome.
    b. The choroid has the highest blood flow of any tissue in the human body.
    c. The vortex veins drain into the central retinal vein.
    d. The retinal pigment epithelium helps form the blood–ocular barrier.

12. All of the following statements regarding potential adverse effects from fluorescein angiography are true, except
    a. Anaphylaxis can occur after fluorescein angiography, but is rare and occurs at the rate of <1 in 100,000 injections.
    b. Urinary discoloration from fluorescein angiography occurs in <1% of patients.
    c. Vasovagal reactions and nausea occur in approximately 10% of injections.
    d. Premedication with antihistamines such as diphenhydramine can reduce the risk of developing an urticarial reaction from sodium fluorescein injection.

13. Which of the following concerning blood pressure–induced choroidal disease is false?
    a. Critical pathophysiologic events lead to occlusion of the choriocapillaris.
    b. Elschnig spots are characteristic.
    c. Exudative retinal detachment may develop as a secondary manifestation.
    d. Hypertensive choroidopathy may be associated with chronic elevation in systemic blood pressure.

14. What is the prevalence of endophthalmitis after an intravitreal triamcinolone injection?
    a. 0%
    b. 0.01% to 0.05%
    c. 0.1% to 0.3%
    d. 0.5% to 1.5%

15. Histopathologic features seen in the retinal vasculature of patients with early diabetic retinopathy include all of the following, except
    a. Loss of arteriolar pericytes.
    b. Thickening of endothelial basement membranes.
    c. Capillary closure and/or nonperfusion.
    d. Medial hyperplasia.

16. Fundus autofluorescence helps evaluate the function of which of the following structures within the eye?
    a. Retinal pigment epithelium.
    b. Bipolar cells.
    c. Ganglion cells.
    d. Retinal photoreceptors.

17. Which of the following regarding diabetic retinopathy is true?
    a. Visual prognosis is generally better in patients with diffuse macular edema than in those with focal macular edema.
    b. One of the definitions of clinically significant macular edema (CSME) from the Early Treatment for Diabetic Retinopathy Study (ETDRS) is the presence of any thickening >500 μm within the macula.
    c. Intraretinal microvascular abnormalities often lead to retinal neovascularization.
    d. Rhegmatogenous retinal detachment (of any type) is uncommon in proliferative diabetic retinopathy.

18. Which factor is most strongly correlated with the development of choroidal effusion following panretinal photocoagulation?
    a. Systemic hypertension.
    b. Increasing age.
    c. Total retinal surface area treated.
    d. Short axial length (<23 mm).

11

19. Each of the following is a valid conclusion of the Diabetes Control and Complications Trial (DCCT), except
    a. Among type 1 diabetics with no retinopathy, intensive treatment can lower the incidence of progressive retinopathy by a factor of five compared with conventional treatment.
    b. Patients with macular edema realize the benefits of intensive control sooner than patients with proliferative retinopathy.
    c. The early worsening seen in patients initiating intensive control has no long-term effect on severity of retinopathy, and the benefit of intensive control is not seen for the first 3 to 5 years of treatment.
    d. The study only tested type 1 diabetics and the conclusions reached may not necessarily apply to type 2 diabetics.

20. All of the following are generally unfavorable clinical prognostic features for visual stabilization following laser treatment of diabetic macular edema, except
    a. Macular nonperfusion.
    b. Cystoid macular edema.
    c. Extensive hard exudation within the fovea.
    d. Focal leakage and thickening.

21. Which one of the following characteristics is felt to confer the greatest protection from the development of proliferative diabetic retinopathy?
    a. Complete posterior vitreous detachment (PVD).
    b. Younger age (<30 years).
    c. Ipsilateral carotid artery stenosis.
    d. No history of hypertension.

22. Which of the following statements regarding diabetic retinopathy is true?
    a. The ETDRS showed that focal laser treatment of clinically significant diabetic macular edema leads to an improvement in vision in twice as many treated patients as untreated patients.
    b. The Diabetic Retinopathy Study (DRS) showed that panretinal photocoagulation (PRP) could reduce the incidence of severe visual loss in certain patients by 50%.

    c. One definition of high-risk proliferative diabetic retinopathy mandating immediate PRP neovascularization is optic disc neovascularization covering greater than half of its area (greater than standard photograph 10A), only if associated with vitreous hemorrhage.
    d. One definition of high-risk proliferative diabetic retinopathy is moderate to severe neovascularization elsewhere, only if associated with vitreous hemorrhage.

23. When performed properly, which of the following is *not* a potential adverse effect of panretinal photocoagulation?
    a. Decreased night vision.
    b. Angle-closure glaucoma.
    c. Iris atrophy.
    d. Decreased reading acuity.

24. Which one of the following concerning hemoglobinopathy and retinopathy is false?
    a. The incidence of proliferative retinopathy is higher in patients with sickle cell thalassemia (Hb SThal) than in patients with SS disease (Hb SS).
    b. The incidence of sickle cell trait (Hb AS) in the African American population is approximately 8% and that of SC disease (Hb SC) in the African American population is <0.5%.
    c. Retinopathy has not been reported in patients with sickle cell trait (Hb AS).
    d. The ocular findings of SC disease (Hb SC) are not limited to the retina.

25. Which of the following statements is false?
    a. Like diabetic retinopathy, the earliest pathophysiologic changes in proliferative (SC) retinopathy include capillary closure and drop out.
    b. Like diabetic retinopathy, SC retinopathy may have both nonproliferative and proliferative forms.
    c. Salmon patches, iridescent deposits, and black sunbursts are hallmarks of proliferative sickle cell retinopathy
    d. Vitreous hemorrhage, parafoveal capillary nonperfusion, retinal detachment, and choroidal neovascularization are all potential causes of severe visual loss in sickle cell disease.

11

26. It is the end of summer, and a 50-year-old diabetic male is hospitalized for encephalitis. He denies recent travel history, but recalls being bitten by many mosquitoes while playing golf last week. He complains of blurred vision in his left eye (image below). Which of the following is most likely true regarding the etiology of this patient's disease?
    a. The etiology of this patient's clinical findings is infectious with cats being the natural host.
    b. These retinal findings are most likely related to diabetic retinopathy and unrelated to the encephalitis.
    c. Vitritis would be an uncommon finding given the clinical scenario.
    d. There is currently no proven systemic treatment for this patient.

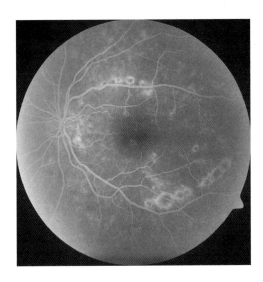

27. Which of the following statements concerning branch retinal vein occlusion (BRVO) is false?
    a. The superotemporal quadrant is the most commonly affected.
    b. Risk factors for BRVO include glaucoma, retinal detachment, and hypertension.
    c. Complications of BRVO include macular ischemia, retinal neovascularization, and rubeosis.
    d. Both long-acting steroid and anti-VEGF intravitreal injections have been effective in managing macular edema secondary to BRVO.

28. Which of the following statements regarding the Branch Vein Occlusion Study (BVOS) is false?
    a. The BVOS documented recovery of a final visual acuity of 20/40 or better in 50% more patients treated with argon macular grid laser (compared with those who were untreated).
    b. Quadrantic scatter photocoagulation reduces the risk of vitreous hemorrhage in eyes with established neovascularization.
    c. Quadrantic scatter photocoagulation reduces the risk of developing neovascularization if the area of retinal ischemia on angiography is at least five disc areas in size.
    d. Large areas of nonperfusion were a significant risk factor for the development of neovascularization, but quadrantic scatter photocoagulation is not recommended in patients solely with areas of retinal nonperfusion (i.e., without retinal neovascularization).

29. Which one of the following concerning solar retinopathy is false?
    a. It is generally associated with sun gazing and, less commonly, arc welding.
    b. The lesion is a photochemical and photothermal insult to the RPE.
    c. Visual acuity loss is generally severe, in the hand motions to counting fingers range.
    d. The lesion appears as a small yellow white spot in the center of the fovea that fades over time, often leaving permanent focal RPE changes.

30. What diagnosis should be considered in a 30-year-old male with a history of bilateral giant retinal tears, cleft palate, severe myopia, severe arthritis requiring a total hip replacement, and a family history of severe arthritis and blindness?
    a. Ehlers-Danlos syndrome.
    b. Marfan's syndrome.
    c. Stickler's syndrome.
    d. Weill-Marchesani syndrome.

31. The key feature on electroretinography distinguishing focal or nonprogressive retinal disease from a diffuse progressive degeneration is an abnormality in the
    a. a-wave amplitude.
    b. b-wave amplitude.
    c. c-wave amplitude.
    d. b-wave implicit time.

11

291

32. The electrooculogram (EOG) may be valuable in evaluating patients with potential retinal toxicity from
    a. Amiodarone.
    b. Chloroquine.
    c. Phenothiazines.
    d. Isoniazid.

33. Which of the following conditions is generally not associated with Purtscher or Purtscher-like retinopathy?
    a. Systemic lupus erythematosus (SLE).
    b. Thrombotic thrombocytopenic purpura (TTP).
    c. Long-bone fractures.
    d. Hepatorenal syndrome.

34. Which of the following is generally not considered a function of visual evoked cortical potential testing?
    a. To help assess visual acuity in infants with a checkerboard stimulus.
    b. To help assess RPE function when retinal function is relatively normal.
    c. To help evaluate visual acuity potential in patients with dense cataracts.
    d. To help identify visual field defects.

35. Which of the following statements is true regarding color vision testing?
    a. Ishihara color plate testing is equally sensitive to Farnsworth Panel D-15 testing in classifying color deficiency, but can be performed significantly faster.
    b. Patients with congenital color deficiencies demonstrate irregular patterns on the D-15 test, whereas patients with acquired optic nerve damage generally demonstrate more classic patterns.
    c. Blue–yellow confusion errors are easily demonstrated with D-15 testing and generally signify congenital disease.
    d. Farnsworth-Munsell 100-hue testing is very sensitive but can be time consuming and cause fatigue.

36. In which of the following subset of patients is central serous chorioretinopathy relatively (CSCR) uncommon?
    a. African Americans.
    b. Type-A middle-aged males.
    c. Patients with elevated corticosteroid levels.
    d. Patients with a family history of CSCR.

37. Which of the following statements regarding indocyanine green (ICG) angiography is false?
    a. ICG angiography is useful in distinguishing between occult choroidal neovascularization and idiopathic polypoidal choroidal vasculopathy.
    b. ICG angiography should not be performed in patients with a known allergy to iodide.
    c. ICG angiography has a lower incidence of side effects than does fluorescein angiography.
    d. ICG angiography is useful in detecting occult diabetic retinopathy.

38. Which one of the following statements concerning Leber's congenital amaurosis (LCA) is false?
    a. In LCA, the infant is typically blind and the electroretinogram is typically minimal or non-recordable at birth.
    b. In LCA, the fundus examination is typically normal at birth.
    c. Gene therapy with complementary DNA using an adenoviral-associated vector has demonstrated improvement in vision in patients with LCA.
    d. The most common pattern of inheritance in LCA is autosomal dominant.

39. Preservation of visual acuity past the age of 45 years in a patient with a retinal degeneration and an X-linked inheritance pattern suggests the diagnosis of
    a. Recessive cone–rod degeneration.
    b. Gyrate atrophy.
    c. Refsum's disease.
    d. Choroideremia.

11

40. Which of the following statements regarding gyrate atrophy is true?
    a. It is inherited on an X-linked recessive basis.
    b. There is a systemic deficiency in ornithine aminotransferase activity.
    c. Serum abnormalities include hyperornithinemia and hyperlysinemia.
    d. Life span is markedly decreased in this disorder.

41. Which of the following concerning fundus flavimaculatus is true?
    a. The pisciform lesions seen in the posterior fundus represent lipofuscin-like deposits at the level of the RPE cells.
    b. 50% of cases are autosomal recessive.
    c. Visual acuity loss is usually severe and most patients become legally blind by the age of 50.
    d. On angiography, about 15% of patients have the finding of a "dark choroid," where the choroid is hypofluorescent.

42. Which form of congenital dyschromatopsia is accompanied by abnormally low visual acuity?
    a. Protanopia.
    b. Deuteranopia.
    c. Tritanopia.
    d. Rod monochromatism.

43. Which of the following statements is false regarding Refsum's disease?
    a. Both infantile and adult forms exist.
    b. Night blindness can be an early symptom in patients.
    c. Phytanic acid levels are typically elevated.
    d. Phytanic acid oxidase activity is increased in cultured fibroblasts.

44. What proportion of patients with intracranial hemorrhage have Terson's syndrome?
    a. 10%.
    b. 33%.
    c. 50%.
    d. 90%.

45. Which of the following regarding familial drusen is false?
    a. The initial fundus manifestations generally appear in the third decade of life.

b. Mutations in the gene EFEMP1 encoding an extracellular matrix protein are responsible for Doyne's honeycomb dystrophy.
    c. Clinical presentation can be quite variable.
    d. The ERG is generally markedly depressed.

46. Which of the following conditions would explain the electroretinogram found in the picture below (assume that the top line represents the right eye and the bottom line represents the left eye)?
    a. Ocular ischemic syndrome.
    b. Retinitis pigmentosa.
    c. Stargardt's disease.
    d. Proliferative diabetic retinopathy

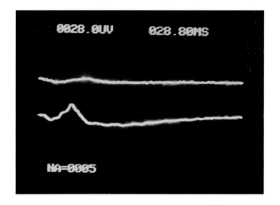

47. Which of the following treatment modalities should be considered in a macular degeneration patient with the fundus as shown?
    a. Monthly intravitreal injections of ranibizumab.
    b. Combination of monthly intravitreal bevacizumab and photodynamic therapy.
    c. Triple therapy: intravitreal bevacizumab, photodynamic therapy, and intravitreal steroid therapy.
    d. Observation.

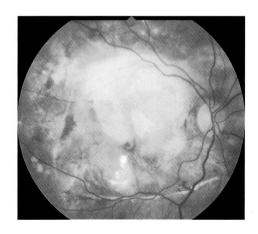

11

59. Which one of the following concerning fluorescein angiography and the blood–ocular barrier is true?
    a. Fluorescein is a high molecular weight compound normally confined to the intravascular space.
    b. Fluorescein absorbs light in the yellow–green range (530 nm) and, once excited, emits light in the blue range (490 nm).
    c. The "red-free" filter is the initial filter through which white light passes before entering the eye.
    d. Autofluorescence images cannot be acquired after intravenous fluorescein injection.

60. Which of the following concerning the characteristics of hyperfluorescence patterns on fluorescein angiography is false?
    a. Staining generally refers to the uptake of fluorescein by solid collagenous tissue.
    b. Transmitted fluorescence, or a window defect, generally implies a focal defect in the retinal pigment epithelium.
    c. Pooling implies collections of fluorescein within fluid-filled spaces.
    d. True leakage consists of early hyperfluorescence that diminishes in late views.

61. Which of the following with regard to the classification of age related macular degeneration (AMD) is false?
    a. Nonexudative AMD accounts for 90% of all patients affected by this disorder.
    b. Exudative AMD accounts for 90% of all patients with severe visual loss (worse than 20/200) who are affected by this disorder.
    c. Patients with either pigment epithelial detachment or choroidal neovascularization should be considered to have exudative AMD.
    d. In patients with nonexudative AMD, those with central geographic atrophy generally preserve the best visual acuity.

62. A randomized clinical trial has documented that vitreous surgery with gas–fluid exchange and prone positioning offers no long-term benefit

relative to observation for which of the following conditions:
    a. Idiopathic macular hole, stage 1.
    b. Idiopathic macular hole, stages 1 and 2.
    c. Idiopathic macular hole, stages 1, 2, and 3.
    d. Idiopathic macular hole, regardless of stage.

63. The prevalence of a full-thickness macular hole in the fellow eye of a patient with an established full-thickness macular hole is approximately
    a. <10%.
    b. 15% to 25%.
    c. 25% to 50%.
    d. >75%.

64. The lesion that is felt to be an immediate precursor to a full-thickness macular hole is
    a. A complete posterior vitreous detachment.
    b. A macular cyst.
    c. A sensory retinal detachment involving the fovea.
    d. A subfoveal pigment epithelial detachment.

65. Which of the following concerning ocular toxicity of hydroxychloroquine and chloroquine is false?
    a. Both hydroxychloroquine and chloroquine have been clearly associated with retinal toxicity and may also be associated with a vortex keratopathy.
    b. Obese patients are generally at lower risk of developing toxicity than "leaner" patients.
    c. Important tests in the evaluation for subclinical chloroquine retinopathy include color vision testing and threshold central visual field testing.
    d. Vision loss from hydroxychloroquine toxicity generally does not recover and can progress even after discontinuation of hydroxychloroquine.

66. Which of the following drugs most likely resulted in the retinopathy shown in the image at the top of the next page?
    a. Thioridazine.
    b. Hydroychloroquine.
    c. Talc.
    d. Tamoxifen.

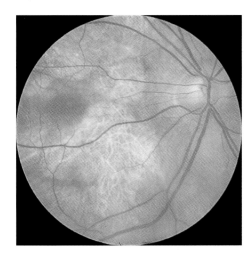

67. A 30-year-old presents with fundus findings demonstrated in the image below as well as peripheral retinal neovascularization. The patient is most likely:
   a. A longstanding intravenous drug abuser.
   b. A young female using oral contraceptives with a history of systemic lupus erythematosus.
   c. A hepatitis C–positive patient with significant abdominal distention.
   d. A patient treated with intravitreal ranibizumab for age-related macular degeneration.

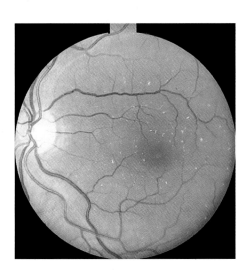

68. Which disease should one suspect in a young boy with vascular attenuation, optic atrophy, peripheral pigmentary loss, seizures, and a history of progressive dementia?
   a. Usher's syndrome.
   b. Retinitis pigmentosa.
   c. Leber congenital amaurosis.
   d. Batten's disease.

69. Which of the following molecules is likely defective in a patient with the fundus photograph shown below?
   a. Hexosaminidase A.
   b. Alpha-galactosidase A.
   c. Apolipoprotein B.
   d. Ornithine aminotransferase.

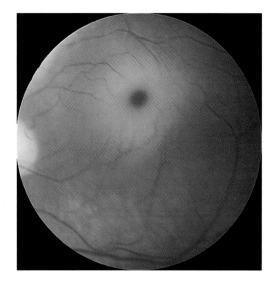

70. The mother of a young Puerto-Rican child with the fundus similar to the one shown below should be queried as to:
   a. Whether her son has asthma or breathing difficulty.
   b. Whether her son bruises easily.
   c. Whether her son has been abusing intravenous drugs.
   d. Whether her son has developmental delay.

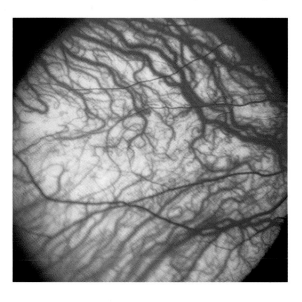

11

297

71. Which of the following disorders is considered a form of congenital stationary night blindness (CSNB)?
    a. Oguchi's disease.
    b. Fundus flavimaculatus.
    c. Retinitis punctata albescens.
    d. Leber congenital amaurosis.

72. Symptoms of cone dystrophies can include all of the following, except:
    a. Progressive loss of visual acuity.
    b. Hemeralopia.
    c. Anisometropia.
    d. Photophobia.

73. Which of the following is not an area of firm vitreoretinal attachment?
    a. The vitreous base.
    b. The edge of retinal scars.
    c. The edge of the optic nerve.
    d. The vortex veins.

74. Which of the following statements regarding posterior vitreous detachments is false?
    a. The prevalence of posterior vitreous detachment (PVD) is higher after intracapsular cataract surgery than after extracapsular cataract surgery.
    b. Less than 20% of patients with a symptomatic PVD actually have a retinal tear.
    c. More than 50% of patients with an acute symptomatic PVD and associated vitreous hemorrhage on clinical examination also have a retinal tear.
    d. OCT has demonstrated that vitreous detachments often start at the optic disc and spread temporally.

75. Which of the following statements regarding lattice degeneration is true?
    a. The prevalence of lattice retinal degeneration in the adult population is approximately between 5% and 10%.
    b. More than 75% of all eyes with a rhegmatogeneous retinal detachment (RRD) exhibit lattice degeneration.

    c. Lattice degeneration is bilateral in over 75% of cases.
    d. Lattice degeneration is much less common in high myopes.

76. A patient with the 3D OCT findings below is seen in your clinic. Which of the following is least likely?
    a. Spontaneous resolution may occur.
    b. Complete posterior vitreous detachment likely occurred in the past.
    c. Surgery may be indicated, depending on symptoms.
    d. Angiography may demonstrate leakage of fluorescein dye from retinal vessels in the macular region as well as from the optic nerve.

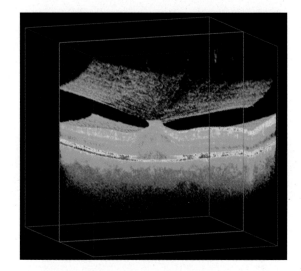

77. A 17-year-old boy presents with complaints of difficulty reading his schoolwork. He is completely healthy. Visual acuities measure 20/80 in the right eye and 20/100 in the left eye. Fundus photographs and angiography are shown at the top of the next page. Which one of the following is false regarding his case?
    a. One of his parents almost certainly has similar findings.
    b. His ERG may be normal.
    c. Examination of his peripheral retina may show yellow–white flecks.
    d. His visual fields may be normal, but he can be counseled to expect further visual loss.

11

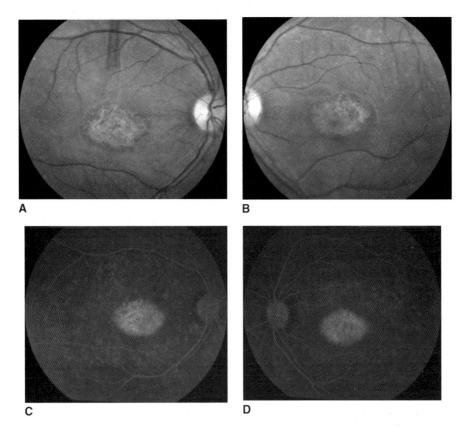

A   B

C   D

78. A 58-year-old man with essential hypertension is referred to a retinal specialist with "rule out cystoid macular edema" 4 weeks after uncomplicated phacoemulsification on his right eye. His best corrected acuity is 20/40 in the right eye and 20/200 in the left eye. Examination of the right eye shows a quiet pseudophakic anterior segment. The vitreous is clear bilaterally. There is a posterior subcapsular cataract in the left eye felt sufficient to account for his acuity. His fundi are shown below. Peripherally, he has bilateral inferior retinal detachments that shift with head position. No retinal breaks are seen. A fluorescein angiogram for the right eye is shown below (angiographic quality for the left eye was poor due to the cataract). Which one of the following regarding this man is true?

a. Therapy should include retrobulbar steroid and a topical nonsteroidal agent.
b. Therapy should include laser photocoagulation of the right macula.
c. Therapy should include oral steroids.
d. The patient should be promptly referred to his internist.

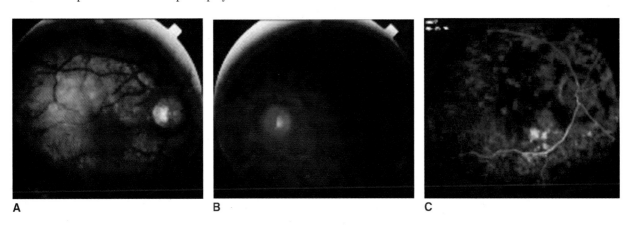

A   B   C

79. A 75-year-old woman presents to you complaining of painless decreased vision in her left eye worsening over the past 6 hours. She denies any other systemic problems and has no other medical history. Blood pressure, measured in your clinic, is 145/90. Ophthalmic examination reveals a visual acuity of 20/20 OD and CF at 6 ft OS. Ophthalmic examination reveals a normal right eye, an RAPD OS, and the left fundus as shown below. Which of the following would be the most appropriate next step?

a. Obtain a serum ANA, ACE, lysozyme, HLA-B27 haplotype testing, and place a PPD.

b. Obtain a serum erythrocyte sedimentation rate and C-reactive protein.

c. If the patient does not have a history of jaw claudication, initiate ASA 325 mg sublingually.

d. Obtain an FTA-Abs and VDRL.

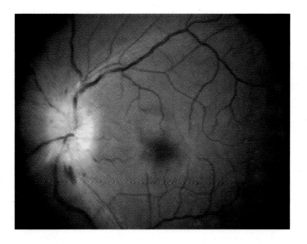

80. A 20-year-old male presents with the findings in image shown at the top of the next column. Which of the following statements with regard to the condition shown above is true?

a. The condition is usually inherited in an autosomal dominant fashion.

b. The retinal pathology is typically in the outer plexiform layer.

c. A late petalloid leakage pattern seen with fluorescein angiography is pathognomonic.

d. Mutations of the gene responsible for this condition lead to Müller's cell degeneration.

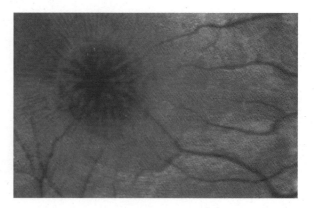

81. A 45-year-old man complains of blurry vision in his right eye that has gradually worsened over the past 2 years. His right fundus is shown below. There are no other abnormalities that you detect in his right eye. Which of the following statements regarding the condition shown is true?

a. The condition is typically bilateral.

b. Patients with this condition generally have a good visual prognosis.

c. Amazingly, the lesions shown generally do not create any visual field deficits.

d. The condition generally is not chronic.

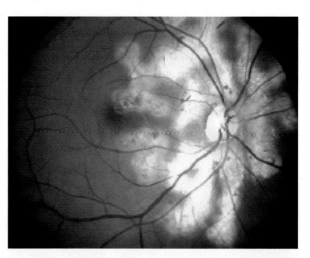

82. Which of the following statements regarding the condition shown (image at the top of the next page) is true?

a. Most cases of this condition are bilateral.

b. Visual acuity in patients with this condition is generally <20/200.

c. The prevalence of this condition is increased in patients with diabetes.

d. The condition is common in young Asian males.

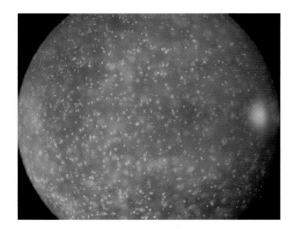

83. A 20-year-old Jewish man complains of blurry vision bilaterally and difficulty driving at night. The fundus of his right eye (shown below) is very similar to the that of his left eye. Which of the following statements regarding the condition shown is false?

   a. The condition can be inherited via several inheritance patterns.

   b. Night blindness is one of the earliest symptoms of the disorder.

   c. An ERG would typically show reduction of both a-wave and b-wave amplitudes.

   d. The presence of bone spicules and chorioretinal atrophy is virtually pathognomonic for the condition.

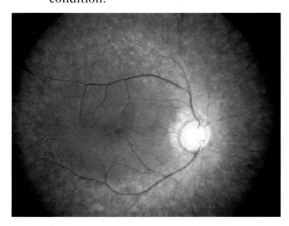

84. An 8-year-old boy is having difficulty seeing in his left eye. His ophthalmic (including funduscopy) examination is normal except for his left fundus. A peripheral photograph of his left fundus is shown at the top of the next column. Which of the following statements is true regarding the patient's condition?

   a. Although not so in this specific case, most cases of this condition are bilateral.

   b. The condition is typically inherited in an X-linked recessive pattern and has a high male preponderance.

   c. The condition can generally be managed with a single session of laser photocoagulation or cryotherapy.

   d. Although it can occur, retinal neovascularization is not common.

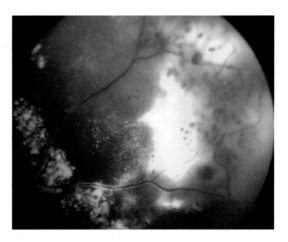

85. A 10-year-old boy is found to have the fundus appearance shown below. Which of the following statements is true regarding the patient's condition?

   a. The condition is typically unilateral and idiopathic.

   b. The ERG is generally normal, and the EOG is abnormal in eyes with this condition.

   c. Visual acuity is generally 20/200 or worse at the stage shown.

   d. To date, the gene responsible for this condition has not been identified.

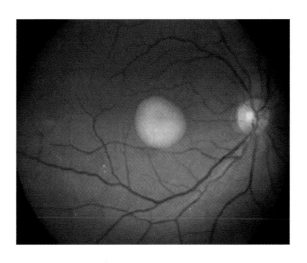

11

86. Which of the following statements regarding the condition shown below is true?
    a. The condition can be a precursor for malignant transformation.
    b. The condition typically leads to rhegmatogenous retinal detachments.
    c. The condition has been associated with nystagmus and amblyopia in the past.
    d. The condition requires cryotherapy or laser in symptomatic patients in order to prevent retinal detachments.

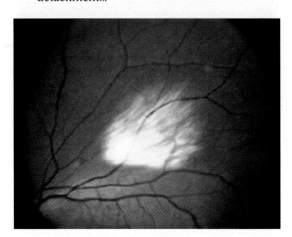

87. Which of the following statements regarding the condition shown below is true?
    a. The most likely diagnosis is an ophthalmic artery obstruction.
    b. An ESR and CRP should be drawn to rule out giant cell arteritis in patients who present with this condition.
    c. The most likely diagnosis is iatrogenic subretinal silicone oil after pars plana vitrectomy.
    d. Sphingolipidoses are usually the cause of this condition.

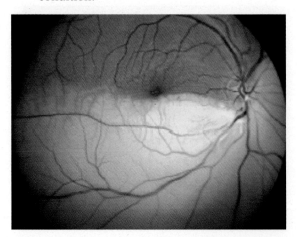

88. Which of the following statements regarding the condition shown below is true?
    a. A defect in the gene for fibrillin is the most common systemic disease associated with the condition.
    b. Photodynamic therapy (PDT) currently has no known role in the treatment of this condition.
    c. Fluorescein angiography of the eye shown above will most likely demonstrate early hypofluorescence followed by late staining.
    d. Up to half of all patients with this condition will have no systemic medical condition.

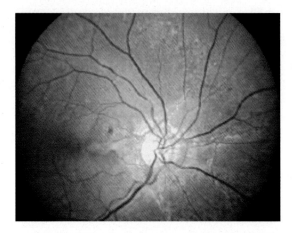

89. A 25-year-old woman complains of blurry vision in her right eye over the past 3 days. She denies any past medical or ocular history. Anterior segment exam is normal bilaterally. Her right fundus and angiogram are shown below and at the top of the next page. Which of the following statements is true?
    a. The condition shown is generally unilateral.
    b. Visual prognosis is generally poor.
    c. The condition can be associated with a fatal vasculitis.
    d. The vast majority of patients have a viral prodrome before visual loss occurs.

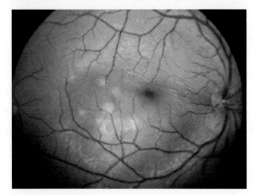

11

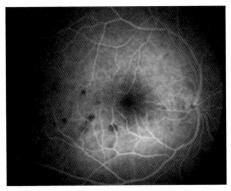

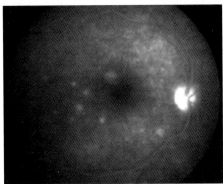

91. Which of the following statements regarding the condition shown in the next column is true?
    a. The condition shown is a posterior staphyloma.
    b. AIDS patients presenting with this condition must obtain neuroimaging.
    c. This particular patient will likely need a prolonged course of steroids to help preserve visual acuity.
    d. Folic acid is used in patients being treated for this condition to protect against thrombocytopenia and leukopenia.

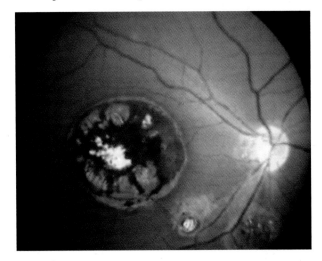

90. Which of the following statements regarding the pathology shown below is true?
    a. Visual acuity in this patient is probably normal.
    b. If this eye is from a type 2 diabetic patient, early vitrectomy may be indicated.
    c. If this eye is from a type 1 diabetic patient with severe proliferative diabetic retinopathy, early vitrectomy may be beneficial.
    d. Hypertension is the most frequent cause of this condition in adults.

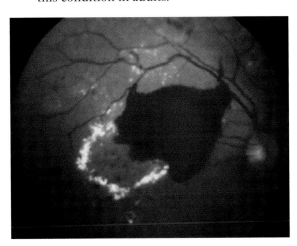

92. A 39-year-old retinal surgeon complains of the onset of blurry vision in his left eye over the past week. Ophthalmic examination is normal bilaterally, except for the left fundus, which is shown in the next page. To confirm your diagnosis, you decide to obtain a fluorescein angiogram, part of which is depicted at the top of the next page. Which of the following statements is true?
    a. The leakage pattern shown on the late frame of the angiogram occurs in most cases and is pathognomonic.
    b. More than half of all eyes with this condition eventually develop permanently reduced visual acuity.
    c. Given his occupational needs, early focal photocoagulation in this patient would be the treatment of choice.
    d. Reduced fluence photodynamic therapy may be of benefit if his symptoms do not resolve.

11

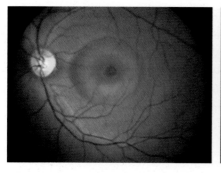
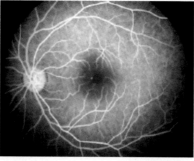
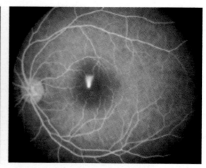

93. Which of the following most likely represents the condition shown below?
    a. Retinitis punctata albescens.
    b. Fundus albipunctatus.
    c. Oguchi's disease.
    d. Enhanced S-cone syndrome.

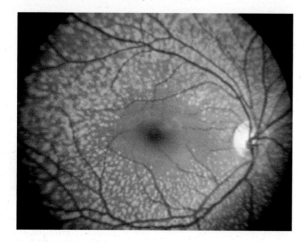

94. A 28-year-old Asian female with perilimbal vitiligo complains of blurry vision bilaterally, which has dramatically worsened over the past 2 days. She denies any past medical or ocular history or any recent history of trauma. Her left fundus is shown below. Two frames from a fluorescein angiogram (FA) are also shown below. Which of the following statements is true?
    a. The patient most likely has sympathetic ophthalmia.
    b. The patient most likely has endophthalmitis.
    c. Most patients with this condition develop Sugiura's sign.
    d. The prognosis of this condition is generally poor.

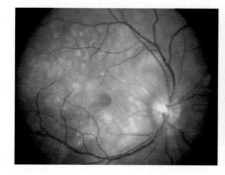
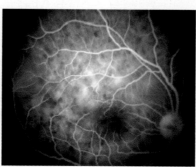
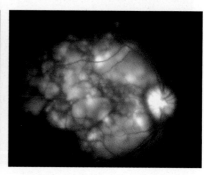

11

95. A 50-year-old man complains of fever, malaise, and visual loss in his right eye 2 weeks ago. The right eye fundus is shown below. Which of the following statements is false?
   a. Given his history, the most likely etiologic agent for his condition is Bartonella henselae.
   b. Oral ciprofloxacin is an effective treatment for this patient.
   c. The patient may have a painful lymphadenopathy as well.
   d. This patient will likely have a chronic recurrent course with poor visual prognosis.

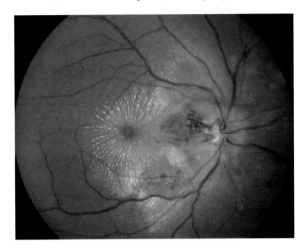

96. Which of the following conditions in a patient with a history of limbal opacities is most likely to represent the fundus shown below?
   a. Hydroxychloroquine retinopathy (retinal crystals and cornea verticillata).
   b. Bietti crystalline corneoretinal dystrophy.
   c. Cystinosis.
   d. Synchysis scintillans.

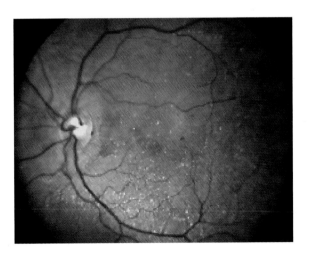

97. A 65-year-old man undergoes uncomplicated phacoemulsification and PCIOL implantation in his right eye. Two months later, he complains of blurry vision in his right eye, but his vision remains 20/20 in that eye. An FA is performed and is shown below. Which of the following statements regarding the patient's condition is false?
   a. The patient has Irvine-Gass syndrome.
   b. The patient's condition will most likely spontaneously resolve.
   c. Angiographic evidence of this condition is more common than clinical evidence.
   d. The peak incidence of this condition is generally within 2 weeks after surgery.

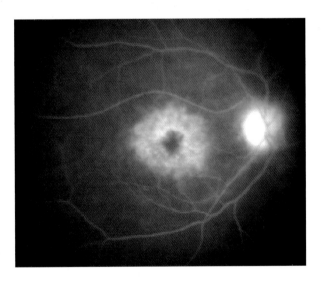

98. A 70-year-old Japanese man complains of visual loss in his left eye. His right eye reveals a few scattered macular drusen. Fluorescein and ICG angiography frames are shown at the top of the next page. Which of the following statements regarding this man's condition is true?
   a. The condition shown usually occurs in women.
   b. Retinal neovascularization commonly occurs as shown by ICG angiography.
   c. This condition often shows serosanguinous detachments of the retina.
   d. Multiple confluent drusen are common in this condition.

11

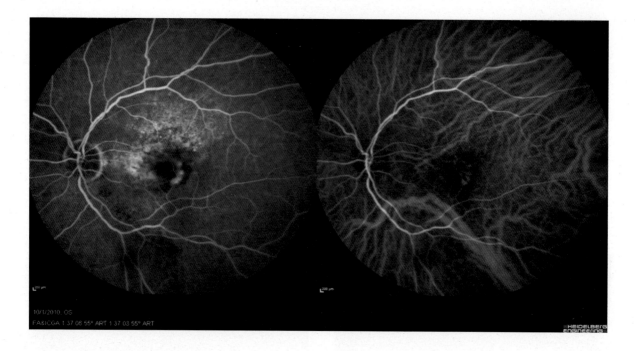

99. Mutations in what gene could result in the angiogram shown below, assuming that the left eye had a very similar appearance?
    a. Peripherin/RDS.
    b. Rhodopsin.
    c. Ornithine aminotransferase.
    d. Guanylate cyclase activator 1A.

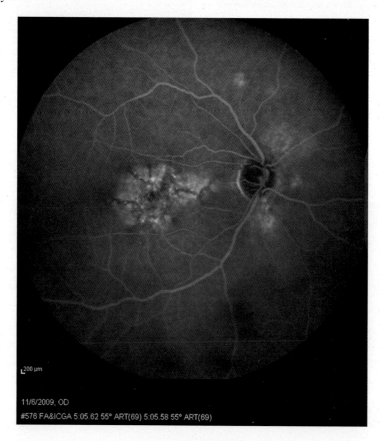

100. A 95-year-old female complains of longstanding severe visual loss in both eyes. Her right eye looks very similar to her left. What would your best recommendation for treatment be?

   a. Monthly bilateral intravitreal ranibizumab.

   b. Reduced fluence photodynamic therapy.

   c. Submacular surgery.

   d. Referral to a low vision specialist.

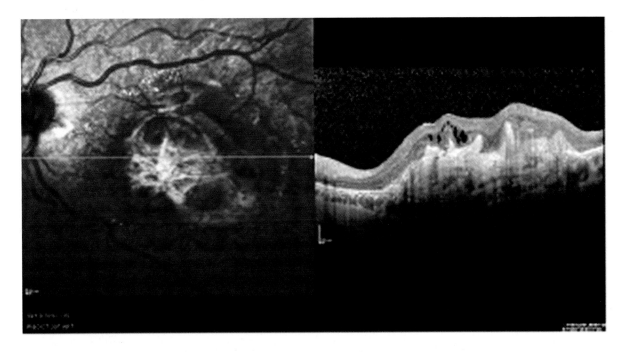

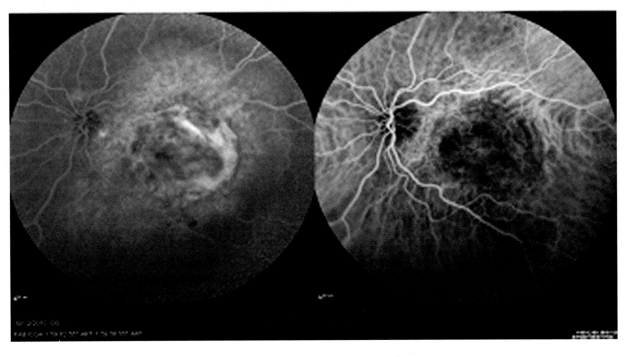

11

101. An 80-year-old female with a history of exudative age-related macular degeneration was receiving intravitreal ranibizumab therapy. After four injections, her choroidal neovascularization regressed and her vision improved from 20/800 pretreatment to 20/60. After her fifth injection, her vision worsened from 20/60 to 20/200. What does the autofluorescence image below most likely represent?

a. A tear in the retinal pigment epithelium.

b. Extension of geographic atrophy from her macular degeneration.

c. The development of subfoveal hemorrhage after intravitreal injection.

d. Recurrence of her choroidal neovascularization refractory of anti-VEGF therapy.

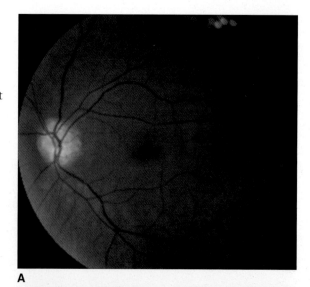

A

B

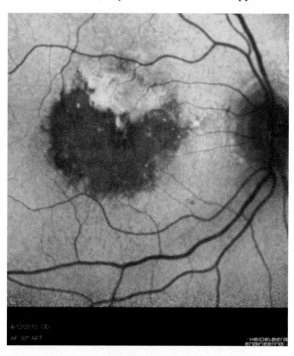

102. A red-free image and an autofluorescence image of a 20-year-old healthy female are shown in images A and B at the top of the next column. Which of the following statements regarding the condition shown is false?

a. This condition rarely affects non-Caucasians.

b. Most patients have some type of visual field defect.

c. Oral acetazolamide has been shown to improve visual field defects in some cases.

d. The condition may be associated with pseudoxanthoma elasticum.

103. A 52-year-old man with a history of hypertension, hyperlipidemia, type 2 diabetes, and previous history of lung cancer (treated with prior chemotherapy with no known metastasis) complains of gradually worsening vision in his right eye. His blood pressure in your clinic measures 170/80. His fundus photograph and autofluorescence image of his right eye are shown at the top of the next page in left column. After your examination, the next appropriate step would be:

a. Referring him to his internist for better hypertension control.

b. Immediately referring him back to his oncologist and obtaining neuroimaging.

c. Obtaining serum ESR and CRP levels.

d. Obtaining serum HLA-A29 testing.

11

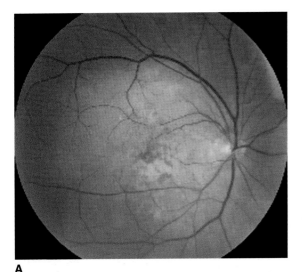

A

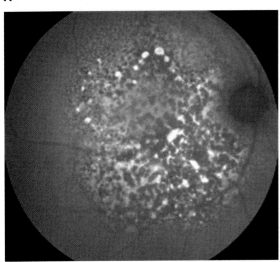

B

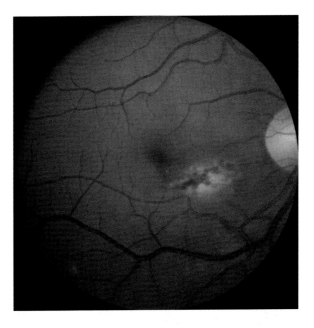

104. A 29-year-old HIV+ male with a CD4 count of <50 cells/mL complains of decreased vision in his right eye and was found to have the presentation at the top of the right column. Which of the following statements is false?
   a. Frosted branch angiitis can be associated with this condition.
   b. After his CD4 count rises, he is at risk for developing CME and cataracts.
   c. More than one-third of patients with his condition develop retinal detachment within 1 year.
   d. Serum IgG titers of the etiologic agent causing this condition are diagnostic.

105. An 80-year-old female presents with sudden loss of vision in her right eye. She specifically complains of difficulty seeing superiorly with her right eye. On clinical examination, she was noted to have macular edema and the fundus as shown below. Which of the following statements is true?
   a. She most likely has an altitudinal defect bilaterally.
   b. Diabetes and glaucoma are significant risk factors for developing this condition.
   c. Long-acting dexamethasone implants have been shown to improve vision in patients with this condition.
   d. Given her extensive retinal ischemia, panretinal photocoagulation (PRP) is indicated to prevent the development of retinal neovascularization.

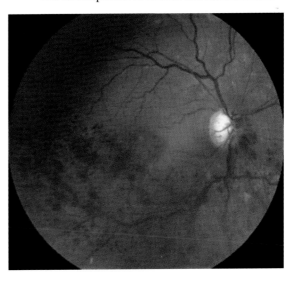

11

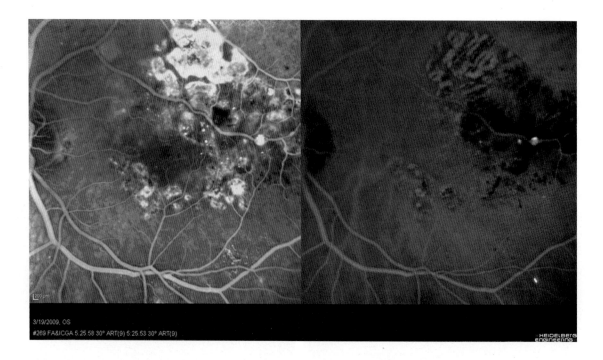

109. A 65-year-old man presents with gradually decreasing vision in his left eye and spectral domain OCT of his left eye is shown below. Which of the following statements regarding this condition is false?

   a. This condition is associated with mutations in the COLA1 gene.
   b. Optic disc leakage would likely be present on fluorescein angiography in this patient.
   c. Pars plana vitrectomy and internal limiting membrane peeling can often improve vision in patients presenting with this condition.
   d. This condition may spontaneously resolve with time.

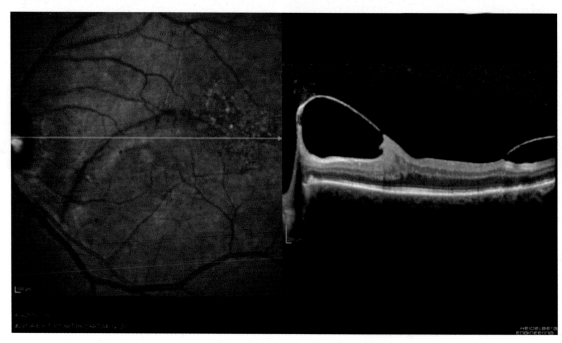

110. The right eye and left eye of a young boy with a history of seizures and cerebral calcification are shown below. Which of the following statements regarding this condition is true?
   a. This condition is generally inherited in an autosomal recessive fashion.
   b. Mental retardation is almost always present.
   c. Lesions from this condition are always present at birth.
   d. Unilateral glaucoma is common in this condition.

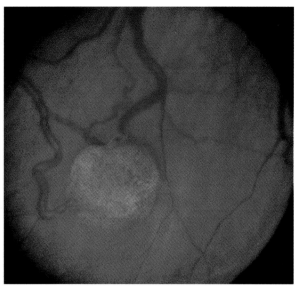

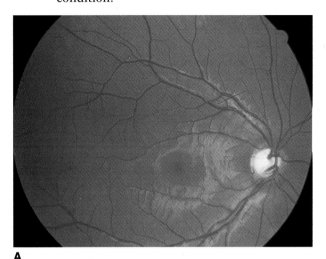

A

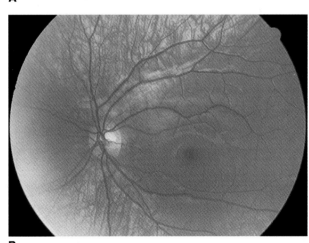

B

111. Which of the following potentially fatal systemic tumors is generally not associated with the lesion shown in the fundus photograph shown at the top of the next column?
   a. Renal cell carcinoma.
   b. Cerebellar hemangioblastoma.
   c. Pheochromocytoma.
   d. Colon adenocarcinoma.

112. The right eye of a patient is very similar to his left eye shown below. His children and his father also exhibit very similar fundus features. Which of the following statements regarding the condition he most likely has is true?
   a. He most likely has a family history of breathing difficulty.
   b. He most likely has esotropia.
   c. Most commonly, the nasal retina fails to vascularize, leading to tractional detachment.
   d. The X-linked variant of this condition is linked to the locus of Norrie's disease.

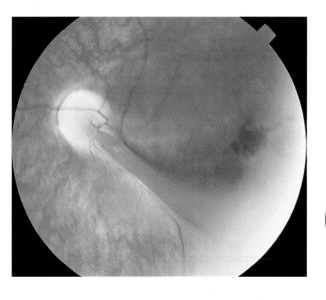

11

113. Which of the following statements regarding bevacizumab is false?
    a. It has been approved for the treatment of colon cancer, but is used intravitreally for the management of age-related macular degeneration.
    b. Although it was developed by the same company that developed ranibizumab, it is significantly less expensive to administer than intravitreal ranibizumab.
    c. It likely has a longer half-life when administered intravitreally compared to that of ranibizumab.
    d. Although it is commonly used by retinal specialists, it has been shown to be less efficacious in the treatment of age-related macular degeneration than ranibizumab as of 2010.

114. Which of the following descriptions of severity of retinopathy of prematurity (ROP) is incorrect?
    a. Stage 1: presence of a flat demarcation line between vascularized and nonvascularized retina.
    b. Stage 2: presence of a demarcation line with height, width, and volume (ridge).
    c. Stage 3: presence of a ridge with fibrovascular proliferation.
    d. Stage 4: total retinal detachment with funnel.

115. Which of the following statements regarding retinopathy of prematurity is correct?
    a. Plus disease is characterized by retinal neovascularization at the posterior pole.
    b. Eyes with ROP only in zone III generally have a good prognosis.
    c. Threshold disease is defined as more than eight contiguous clock hours of extraretinal neovascularization or 12 cumulative clock hours of extraretinal neovascularization in association with plus disease and location of retinal vessels in zone I or zone II.
    d. Spontaneous regression of ROP occurs in <50% of patients.

116. Which of the following systemic disorders is not associated with CRVO?
    a. Diabetes.
    b. Glaucoma.
    c. Hypertension.
    d. Cataracts.

117. Which of the following statements regarding phakomatoses is true?
    a. An ophthalmologist treating a retinal hemangioma may expect temporary worsening of exudation following successful treatment.
    b. Both congenital arteriovenous malformations of the retina (racemose angioma) and cavernous hemangiomas of the retina are distinguished from the vascular malformations of von Hippel's disease by the lack of exudation and subretinal fluid.
    c. The most common complication of retinal cavernous hemangioma is increased episcleral venous pressure.
    d. Sturge-Weber syndrome is inherited in an autosomal recessive fashion.

118. Which of the following factors supports an etiologic connection between Histoplasma infection and the presumed ocular histoplasmosis syndrome (POHS)?
    a. Over 90% of patients with POHS have a positive histoplasmin skin reaction.
    b. The highest prevalence of POHS is among the populations of the southwest states such as New Mexico, Arizona, and California.
    c. In biopsies of patients with vitritis, Histoplasma organisms have been recovered from the human vitreous.
    d. Systemic treatment with antifungal agents leads to resolution of the ocular findings.

119. Which of the following is not a method of treatment of choroidal neovascularization secondary to ocular POHS?
    a. Intravitreal bevacizumab.
    b. Systemic antifungal medications.
    c. Photodynamic therapy.
    d. Argon laser photocoagulation.

11

120. The best predictor of future contralateral visual loss in a patient with a disciform macular scar from POHS is the presence or absence of
    a. A focal macular scar in the better eye.
    b. Peripapillary scarring in the better eye.
    c. Active vitritis in the better eye.
    d. Symmetric peripheral punched-out lesions of each eye.

121. Which of the following concerning angioid streaks is true?
    a. They always extend in continuity from the optic nerve head.
    b. They appear as window defects on fluorescein angiography.
    c. The typical pattern forms concentric circles around the optic nerve head.
    d. Histopathologically, they represent discontinuities in a thickened, abnormal choroid.

122. Which of the following statements regarding idiopathic epiretinal membranes is false?
    a. They are bilateral in 20% of patients.
    b. They are found in 20% of patients over the age of 75.
    c. The majority of patients with idiopathic epiretinal membranes maintain vision better than 20/50.
    d. They are more common in women.

123. What radiation dosage level may be considered a threshold for the development of radiation retinopathy?
    a. 500 rad.
    b. 1,000 rad.
    c. 3,000 rad.
    d. 5 Gy.

124. Which of the following concerning the distribution of photoreceptors in the normal human retina is true?
    a. The ratio of rods to cones is approximately 4:1.
    b. There are far more cones than rods in the central 18° of the macula.
    c. Cone density is maximal in a ring 20° to 40° eccentric to the foveola.
    d. Nearly half of all cones lie outside the macula.

125. Which of the following statements regarding giant retinal tears and retinal dialyses is false?
    a. A giant retinal tear is a circumferential retinal break of 90° or greater (three clock hours or more).
    b. Eyes with retinal dialyses usually have associated posterior vitreous detachments (PVDs).
    c. Idiopathic giant retinal tears are the most common form of giant retinal tears, and they mostly occur in males.
    d. Retinal dialyses generally occur either at or slightly posterior to the ora serrata.

126. Which of the following statements regarding electroretinograms (ERG) is true?
    a. A blue flash of light in a dark-adapted patient will generate an ERG with rod input only.
    b. A blue flash of light in a light-adapted patient will generate an ERG with cone input only.
    c. Increasing the intensity of the stimulus flash in a scotopic ERG will result in a decrease in both implicit time and amplitude of the b-wave.
    d. In order to truly isolate cone function, it is necessary to present a light stimulus as flicker flash at a minimum of 5 Hz.

127. Which of the following statements concerning electrooculography (EOG) is true?
    a. The corneal surface or vitreal space is positive relative to sclera.
    b. Amplitudes generally diminish with light adaptation and increase with dark adaptation.
    c. Amplitudes are typically measured by alternating vertical gaze from up to down.
    d. An EOG is generally considered abnormal if the dark-peak to light-trough is <3.5.

128. Both electrooculography (EOG) and electroretinography (ERG) are similarly depressed for all of the following conditions, except:
    a. Choroideremia.
    b. Gyrate atrophy.
    c. Oguchi's disease.
    d. Best's disease.

315

129. Which of the following is not a reported complication from intravitreal injection?
    a. Retinal detachment.
    b. Anaphylaxis.
    c. Retinal pigment epithelium tear.
    d. Transmission of HIV.

130. The most common pattern of congenital dyschromatopsia is:
    a. Deuteranomaly.
    b. Protanomaly.
    c. Protanopia.
    d. Deuteranopia.

131. Which of the following statements regarding retinitis pigmentosa is true?
    a. The vast majority of severe hearing loss associated with retinitis pigmentosa (RP) is acquired.
    b. Usher's syndrome describes any combination of pigmentary retinopathy and partial or complete acquired deafness.
    c. Many patients with Usher's syndrome may have cerebellar and/or vestibular abnormalities.
    d. Unilateral retinitis pigmentosa is generally inherited in an X-linked recessive fashion.

132. Which of the following is not true with regard to a patient presenting with the condition shown at the top of the next column?
    a. Visual acuity is almost always normal in patients presenting with this finding.
    b. A central core of white glial tissue occupies the position of the normal cup.
    c. Serous retinal detachments can occur in approximately one-third of affected patients, but the source of the subretinal fluid is unknown.
    d. These ocular findings have been associated with basal encephalocele in patients with midfacial anomalies.

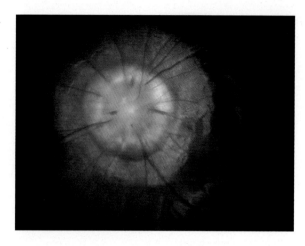

133. A relative lightening of the fundus and RPE after 4 hours of dark adaptation is a feature of which of the following disorders?
    a. Fundus albipunctatus.
    b. Oguchi's disease.
    c. Retinitis pigmentosa
    d. Fundus flavimaculatus.

134. Foveal hypoplasia may be associated with all of the following disorders, except:
    a. Albinism.
    b. Congenital cytomegalovirus disease.
    c. Aniridia.
    d. Persistent hyperplastic primary vitreous

135. Which of the following statements regarding diabetic retinopathy is false?
    a. Diabetic retinopathy is rarely found in individuals under the age of 10.
    b. After 20 years of type 2 diabetes, nearly 99% of patients had some degree of diabetic retinopathy.
    c. Diabetic macular ischemia is a common cause of moderate vision loss in patients with diabetic retinopathy.
    d. Patients with proliferative diabetic retinopathy are at increased risk of myocardial infarction and cerebrovascular accidents.

136. The finding most frequently associated with degenerative retinoschisis is
    a. Peripheral cystoid degeneration.
    b. Bullous retinoschisis.
    c. Reticular retinoschisis.
    d. Rhegmatogenous retinal detachment.

137. Which of the following statements regarding retinoschisis is true?
    a. Typical degenerative retinoschisis is associated with an increased risk of retinal detachment.
    b. The majority of patients with retinoschisis are hyperopic and have bilateral retinoschisis.
    c. The absolute scotoma caused by posterior extension of retinoschisis is highly symptomatic.
    d. Retinoschisis is almost always associated with retinal dialysis.

138. In a patient with leukocoria, all of the following findings are more likely to indicate persistent fetal vasculature (PFV) and not retinoblastoma except:
    a. Unilaterality.
    b. Presence of microphthalmos.
    c. Presence of cataract.
    d. Presence of calcification.

139. Which one of the following concerning asteroid hyalosis is false?
    a. It is more common with aging and is more commonly bilateral.
    b. It is generally associated with no decrease in visual acuity.
    c. The vitreous is otherwise normal.
    d. The particulate matter seen clinically consists of calcium soaps.

140. Findings consistent with exudative detachment rather than rhegmatogeneous retinal detachment include all of the following, except:
    a. Shifting fluid.
    b. A lack of "tobacco dust."
    c. Smooth, domed appearance of the retina.
    d. Undulation of the retina with eye movements.

141. The key prognostic factor in predicting postoperative visual acuity following surgical repair of rhegmatogeneous retinal detachment is:
    a. The size of the largest retinal break.
    b. The number of retinal breaks.
    c. The presence and duration of macular detachment.
    d. The presence or absence of myopia.

142. All of the following conditions may increase the risk of rhegmatogenous retinal detachment (RRD), except:
    a. Lattice degeneration.
    b. Retinal holes
    c. Meridional complexes.
    d. Cobblestone degeneration.

143. Which of the following is not a risk factor for the development of age-related macular degeneration (AMD)?
    a. A history of smoking.
    b. A family history of AMD.
    c. Advanced age.
    d. A history of type 2 diabetes.

144. Which of the following statements regarding AREDS supplementation is false?
    a. There may be an increased risk of developing lung cancer in smokers taking beta-carotene.
    b. Patients with a strong positive family history of AMD should consider taking AREDS supplementation even if they do not yet have AMD.
    c. Cupric oxide was included in AREDS supplementation to prevent zinc-induced anemia.
    d. Patients taking AREDS supplementation demonstrated a decreased risk of developing AMD even 10 years after starting supplementation.

145. What is the most common complication of vitrectomy surgery?
    a. Cataract.
    b. Endophthalmitis.
    c. Retinal detachment.
    d. Vitreous hemorrhage.

146. What is the most common fungus causing chronic postoperative endophthalmitis?
    a. Candida.
    b. Histoplasma.
    c. Aspergillus.
    d. *Propionibacterium acnes.*

11

147. The EVS has documented which one of the following?
    a. Intravenous ceftazidime reduces the duration of severe visual loss in acute postoperative bacterial endophthalmitis, but does not improve long-term visual outcome.
    b. Intravenous ceftazidime reduces the duration of severe visual loss and improves long-term visual outcome in patients with acute postoperative bacterial endophthalmitis.
    c. Intravenous amikacin reduces the duration of severe visual loss in acute postoperative bacterial endophthalmitis, but does not improve long-term visual outcome.
    d. Neither intravenous ceftazidime nor amikacin offers any therapeutic advantage in acute postoperative bacterial endophthalmitis.

148. Findings of the CVOS include each of the following, except:
    a. Grid pattern photocoagulation does not significantly reduce cystoid macular edema (CME) associated with CRVO.
    b. Grid pattern photocoagulation does not significantly alter visual outcome in patients with CME associated with CRVO.
    c. Roughly 25% to 30% of patients with at least 10 disc areas of nonperfusion will develop iris or angle NV within 3 years.
    d. Prophylactic scatter laser showed a trend toward reducing the incidence of iris or angle NV, but baseline differences in the treatment versus no treatment groups eliminated any statistical significance.

149. Which of the following statements regarding optical coherence tomography (OCT) is false?
    a. OCT uses a combination of infrared light and sound waves to create images.
    b. Images created with OCT have much better resolution than standard 10 MHz B-scan ultrasound.
    c. OCT image quality will decrease as the amount of vitreous hemorrhage increases.
    d. Ultrahigh resolution OCT can create images with resolutions of 2 to 3 μm.

150. Regarding the surgical treatment of proliferative vitreoretinopathy, which one of the following is false?
    a. Silicone oil and SF6 gas are equally effective tamponade agents.
    b. Silicone oil and C3F8 gas are equally effective tamponade agents.
    c. When silicone oil is used as tamponade in PVR, there is no significant difference in outcomes between eyes undergoing primary (i.e., their first) vitrectomy and previously vitrectomized eyes.
    d. When C3F8 is used as tamponade in PVR, there is no significant difference in outcomes between eyes undergoing primary (i.e., their first) vitrectomy and previously vitrectomized eyes.

11

Answers

1. **a.** The membrane may be thought of as an elastin sandwich—the bread is collagenous zones and basement membrane on either side.

2. **d.** The vitreous typically occupies 80% of eye volume, and is most firmly attached to the vitreous base. Vitreomacular traction syndrome generally results with an incomplete PVD with traction on the macula.

3. **a.** The retinal vasculature generally supplies only 5% of the oxygen required by the fundus. The remainder is supplied by the choroidal circulation. Bipolar cells generally synapse with ganglion cells. The macula, histologically, generally has ganglion cells that are two or more layers thick.

4. **c.** Treatment is generally reserved for (a) occupational or other demands for rapid recovery of binocular function (unless the lesion has significant proximity to the fovea in which laser treatment can cause permanent vision loss), (b) persistent serous detachment (>4 months), (c) prior episodes of CSCR that have been associated with permanently decreased visual acuity, and (d) permanent visual loss due to CSR in the contralateral eye.

5. **a.** The image shows a retinal capillary hemangioma fed and drained by prominent dilated tortuous retinal blood vessels. Superior to the lesion is an area of chorioretinal atrophy subsequent to prior cryotherapy of another retinal capillary hemangioma. These lesions are found in von Hippel-Lindau disease. Café-au-lait spots are characteristic of neurofibromatosis and are not seen as part of von Hippel-Lindau disease.

6. **b.** Intraocular lens implantation at the time of extracapsular cataract extraction does not change the incidence of CME.

7. **c.** Eales' disease is an idiopathic retinal vasculitis in young boys or men (most commonly from India) and is generally bilateral. The original syndrome was defined as retinal vasculitis in a young man with associated epistaxis, constipation, and positive reaction to dermal purified protein derivative (PPD). A potentially lethal cerebral vasculitis also has been recognized as an occasional finding. Neovascularization can be treated with scatter photocoagulation and visual prognosis is generally good with prompt appropriate therapy.

8. **d.** Fourier-domain OCT offers significantly increased resolution with the added benefit of shorter scan times.

9. **b.** In Stargardt's disease, defects in the ATP-binding cassette transporter of the retina (or ABCR) protein lead to an excess of all-trans retinol in the outer segment discs (which are part of the photoreceptor rods).

10. **b.** Breaks within Bruch's membrane result in this clinical appearance of angioid streaks. A number of systemic disorders are associated with angioid streaks, including pseudoxanthoma elasticum ("P"), Ehlers-Danlos syndrome ("E"), Paget's disease of bone ("P"), sickle cell disease and sickle cell trait ("S"), and idiopathic ("I") causes—remember these by the acronym "PEPSI." About 50% of cases of angioid streaks are idiopathic.

11. **c.** The vortex veins drain into the superior ophthalmic vein.

12. **b.** Urinary discoloration occurs in almost all patients injected with fluorescein sodium. Reduced fluorescein doses should be administered in patients with renal compromise. Finally, pregnant women should generally not receive fluorescein angiography (although its potential teratogenicity has not been identified).

11

photocoagulation recovered 20/40 or better vision (60% vs. 34%). Quadrantic scatter photocoagulation treatment is generally not undertaken until signs of neovascularization are evident because the long-term incidence of severe visual loss in patients with extensive nonperfusion is low (only a subset of these actually develop neovascularization). This risk increases once neovascularization occurs. Greater than five disc diameters of ischemia was found to be associated with a 31% risk of developing neovascularization.

29. **c.** Visual acuity in solar retinopathy is generally not reduced below 20/200 and is frequently only minimally reduced.

30. **c.** The description is classic for Stickler's syndrome, or hereditary arthroophthalmopathy. It is inherited in an autosomal dominant fashion and is characterized by progressive myopia with a high incidence of retinal detachment and abnormal epiphyseal development with premature degenerative changes to various joints. Most cases are secondary to premature termination codons in COL2A1—the gene for type II collagen that is a major constituent in both cartilage and vitreous.

31. **d.** Although the b-wave amplitude can be decreased in focal or stationary retinal disease, the b-wave implicit time is increased only in diffuse, progressive retinal disease.

32. **b.** An abnormally low light-peak–to–dark-trough ratio on EOG has been found to occur in retinal toxicity from hydroxychloroquine and chloroquine.

33. **d.** All of the other answers have been associated. Hepatorenal syndrome is generally not associated with Purtscher retinopathy. Chronic renal failure has also been associated with Purtcher-like retinopathy.

34. **b.** The electrooculogram (EOG) can help assess RPE function when retinal function is normal. Visual evoked cortical potential (VECP) testing can be abnormal whenever there is a defect in the visual pathway anywhere from the retina to the cortex.

35. **d.** Blue–yellow errors generally signify acquired disease. D-15 testing is more sensitive than Ishihara color plate testing in classifying color vision deficiencies. Patients with congenital disease generally demonstrate classic patterns of error on the D-15 test, whereas patients with acquired disease (e.g., from optic nerve damage or retinal damage) generally demonstrate more irregular patterns.

36. **a.** African Americans have a lower incidence of CSCR compared to other races. Type-A middle-aged males and patients with elevated corticosteroid levels are at increased risk of developing CSCR.

37. **d.** ICG angiography is very useful in helping distinguish between occult CNV and polypoidal lesions. It can also be quite helpful in patients with CSCR. Although it generally is much better tolerated than fluorescein angiography, it should not be used in patients with a known history of iodide allergy as ICG contains 5% iodide. ICG is not useful in diabetics as these patients have pathology that is generally limited to the retina (as opposed to deeper in the choroid).

38. **d.** Most forms of Leber's congenital amaurosis are autosomal recessive. Gene therapy using an adenoviral vector has shown some promise in helping patients with this debilitating disease.

39. **d.** The other syndromes are autosomal recessive. With choroideremia, central acuity is spared until later in life relative to X-linked RP.

40. **b.** Gyrate atrophy is an autosomal recessive deficiency in ornithine aminotransferase activity. This deficiency causes an increase in serum ornithine levels and a decrease in serum lysine levels. Gyrate atrophy generally does not affect intelligence or lifespan.

11

41. **a.** Although the inheritance in Stargardt's disease/fundus flavimaculatus is generally autosomal recessive, autosomal dominant pedigrees also have been documented. Approximately 80% of patients with Stargardt's disease have a dark choroid. Most patients do not become legally blind (e.g., severe visual loss in both eyes).

42. **d.** Rod monochromats (true color blindness) typically have nystagmus, visual acuity in the 20/200 range, and see the world in shades of gray. Blue-cone monochromats have variable nystagmus and acuities in the 20/40 to 20/200 range.

43. **d.** Diagnosis of Refsum disease is made by demonstrating elevated plasma levels of phytanic acid or reduced phytanic acid oxidase activity in cultured fibroblasts. Refsum disease is characterized by ataxia, polyneuropathy, anosmia, pigmentary retinopathy, deafness, and cardiac myopathy. Dietary restriction of phytanic acid precursors may slow retinal degeneration.

44. **b.** Up to one-third of patients with intracranial hemorrhage will have intraocular hemorrhage (the presence of both simultaneously is termed Terson's syndrome).

45. **d.** Familial drusen are an autosomal dominant disorder that begins with asymptomatic retinal changes generally observed in the third decade of life. Doyne's honeycomb dystrophy and Malattia Leventinese are two forms caused by mutations in the EFEMP1 gene on chromosome 2. The ERG is usually normal or mildly decreased.

46. **a.** The ERG shows significant attenuation of both the a and b waves consistent with ocular ischemic syndrome. The other entities listed are generally bilateral diseases.

47. **d.** Patients with severe disciform scarring, as shown in this question, demonstrate little benefit with intravitreal anti-VEGF therapy or photodynamic therapy given the extensive damage to the macula.

48. **b.** The image reveals peau d'orange, angioid streaks, and choroidal neovascularization classic for pseudoxanthoma elasticum, which is generally autosomal recessive and caused by a mutation in the ABCC6 gene. Mutations in the ABCR gene are associated with fundus flavimaculatus. VMD2 and TIMP3 gene mutations are associated with Best disease and Sorsby macular dystrophy, respectively.

49. **a.** The condition in this image most likely represents presumed ocular histoplasmosis syndrome (POHS), which is characterized by punched out chorioretinal lesions in the retina, peripapillary atrophy, and choroidal neovascularization. Vitritis is not present in POHS.

50. **a.** Figure B shows significantly reduced choroidal perfusion typical of standard fluence photodynamic therapy. The other treatments listed will generally not give you a circular area of hypoperfusion as shown.

51. **b.** Usher's syndrome is the presence of congential hearing loss and retinitis pigmentosa. The hearing loss generally remains stable over time. Epiretinal membrane formation is common in patients with Usher's syndrome.

52. **b.** This is a fundus photograph of a patient with pathologic myopia. Characteristic findings include peripapillary atrophy, a tilted optic disc, lattice degeneration with associated retinal holes, and lacquer cracks. Lacquer cracks are breaks in Bruch's membrane that appear yellowish white.

53. **d.** The fundus image shown is one of Purtscher-like retinopathy, which can result from various etiologies. Although cotton wool spots can occur with proliferative diabetic retinopathy (PDR), PDR is almost always associated with other retinal findings as well, including retinal neovascularization, dot-blot hemorrhages and microaneurysms.

54. **c.** Branch retinal artery occlusion (BRAO) can be caused by embolization or thrombosis of the

11

involved vessel with emboli from cholesterol, fibrin-platelet complexes from arteriosclerotic vessels, and calcific emboli. Uncommon causes of emboli include fat emboli, cardiac myxoma, talc emboli in intravenous drug abusers, and septic emboli from endocarditis. Oral contraceptive use, mitral valve prolapse, vasculitides, and connective tissue disorders also have been associated with BRAO. Thrombocytopenia is not associated with BRAOs.

55. **d.** Group 1 is likely a forme fruste of Coats' disease, is unilateral, and generally occurs in males, but Groups 2 and 3 are bilateral and occur in both sexes. Microscopically, the structural abnormalities in IJT are similar to diabetic microangiopathy, rather than a true telangiectasia. Unlike diabetes, there is no stimulus for retinal neovascularization. Exudation in type I may respond to laser photocoagulation. Choroidal neovascularization (CNV) can lead to visual loss, but geographic atrophy also occurs in IJT (though rare). OCT can appear "normal" with IJT, but fluorescein angiography generally shows telangiectasia in the early frames and leakage on late frames.

56. **c.** Retinal telangiectasia (Coats' disease, Leber's miliary aneurysms) is defined by the presence of an exudative retinal detachment with associated vascular anomalies. This condition is not hereditary and is not associated with systemic vascular abnormalities. Usually, only one eye is involved, and there is a significant male predominance.

57. **b.** Clinically, the macula is 5 to 6 mm in diameter, centered between the temporal vascular arcades. In this region, ganglion cells form two or three sublayers within the ganglion cell layer.

58. **c.** The retinal vessels supply the nerve fiber layer, the ganglion cell layer, the inner plexiform layer, and the inner third of the inner nuclear layer. The choroidal vasculature supplies the outer two-thirds of the inner nuclear layer, the outer plexiform layer, the outer nuclear layer, the photoreceptors, and the retinal pigment epithelium.

59. **d.** In fluorescein angiography, white light from the camera first passes through a blue filter. The blue light (wavelength 490 nm) is absorbed by the fluorescein molecules in the retinal and choroidal vasculature, stimulating them to emit yellow–green light (530 nm). A yellow–green filter is placed to block the blue light reflected from the eye, allowing the yellow–green light into the camera. Fluorescein molecules (not bound to albumin), with a molecular weight <600 Da, can easily pass through the spaces between endothelial cells of the choriocapillaris but normally cannot leak through the tight junctions of the RPE or retinal vascular endothelium (blood–retinal barrier). Anaphylactic shock is thought to occur at a rate of <1 in 100,000 procedures. Autofluorescence images can only be acquired before fluorescein injection.

60. **d.** Leakage appears as an area of early hyperfluorescence that gradually increases in size and intensity throughout the angiogram.

61. **d.** Findings in the nonexudative form of AMD include pigmentary changes, drusen, and areas of geographic atrophy. Patients with central geographic atrophy generally have a guarded visual prognosis.

62. **a.** The first study of surgery for macular holes evaluated patients with the earliest stage, stage I. The natural history of the disorder, with up to 50% experiencing spontaneous improvement, is at least as favorable as, if not superior to, surgical intervention.

63. **a.** Because a significant proportion of early holes spontaneously resolve, only a small fraction, 5%, develop bilateral full-thickness defects.

64. **c.** Idiopathic macular holes are believed to arise due to both tangential and anteroposterior vitreous traction. The earliest change is loss of the

normal foveal depression due to elevation of the fovea itself off the RPE, thus constituting a tiny sensory retinal detachment. This appears clinically as a yellow dot or ring (stages IA and IB, respectively).

65. **b.** Although hydroxychloroquine is thought to be less toxic, both hydroxychloroquine and chloroquine have a significant risk of retinal toxicity leading to atrophic bull's-eye maculopathy. Color vision testing and threshold central visual field testing (with a 10-2 red target visual field) are important in assessing subclinical retinopathy. The EOG is not the most sensitive parameter in detecting chloroquine retinopathy, although it does reflect pathophysiology (RPE damage) when abnormal. Obese patients are at higher risk of toxicity because of their likely higher dosage of medication. Because of their slow excretion, toxic effects of chloroquine and hydroxychloroquine may progress despite cessation of the drug. Any abnormalities caused by these medications are probably permanent, although mild deficits may be reversible.

66. **a.** Thioridazine (Mellaril) is more likely to cause retinal pigment stippling or widespread atrophy of the pigment epithelium and choriocapillaris as shown in this image.

67. **a.** Chronic intravenous drug abusers can develop talc retinopathy (as shown) with talc emboli leading to multiple branch retinal artery occlusions as well as peripheral retinal neovascularization.

68. **d.** Juvenile neuronal ceroid lipofuscinoses, or Batten disease, is the most common type of neuronal ceroid lipofuscinoses (NCL) in the United States. Juvenile visual loss can often manifest as a patient's first symptom. Death usually occurs by the fourth decade.

69. **a.** The fundus above shows a classic cherry-red spot found in patients with Tay-Sachs disease, the most common ganglioside storage disease. Ganglioside accumulates within parafoveal ganglion cells leading to the cherry-red spot appearance. Mutations in the alpha-galactosidase A gene result in Fabry's disease, which is associated with retinal vascular tortuosity and dilatation. Apolipoprotein B is not made in patients with abetalipoproteinemia leading to vitamin A deficiency and retinal degeneration. Patients with mutations in ornithine aminotransferase develop gyrate atrophy.

70. **b.** Hermansky-Pudlak syndrome is a rare autosomal recessive form of oculocutaneous albinism that can be lethal and must be recognized. It is associated with easy bruising and bleeding secondary to platelet dysfunction and is more common in Puerto-Ricans.

71. **a.** Oguchi disease and fundus albipunctatus are forms of congenital stationary night blindness with abnormal fundus findings. Fundus flavimaculatus (or Stargardt's disease) is a condition with abnormal lipofuscin deposition in the RPE. Functional problems in this syndrome are not limited to night blindness and vision loss can be progressive. Retinitis punctata albescens is a phenotype of retinitis pigmentosa (RP) with deep retinal white dots or flecks. Leber congenital amaurosis is a form of infantile RP, not CSNB.

72. **c.** Cone dystrophies generally lead to progressive loss of color vision and visual acuity. Patients with cone dystrophy may also complain of difficulty with night driving, as urban night driving is generally performed with background illumination at low photopic intensities. Hemeralopia (day blindness) and photophobia (sensitivity to light) are common symptoms as well.

73. **d.** Other areas of firm vitreoretinal attachment include the major retinal vessels/arcades. The vortex veins represent a firm point of attachment between the choroid and sclera.

74. **d.** Removal of the lens and posterior capsule allows the hyaluronic acid in the vitreous to diffuse into the anterior chamber and out of the

11

eye, leading to higher prevalence of PVD after intracapsular cataract extraction. Hemorrhage or vitreous cells ("tobacco dust") are suggestive of retinal breaks. OCT (especially spectral domain imaging) has shown that PVDs often originate in the perifoveal macula.

75. **a.** Although 5% to 10% of the general population has lattice degeneration, only a small subset will develop a retinal detachment. Lattice degeneration is present in 20% to 30% of eyes with an RRD. Important histologic features of lattice degeneration include discontinuity of the internal limiting membrane and a pocket of liquefied vitreous overlying the degeneration. Vitreoretinal condensation and adherence occur at the margin of the lesion. Other features include sclerosis of the vessels and variable degrees of retinal atrophy. Lattice degeneration is more common in myopes and is bilateral in one-third to one-half of affected patients.

76. **b.** This patient has vitreomacular traction syndrome (VMT). The incomplete separation and abnormal adherence of the vitreous that remains attached to the posterior pole leads to traction on the macula. Leakage on angiogram can occur at the fovea or optic nerve. While this may resolve spontaneously with complete separation of the vitreous, surgery is often indicated if the vision is significantly decreased or distorted.

77. **a.** The fundus images show a symmetric pigmentary maculopathy with an evolving "bull's-eye" appearance. In a young man with no history of treatment with hydroxychloroquine or chloroquine, the differential diagnosis is limited to a few macular dystrophies. The two most commonly associated with bull's eye maculopathy are cone dystrophy and Stargardt disease (juvenile macular degeneration). The fluorescein shows the "dark choroid" classically seen in Stargardt disease. This is usually inherited on an autosomal recessive basis, meaning his parents are likely carriers with no detectable ophthalmoscopic changes. ERG and visual fields are typically preserved or

minimally affected. The pisciform yellow–white flecks are abnormal lipofuscin deposition in the RPE. Typically, both eyes of affected patients stabilize at around 20/200 visual acuity.

78. **d.** The patient's history and clinical findings are classic for an unusual paraneoplastic syndrome, bilateral diffuse uveal melanocytic proliferation. The syndrome is seen in patients with cancer, often undiagnosed. In men, lung and colon primaries predominate. In women, neoplasms of the reproductive system (ovarian, uterine) have been reported. The hallmarks of the syndrome, as defined by Gass, include focal red patches at the level of the RPE in the posterior pole (which hyperfluoresce) multiple pigmented and nonpigmented melanocytic "tumors" as well as diffuse proliferation of choroidal melanocytes, exudative retinal detachment, and rapidly developing cataract. Visual loss is initially secondary to cataract and may precede the diagnosis of the cancer. Subsequent photoreceptor loss leads to inexorable, severe visual loss. This is reflected in the ERG as a rod greater than cone degeneration (scotopic greater than photopic loss). The underlying cause is not known but is felt to be due to hormonal effects of the primary carcinoma on preexistent uveal nevus cells. The angiogram shows multiple window defects, reflecting widespread RPE damage corresponding to the red patches and some of the melanocytic deposits. Unfortunately, no treatment is effective at stopping the visual decline. Because there is no serologic test, the diagnosis is made on a completely clinical basis.

79. **b.** The history and the fundus findings are consistent with a diagnosis of anterior ischemic optic neuropathy, a condition presenting with acute painless visual loss and typically with optic disc edema and pallor. Anyone with AION should be ruled out for arteritic AION (AAION) secondary to giant cell arteritis (GCA), as this is a potentially fatal condition. The best initial way to rule out GCA is with an ESR and CRP, as up to 20% of patients with AAION can present with no systemic symptoms (e.g., jaw claudication,

11

scalp pain, fever, and malaise). ESR and CRP (when both are abnormal) have a 97% specificity for AAION. The gold standard for diagnosing GCA is a temporal artery biopsy. Steroids can be initiated prior to the biopsy (which should be performed within 1 week).

80. **d.** The condition shown is congenital X-linked retinoschisis (XLRS), a condition that is inherited on an X-linked recessive basis. Splitting of the retina occurs at the nerve fiber layer. Foveal schisis as shown is almost always observed. There is no leakage observed with fluorescein angiography. Mutations in the adhesion protein retinoschisin, which is responsible for XLRS, result in Müller's cell degeneration.

81. **a.** The condition shown is serpiginous chorioretinopathy, a bilateral condition that usually spreads outward from the optic nerve and/or macula in a serpentine fashion. Serpiginous chorioretinopathy is chronic and recurrent with poor visual prognosis and scotomata affecting the areas of involvement. Treatment with potent immunosuppressives may slow down the disease in some cases, but generally the visual prognosis is poor, especially with macular involvement.

82. **c.** The condition shown is asteroid hyalosis, a benign condition that is usually unilateral (75% of cases), with good visual acuity. There is a clear association of this condition in diabetic patients. It usually occurs in patients over age 50, and vitrectomy may sometimes be used to help visualize other retinal conditions (e.g., diabetic retinopathy) that are difficult to assess because of the asteroid hyalosis.

83. **d.** The condition shown is retinitis pigmentosa. Although it can be inherited via several inheritance patterns, X-linked inheritance usually has the worst prognosis. ERG should be performed on all suspected patients to confirm the diagnosis, as the presence of bone spicules and chorioretinal atrophy can occur in a variety of conditions, including severe uveitis, syphilis, chloroquine toxicity, etc.

84. **d.** The condition shown is Coats disease. Coats disease is not inherited and is generally unilateral. The diagnosis of Coats disease requires the presence of retinal telangiectasia (small anomalous vessels) as shown. It can recur and must be watched carefully, with difficult cases requiring multiple photocoagulation or cryotherapy treatments. Retinal detachments can be late sequelae of the disease. The yellow material is lipid exudate. Posterior retinal neovascularization is not common.

85. **b.** The condition shown is Best disease (or vitelliform dystrophy). It is inherited in an autosomal dominant fashion and is secondary to a mutation in the vitelliform macular dystrophy (VMD2) gene (bestrophin) on chromosome 11. Visual acuity in the "sunny side up" stage shown is generally good. The ERG is usually normal, whereas the EOG is generally abnormal in Best disease.

86. **c.** The condition shown is a myelinated nerve fiber layer (MNFL), a benign condition. It has been associated with nystagmus and amblyopia, but retinal detachment is not associated with MNFL.

87. **b.** The condition shown is a hermiretinal artery occlusion, manifested by nerve fiber layer edema. Atherosclerotic emboli are often the cause, and GCA is discovered in 1%–2% of cases.

88. **d.** The fundus photograph shown demonstrates angioid streaks, which can be associated with several diseases (think "PEPSI"). Up to half of all cases are idiopathic, however. Angiography generally shows a window defect representing the breaks in Bruch's membrane, through which choroidal neovascularization can migrate. Both PDT and intravitreal anti-VEGF therapy have been shown to be of benefit in subfoveal choroidal neovascularization secondary to angioid streaks.

11

89. c. The condition shown is acute posterior multifocal placoid epitheliopathy (APMPPE). It is usually bilateral, and has a good visual prognosis. Up to one-half of patients have a viral prodrome. Fluorescein angiography often demonstrates early hypofluorescence (indicated blockage of the choroidal pattern) with late hyperfluorescence (as shown in the angiogram frames). While APMPPE is generally benign, it can be rarely associated with a fatal cerebral vasculitis.

90. c. The fundus photograph reveals preretinal/vitreous hemorrhage overlying the fovea, with likely significantly decreased visual acuity. The most common cause of vitreous hemorrhage is diabetic retinopathy in adults. The Diabetic Retinopathy Vitrectomy Study (DRVS) demonstrated the benefit of early vitrectomy (within 1 to 6 months after vitreous hemorrhage) in type 1 diabetic patients or those patients with vitreous hemorrhage and severe proliferative diabetic retinopathy.

91. b. The condition shown is toxoplasmic retinochoroiditis (a posterior staphyloma generally would not have satellite lesions). The lesions appear inactive and old in this patient and antibiotic therapy and steroids are of no use in this patient (unless the condition recurs). Immunocompromised patients (including AIDS patients) presenting with toxoplasmic retinochoroiditis must obtain neuroimaging to rule out cerebral lesions. Folinic acid (not folic acid) is used in combination with pyrimethamine to protect against iatrogenic thrombocytopenia and leukopenia.

92. d. The condition shown is central serous chorioretinopathy (CSCR), a condition usually affecting males between the ages of 30 and 50 years, typically with type A personalities. The smokestack presentation shown in the angiogram only occurs in approximately 10% of cases of CSCR. Most eyes with this condition recover visual acuity within 6 months. Early focal photocoagulation in this particular patient (a retinal surgeon) would be contraindicated, given the lesion's proximity to the center of the macula and the potential for a permanent visual scotoma with focal photocoagulation. Waiting for spontaneous remission would be the most appropriate treatment option. If spontaneous remission does not occur within 6–10 weeks, then reduced fluence photodynamic therapy can be considered as it has been shown to be quite successful in patients with this condition.

93. b. The condition shown is fundus albipunctatus. It can be differentiated from retinitis punctata albescens because of the normal vasculature (typically attenuated in retinitis punctata albescens, an RP variant). Familial drusen would appear similar, although the lesions would not be as uniform in size and would form grape-like clusters. Patients with this condition may have good visual acuity and night blindness may be their only symptom.

94. c. Based on the history, the fundus appearance, and the FA, the patient most likely has Vogt-Koyanagi-Harada syndrome (VKH), which is a bilateral condition characterized by granulomatous panuveitis. VKH is a systemic condition with both neurologic and dermatologic manifestations. The FA clearly demonstrates multiple areas of hyperfluorescence with late leakage into the subretinal space. Sugiura's sign, or perilimbal vitiligo, occurs in 75% of cases. Given the lack of trauma and the overall health of the patient prior to examination, both sympathetic ophthalmia and endophthalmitis are unlikely. VKH generally has a good prognosis when effectively and rapidly treated with steroids and immunosuppressives.

95. d. The condition shown is neuroretinitis, which, along with a painful lymphadenopathy, can be a manifestation of cat-scratch disease caused by Bartonella henselae. Neuroretinitis, however, can have a variety of different infectious and immunologic causes, and consequently, a thorough history should be obtained from the patient. Both erythromycin and ciprofloxacin can be used to treat cat-scratch disease. The visual prognosis is generally good with the disease being self-limited.

96. b. The condition described is Bietti crystalline corneoretinal dystrophy, which is characterized by limbal corneal opacities and tapetoretinal dystrophy. Plaquenil retinopathy typically causes a bull's-eye maculopathy. Synchysis scintillans is a condition of cholesterol crystals within the vitreous. Cystinosis typically causes corneal crystals. Fleck retina of Kandori is a disorder similar to fundus albipunctatus with characteristic night blindness.

97. d. The patient has Irvine-Gass syndrome (e.g., cystoid macular edema developing after cataract surgery). The incidence of Irvine-Gass is higher after intraoperative complications, but most cases spontaneously resolve. Peak incidence is 6 to 10 weeks postoperatively.

98. c. The condition shown is idiopathic polypoidal choroidal vasculopathy. In people of Chinese and Japanese origin, it is usually unilateral and generally affects males. In Caucasians, it is more often bilateral and generally affects females. It is characterized by serosanginous detachments of the RPE and retina and can also have associated choroidal neovascularization.

99. a. The angiogram above is from a patient with butterfly pattern dystrophy, which is associated with mutations in the peripherin/RDS gene.

100. d. The patient has bilateral subfoveal disciform scars secondary to advanced exudative age-related macular degeneration. Despite the intraretinal fluid present on spectral domain OCT (SD-OCT), intravitreal anti-VEGF therapy is of very limited benefit in these cases, and no treatment has been clinically proven in this setting. Referral to a low vision specialist is the most appropriate treatment at this point.

101. a. The autofluorescence image represents a tear in the RPE, which can occur after intravitreal injection. The sharp demarcation between the darker area and the lighter area represents the location of the RPE tear.

102. c. Optic disc drusen (ODD) as shown demonstrate autofluorescence (which is shown in the image above). ODD rarely affects non-Caucasians and most patients with ODD have some type of visual field defect. ODD can be associated with pseudoxanthoma elasticum and retinitis pigmentosa. No treatment has been shown to improve visual field defects in patients with ODD.

103. b. This patient had a large chorioretinal metastasis secondary to his lung cancer. Urgent referral to his oncologist and obtaining neuroimaging (in conjunction with the patient's oncologist) is appropriate given that any chorioretinal metastasis is by definition considered a CNS metastasis. The most common primary tumors in patients with chorioretinal mets are lung CA in men (40% of cases) and breast CA in women (almost 70% of cases). Uveal metastases imply a poor prognosis.

104. d. This patient has CMV retinitis, which often occurs in HIV+ patients with low CD4 counts. Treatment is with systemic ganciclovir, intravitreal ganciclovir, or foscarnet. Raising his CD4 count with highly active antiretroviral therapy (HAART) can also eliminate the need for specific anti-CMV treatment. Given that many individuals are seropositive for CMV, serum IgG titers are generally not helpful.

105. c. This patient has a hemiretinal vein occlusion, which is generally unilateral and associated with glaucoma (and not diabetes). Long-acting intravitreal dexamethasone implants, intravitreal anti-VEGF agents, and focal laser treatment have been shown to improve vision in these patients. PRP should be reserved for patients that actually demonstrate retinal neovascularization.

106. a. This patient has multifocal central serous chorioretinopathy as demonstrated by multiple scattered areas of staining (which represent old areas of CSCR) along with new areas of leakage in his left eye.

11

CHAPTER 12

High-Yield Review: Facts and Mnemonics

Glaucoma

-ICE Syndrome:
Iris Nevus (Cogan-Reese)
Chandler's syndrome
Essential iris atrophy

DDx of glaucoma + uveitis: herpetic disease, Posner-Schlossman, Fuchs heterochromic iridocyclitis, sarcoid, toxoplasmosis, syphilis.

ISNT rule (nerve thickness from most to least)–
Inferior rim, Superior, Nasal, Temporal.

Pathology

-Homer-Wright rosette is like a jelly donut that Homer Simpson would eat – the rosette has a filled center, no lumen (as opposed to Flexner-Wintersteiner rosette).

Neuro

Parinaud's syndrome: PARINAUDS
Papilledema
Accommodative insufficiency
Retraction of lid (Collier's sign)
Insufficient convergence
Nystagmus
Aqueductal stenosis
Upgaze deficit
Dissociation of light-near response
Skew deviation

Hereditary optic neuropathies: Kjer's, Behr's, and Leber's

Unilateral caloric stimulation (direction of fast jerk): COWS–Cold Opposite Warm Same.

Oculoplastics

Nerves LeFT out of the annulus of Zinn - LFTs:
Lacrimal
Frontal
Trochlea
Superior ophthalmic vein

Rhyme: "3, 4, SO, V_1, 6…Through the SO Fix" – cranial nerves 3, 4, sympathetics, superior ophthalmic vein, branches of V_1, cranial nerve 6.

Muscles affected by thyroid (in order of frequency): "I M Stuart Little."
Inferior
Medial
Superior
Lateral

Uveitis

Nodules
KoePpe nodules – Pupillary border
Busacca nodules – Mid Periphery
Berlin nodules – Iris Angle

Reiter's Syndrome Can't see, Can't pee, Can't climb a tree: Conjunctivits/irtis, urethritis, polyarthritis.

334

HLA Associations:
A11: Sympathetic Ophthalmia
A29: Birdshot
B5/B12: Behcet's
B7: POHS, Serpiginous, Ankylosing spondylitis
B8: Sjogren's, Sarcoidosis, intermediate uveitis
B12: OCP
B27: Ankylosing spondylitis, Reiter's, IBD, Psoriatic arthritis
Bw54: Posner-Schlossman syndrome
DR4: VKH, OCP

JRA: ANA+, RF- (pauciarticular, females)

Meds that cause anterior uveitis/hypopyon:
Rifabutin, cidofovir

DDx of hypopyon: HLA-B27 uveitis, infection (keratits/endophthalmitis), foreign body, Behcet's (rolling hypopyon), malignancy (leukemia, retinoblastoma), toxic (rifabutin)

Granulomatous uveitis: GLiB SHoTS
Granulomatous uveitis
Leptospirosis/Lyme
Brucellosis
Sarcoid
HSV
TB
Syphilis

DDx of iris heterochromia: Fuchs' heterochromic iridocyclitis, trauma, retained IOFB, congenital Horner's, iris melanoma, Posner-Schlossman, herpetic disease (iris atrophy), medications (prostaglandins), oculodermal melanocytosis

Optics

RAM GAP for duochrome test: if patient sees the Red half clearer, Add Minus. If the Green side is clearer, Add Plus.

Cornea

Cloudy cornea at birth: Don't get STUMPED!
Sclerocornea
Trauma
Ulcer
Mucopolysaccharidosis
Peters anomaly
Endothelial dystrophy (CHED)
Dermoid

Marylin Monroe Always Gets Her Man in L.A. County (corneal dystrophies)
Macular
Mucopolysaccharide
Alcian blue

Granular dystrophy
Hyaline
Masson trichrome

Lattice
Amyloid
Congo red

-Bacteria that can penetrate intact corneas (they create "CANALS")
Corynebacteria
Aegyptus (Hemophilus)
Neisseria
Acanthaomoeba
Listeria
Shigella

Band keratopathy happens at the level of Bowman's membrane

Terrien's in Teens at Twelve: Terrien's marginal degeneration occurs in the Teens and twenties and starts superiorly (at Twelve o'clock)

BIGH3 gene is LARGe (corneal dystrophies)
Lattice
Avellino
Reis-Bucklers
Granular

Interstitial Keratitis (IK): In Kenya, Cogan Saw Two Laughing Hyenas Making Love
IK
Cogan's syndrome
Syphilis
TB
Lyme/leprosy
Herpetic
Measles/Mumps
LGV/Leishmaniasis

-Fungal Keratitis demographics
North: Candida in Canada
South: Fusarium in Florida

DDx for Blue Sclera: Hurlers, Turner, Marfans, osteogenic imperfecta, staphyloma, oculodermal melanocytosis, Ehlers-Danlos, scleromalacia perforans

12

Keratoconus findings: CONES
Central scarring
Oil drop reflex
Nerves prominent
Excessive bulging
Striae – Vogt's

Pediatrics

-MALE: transposition of muscles for A and V patterns
Medial rectus toward the Apex
Lateral rectus toward the Empty space

Hermansky-Pudlak: Platelet defect, Puerto Ricans

Retina

-PEPSI: Angioid Streaks
Pseduoxanthoma elasticum
Ehlers Danlos
Paget's disease of the bone
Sickle cell anemia
Idiopathic

-StARgARdt's disease: Autosomal Recessive (AR)

-Female CARrier states (retinal changes): CAR
Choroideremia
Albinism
Retinitis pigmentosa

-Tuberous Sclerosis: Zits, Fits, Twits: sebaceous adenoma, seizures, mental retardation

-Melanoma: To Find Small Ocular Melanoma: (likelihood of melanoma vs. nevus, 1 factor then 30% chance of progression, 3 factors then 50% chance of progression)
Thickness >2 mm
Fluid
Symptoms
Orange pigment
Margin of optic nerve

-Stages of sickle retinopathy: NASVaR (like NASCaR)
Nonperfusion
AV anastomoses
Sea-fan neovascularization
Vitreous hemorrhage
Retinal detachment

-Best's disease: Chromosome 11 – imagine an egg yolk-like macular lesion with two strips of bacon (for the number 11).

-Choroidal folds: THIN RPE
Tumors
Hypotony
Inflammation/Idiopathic
Neovascular membrane
Retrobulbar mass
Papilledema
Extraocular hardware

-Crystalline retinopathy: (hydroxy–)chloroquine, tamoxifen, canthaxanthine, talc, methoxyflurane, Bietti's, idiopathic juxtafoveal telangiectasia

-CME without leakage on FA: nicotinic acid maculopathy, Goldmann-Favre, retinoschisis

Figure Credit List

Chapter 1, General Medicine

Question 87 (Figure A)
From Berg D, Worzala K. *Atlas of Adult Physical Diagnosis*. Philadelphia, PA: Lippincott Williams & Wilkins; 2006.

Questions 87 (Figure B) and 100
From Goodheart HP. *Goodheart's Photoguide of Common Skin Disorders*. 2nd ed. Philadelphia, PA: Lippincott Williams & Wilkins; 2003.

Chapter 3, Optics

Answers 32, 45, 46, and 52
From Rama D. Jager and Jeffrey C. Lamkin, *Massachusetts Eye and Ear Infirmary Review Manual for Ophthalmology*. 3rd ed. Philadelphia, PA: Lippincott Williams & Wilkins; 2006.

Chapter 4, Ocular Pathology

Questions 31–37, 41, 66, 69, 70, 72, 74, 75, 78, 79, 81, 82 (Figures A and B), 84, 86, 87, 89, 91 (Figures A–C), 93 (Figures A and B), 95, and 97
Copyright Marcus M. Marcet, MD

Question 96 (Figures A and B)
From Jager RD, Lamkin JC. *Massachusetts Eye and Ear Infirmary Review Manual for Ophthalmology*. 3rd ed. Philadelphia, PA: Lippincott Williams & Wilkins; 2006.

Chapter 5, Neuroophthalmology

Question 73
Courtesy of Veeral S. Sheth, MD.

Question 31 (Figures A and B)
From Campbell WW. *DeJong's the Neurologic Examination*. Philadelphia, PA: Lippincott Williams & Wilkins, 2005.

Question 134
From Gold DH, Weingeist TA. *Color Atlas of the Eye in Systemic Disease*. Baltimore, MD: Lippincott Williams & Wilkins; 2001.

Question 141 (Figure A)
From *Dr. Robert Hepler, Department of Ophthalmology, UCLA Center for the Health Sciences, Los Angeles.*

Questions 74, 98, 136, 138, 140, 141 (Figure B)–143
From Jager RD, Lamkin JC. *Massachusetts Eye and Ear Infirmary Review Manual for Ophthalmology*. 3rd ed. Philadelphia, PA: Lippincott Willliams & Wilkins; 2006.

Questions 20 (Figures A and B), 54, 72, 76, 79, and 108 (Figures A and B)
From Tasman W, Jaeger E. *The Wills Eye Hospital Atlas of Clinical Ophthalmology*. 2nd ed. Philadelphia, PA: Lippincott Williams & Wilkins; 2001.

Chapter 6, Oculoplastics

Questions 1, 2, 6 (Figures A and B), 8 (Figures A and B), 9 (Figures A–C), 10, 16, 19, 22, 25, 29 (Figures A–C), 31, 37 (Figures A and B), 47 (Figures A and B), 51 (Figures A–C), 60, 66, 67, 78, 81, 83, 84 (Figures A and B), 86, 88, 90 (Figures A–C), 110, 114, 116, 125, 127, 132 (Figures A and B), 137, 145 (Figures A and B), 148, and 150
Copyright Marcus M. Marcet, MD.

Chapter 7, Intraocular Inflammation and Uveitis

Question 68 (Figures A and B), 84 (Figures A and B), 91, and 118 (Figures A and B).
Credit to Lee Jampol, MD of Northwestern University for donation photo.

Question 99
Credit to Dr. Manjot Gill of Northwestern University for donation of photo.

Question 67
From Neville BW, Damm DD, White DK. *Color Atlas of Clinical Oral Pathology*. 2nd ed. Baltimore, MD: Williams & Wilkins; 1998.

Questions 27, 40, 53, 61–64, 98, 108 (Figures A and B), 112, and 117.

From Tasman W, Jaeger E. *The Wills Eye Hospital Atlas of Clinical Ophthalmology*. 2nd ed. Philadelphia, PA: Lippincott Williams & Wilkins; 2001.

Chapter 8, Glaucoma, Lens, and Anterior Segment Trauma

Question 121

From Gold DH, Weingeist TA. *Color Atlas of the Eye in Systemic Disease*. Baltimore, MD: Lippincott Williams & Wilkins; 2001.

Questions 53 (Figures A and B) and 81

From Ehlers JP, Shah CP. *The Wills Eye Manual*. 5th ed. Philadelphia, PA: Lippincott Williams & Wilkins; 2008.

Question 84

From O'Doherty N. *Atlas of the Newborn*. Philadelphia, PA: JB Lippincott; 1979.

Questions 105 (Figures A and B) and 106 (Figures A and B)

From Jager RD, Lamkin JC. *Massachusetts Eye and Ear Infirmary Review Manual for Ophthalmology*. 3rd ed. Philadelphia, PA: Lippincott Willliams & Wilkins; 2006.

Questions 49, 55, and 137

From Tasman W, Jaeger E. *The Wills Eye Hospital Atlas of Clinical Ophthalmology*. 2nd ed. Philadelphia, PA: Lippincott Williams & Wilkins; 2001.

Chapter 9, Cornea, External Disease, and Refractive Surgery

Question 112

From Gold DH, Weingeist TA. *Color Atlas of the Eye in Systemic Disease*. Baltimore, MD: Lippincott Williams & Wilkins; 2001.

Question 48

From Goodheart HP. *Goodheart's Photoguide of Common Skin Disorders*. 2nd ed. Philadelphia, PA: Lippincott Williams & Wilkins; 2003.

Question 99

From Jager RD, Lamkin JC. *Massachusetts Eye and Ear Infirmary Review Manual for Ophthalmology*. 3rd ed. Philadelphia, PA: Lippincott Williams & Wilkins; 2006.

Questions 1, 8, 57, 94, 132, 136, 138–141, 145, and 199

From Tasman W, Jaeger E. *The Wills Eye Hospital Atlas of Clinical Ophthalmology*. 2nd ed. Philadelphia, PA: Lippincott Williams & Wilkins; 2001.

Chapter 10, Pediatric Ophthalmology and Strabismus

Question 74

Courtesy of Dean John Bonsall, MD.

Question 108

From Gold DH, Weingeist TA. *Color Atlas of the Eye in Systemic Disease*. Baltimore, MD: Lippincott Williams & Wilkins; 2001.

Question 100

From Goodheart HP. *Goodheart's Photoguide of Common Skin Disorders*. 2nd ed. Philadelphia, PA: Lippincott Williams & Wilkins; 2003.

Questions 7, 35, 98, 146 (Figures A and B), and 150

From Tasman W, Jaeger E. *The Wills Eye Hospital Atlas of Clinical Ophthalmology*. 2nd ed. Philadelphia, PA: Lippincott Williams & Wilkins, 2001.

Chapter 11, Retina and Vitreous

Question 77 (Figures A-D)

Courtesy of Paulpoj Chiranand, MD.

Questions 98 (Figures A and B)–101, 103 (Figures A and B)–105, 106 (Figures A–C)–109

Courtesy of Jager RD.

Questions 26, 76, and 132

Courtesy of Veeral S. Sheth, MD.

Questions 10, 72, 110 (Figures A and B), and 111

From Gold DH, Weingeist TA. *Color Atlas of the Eye in Systemic Disease*. Baltimore, MD: Lippincott Williams & Wilkins; 2001.

Questions 78–79 and 81–96

From Jager RD, Lamkin JC. *Massachusetts Eye and Ear Infirmary Review Manual for Ophthalmology*. 3rd ed. Philadelphia, PA: Lippincott Willliams & Wilkins; 2006.

Questions 5, 46–49 (Figures A and B), 50, 52, 53, 66, 67, 69, 80, and 112

From Tasman W, Jaeger E. *The Wills Eye Hospital Atlas of Clinical Ophthalmology*. 2nd ed. Philadelphia, PA: Lippincott Williams & Wilkins; 2001.

Index